T0155212

SHEEP KEEPING

The Professional Smallholder Series

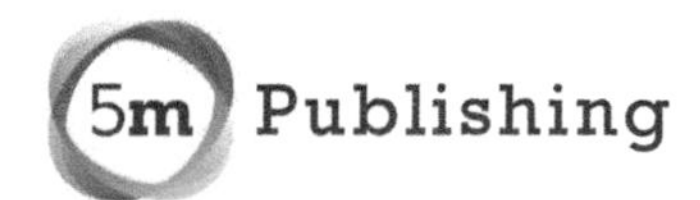

SHEEP KEEPING

The Professional Smallholder Series

PHILLIPA PAGE AND KIM HAMER

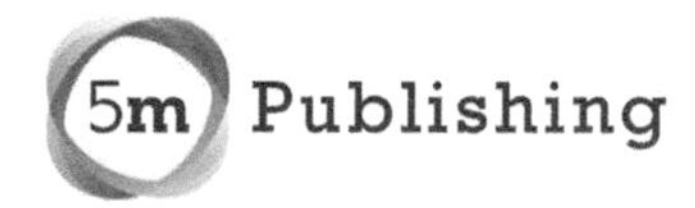

First published 2017

Published by
5M Publishing Ltd,
Benchmark House,
8 Smithy Wood Drive,
Sheffield, S35 1QN, UK
Tel: +44 (0) 1234 81 81 80
www.5mpublishing.com

A Catalogue record for this book is available from the British Library

ISBN 9781910455937

Book layout by
Keystroke, Neville Lodge, Tettenhall, Wolverhampton

Printed by CPI Antony Rowe Ltd, UK

Photos by the authors unless otherwise indicated.
Photo facing page 1, Helen Grimshaw.

CONTENTS

THE PROFESSIONAL SMALLHOLDER SERIES

The Professional Smallholder series provides expert veterinary level information to smallholder farmers, backyard animal keepers and animal enthusiasts on a wide range of topics to help keep your animals happy, healthy, productive and well cared for. Pigs, poultry, sheep and goats and other commonly farmed animals are covered as well as less commonly farmed animals such as camelids.

The books in the series are written by vets and experts for animal keepers, with the aim of providing higher level follow-on information. The books are accessible and the content is practical and current, including subjects like behaviour, health management, anatomy, reproduction and breeding, diseases and disorders, equipment, business matters and organic farming.

The level of the content is directed at the informed owner and is suitable for experienced animal keepers and new farmers. It is also relevant to people with a few hobby animals and more extensive livestock keeping systems. The coverage is useful to and of interest to animal keepers worldwide.

Informed and informative to read, with personal insights from the authors, these books will be beneficial to smallholder farmers of large and small enterprises, agricultural students and potential smallholders.

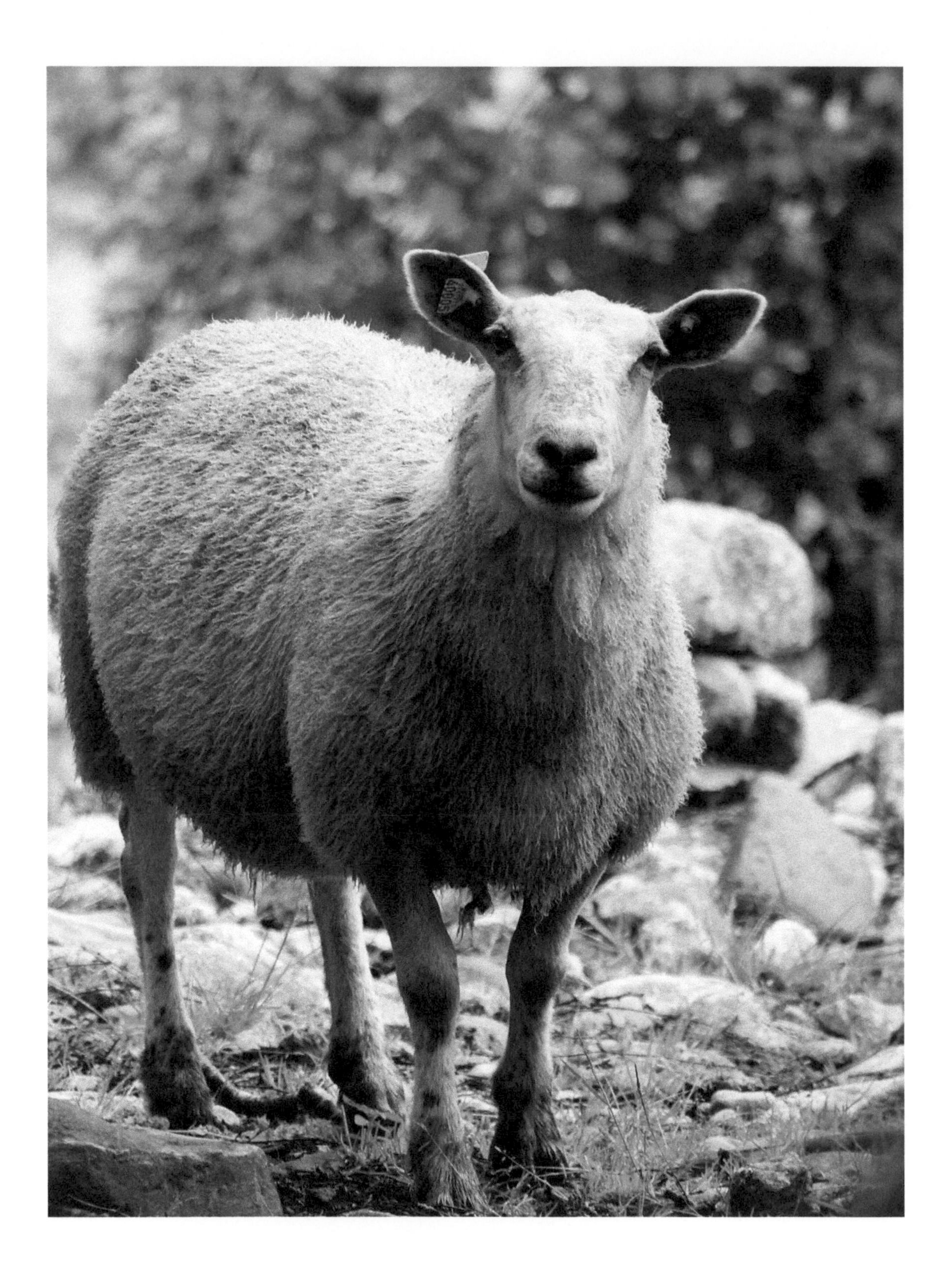

KEEPING SHEEP 1

Sheep are fascinating. They are often viewed as the characteristic grazing animal of the countryside and complement green pastures. They provide the traditional farming scene to people enjoying the outdoors. On closer inspection by their shepherds, farmers and people with an interest in keeping sheep, they are far more than the obligatory addition to the landscape.

Sheep are interesting, both physiologically and behaviourally. They can convert grass, an otherwise indigestible food source to humans into digestible protein. These proteins are then made available to humans in the form of meat and milk. Wool is also an important utilised product. Uniquely, these products can be produced extensively on pasture with minimal input and cultivation.

A thorough understanding of their husbandry needs is required to maintain a healthy and productive flock. Creating optimal health and welfare will ensure that keeping sheep is an enjoyable experience both for you and the sheep.

The aim of this book is to help demonstrate and explain sheep husbandry and health care. It will hopefully provide a sound veterinary reference guide for the common diseases, with suggested treatments and when to call for veterinary advice. The book should also stimulate your interest in the physiological and behavioural characteristics of the ovine species.

Sheep are stoical animals – a feature which has developed from their 'prey' animal existence. They can mask disease, pain and stress very well and to the untrained eye many of these afflictions may be missed. Therefore, they can be challenging and interesting to work with. Once the skill of keeping sheep has been developed and a deep understanding of their behaviour has been acquired, it becomes very satisfying to use your shepherding skills to keep sheep healthy.

Understanding sheep behaviour is an instinct as much as a learned skill. Many livestock farmers have the benefit of generations of family farming to pass this knowledge on. They also have a lot of practice and the familiarity of working with sheep daily.

For those of us who have not been fortunate to have this experience handed down to us, there is plenty we can learn. This book will hopefully inspire and help you to be sure that you are able and willing to look after a flock of sheep responsibly.

WHY KEEP SHEEP?

Traditionally, sheep were kept for their produce: lamb or mutton and milk to make cheese. Their wool is used for clothing and commonly now for carpets, plus their skins for rugs. Sheep farming systems across the world supply the demand for these essential commodities.

To complement and support commercial sheep farming systems, there needs to be sheep enterprises with an emphasis on the genetic development of pedigree rams and ewes. These systems focus on producing suitable pedigree animals with desired genetic traits for commercial production as well as maintaining native breeds and genetic variation.

In the United Kingdom, there is a hugely diverse stratified sheep breeding pyramid. As an example, the upland and hill areas breed and create cross-bred sheep for use with commercial rams on lowland or improved pasture.

These cross-bred ewes such as the North of England Mule, Welsh Mule and the Scotch Mule, are used for their prolificacy, milk yield and mothering ability. In commercial systems, they can be mated to genetically superior rams, from flocks that have used recording systems to improve the breeding potential and quality of finished lamb carcasses.

This is one example of a sheep breeding enterprise. There are many other breeding systems that have adapted to the land and area of sheep production. The outputs from pedigree or cross-bred stock differ depending on whether they are produced for pedigree or commercial lamb production. On many farms there will be more than one type of sheep enterprise.

Other non-commercial reasons for keeping sheep are now prominent in certain areas of the world, particularly the developed world. For example:

- As a hobby flock
- On small paddocks to act as 'lawnmowers' to keep land tidy
- As unusual pets
- On moving to the countryside to experience farming life
- To provide home-grown meat
- To produce pedigree sheep
- At the request of keen, enthusiastic children

Before embarking upon purchasing your first flock, it is important to consider why you would like some sheep and to make sure that you have a good understanding of their husbandry requirements. Failure to consider these factors can be detrimental to the health and welfare of the sheep.

The Farm Animal Welfare Council (FAWC) have produced a guidance document for all livestock farmed species which can be accessed on the UK government website www.gov.uk/guidance/animal-welfare. Understanding the welfare requirements in this document benefits all sheep keepers and their sheep. The welfare of sheep is protected by the Animal Welfare Act 2006 and the Welfare of Farmed Animals (England) Regulations 2007.

Preparation and continued commitment to gaining knowledge helps novice flock keepers to avoid unnecessary lapses in welfare. It is encouraging that you are reading this book to help you keep sheep successfully.

DO YOU HAVE SUITABLE FACILITIES FOR KEEPING SHEEP?

Sheep have an in-built desire to be with and live with other sheep as a flock. As previously described, they are a prey species and so flock together to feel safe. They have not been domesticated enough to live alone. They must be kept with a companion, and ideally with a minimum of three or four in case one dies.

As sheep are grazing animals, the obvious requirement is an area for grazing. Knowing how much land you have available for grazing will help you to plan the size of your flock. This will allow you fence and 'rest' areas of grazing. This will improve parasite control and the nutritional content of the grass, both of which will be discussed later in the book.

The general stocking rate for sheep (number of sheep that can be kept on an area of land) is four adult ewes to an acre of land. At this rate, the sheep should be able to be grazed all year round and depending on the quality of grazing they should need little extra feed. However, it must be considered that if you are going to put the ewes to a ram then the stocking rate will increase once the lambs are born.

In small flocks, it may be better to understock your available pasture so that you can 'rest' land and have an 'isolation' paddock for buying in new sheep. The grazing requirement can be reduced if you are prepared to feed the sheep hay or silage for longer periods during the year.

In certain weather conditions, the grazing will need protecting from poaching and damage and so it will be necessary to be able to rotate where you graze the sheep. Therefore, good fencing is essential. Sheep are inquisitive and will attempt to break out of a field for numerous reasons. Often, it is because they have become short of grass and want to look elsewhere.

Sheep will also 'escape' if they are very well fed and fit and have lots of energy to take themselves off to explore. Younger lambs escape for fun and itchy sheep escape by mistake if they lean and scratch against a poorly secured gate.

Like many other animals, they display a range of personalities and there are sheep that will insist on trying to break out of a field regardless of what you do. These troublemakers can be a problem in leading others astray. It is wise to ensure that you are covered by insurance in case they wander or stray and cause an accident or damage to property.

Fencing

A thick-bottomed hedge is a good type of field boundary as it will provide shelter in bad weather as well as keeping sheep in. If, however, brambles are present, you will find that inquisitive sheep will get caught in brambles and may frequently need removing at your discomfort unless you have very thick gloves. Fields with hedgerow fences need the boundary checking daily to ensure that no sheep have become trapped.

Post and rail fencing is good but will not keep small lambs in unless you adapt the lower part of the fence. Most sheep farms are fenced using posts and pig wire fencing (Fig. 1.1). This is cheaper compared to post and rail fencing and is stock-proof if constructed correctly. The only issue to note here is that lambs with horns will get caught in the fence.

Electric fencing is also used in many sheep systems as it provides a means of being able to fence off areas of grazing to help with rotations. It can also be used where the permanent fencing is not stock-proof and as a quick measure to keep sheep in.

It is important that sheep are 'trained' to the electric fence as otherwise they will not respect it and cause a lot of extra work when they go through it and destroy your hard efforts. The

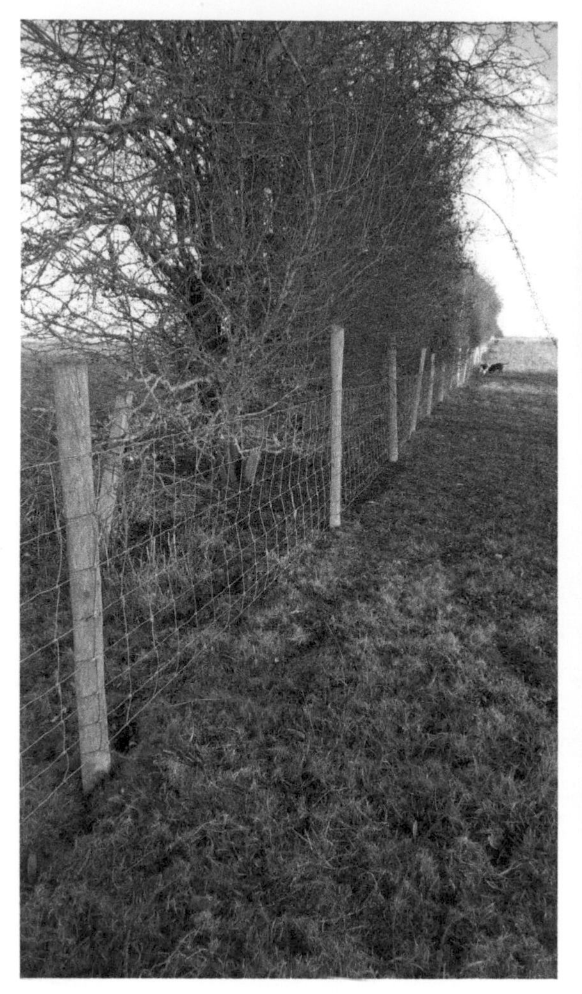

FIGURE 1.1 An example of suitable fencing for sheep.

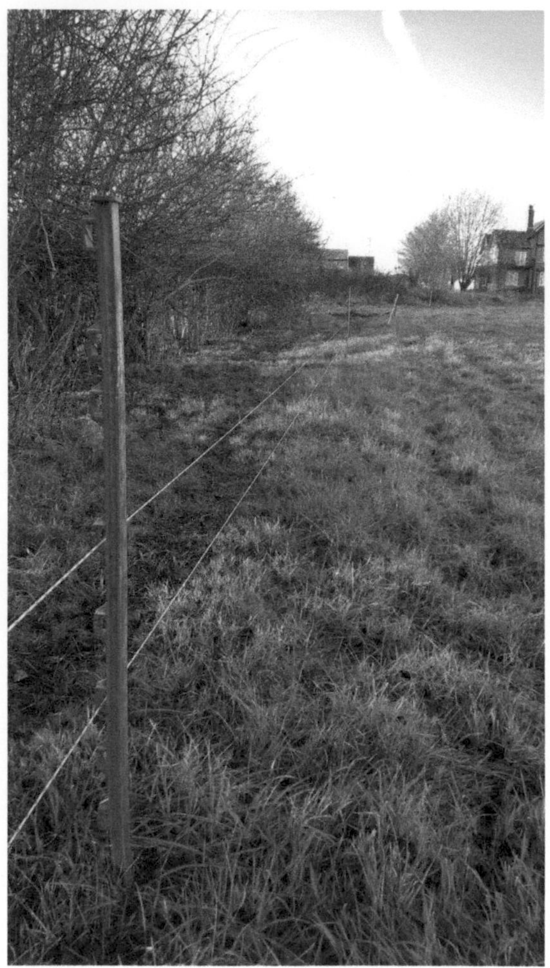

FIGURE 1.2 Electric fencing against a permanent fence to 'train' sheep.

best way of doing this is to place an electric fence along one side of a stock-proof field and make sure it is always fully electrified whilst sheep are in the field. They will then be able to test it and learn without escaping and causing too much damage (Fig. 1.2). Note that Figure 1.2 shows two strands of electric fence. Sheep need three strands of electric fence, especially when being trained for the first time.

Shelter

Sheep are hardy animals with respect to the weather. Their fleece repels water and keeps their skin dry. This only works well, however, if they remain still during periods of rain and snow and if they remain in their own space and not close together with other sheep. Therefore, during wet weather, you will see sheep stood with their backs to the direction of the rain. The fleece will be doing an excellent job of stopping the

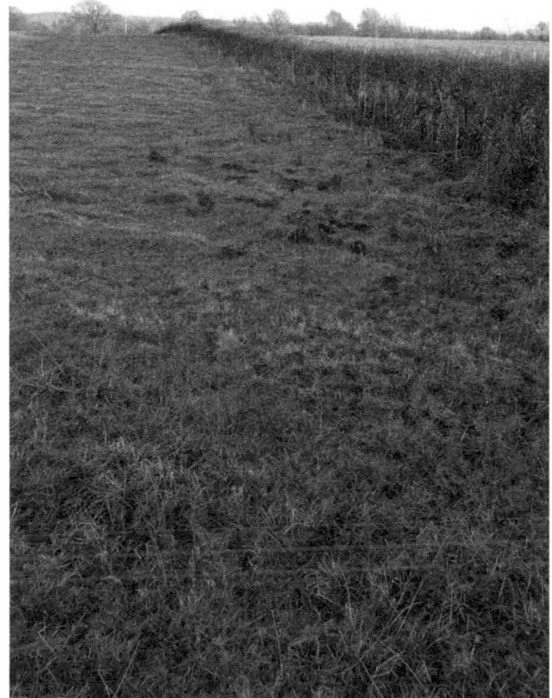

FIGURE 1.3 Hedgerows provide excellent shelter for sheep.

water from moving down the fleece to the skin, but this is disrupted if they start moving. Farmers will refrain from gathering sheep together during rain or when wet, as once they stand touching other sheep the fleece will fail in its attempts to repel water and the skin will become wet.

Where possible, sheep will shelter from the weather and it is a requirement that shelter is provided. In large flocks out at pasture, trees and hedgerows provide excellent shelter spots (see Fig. 1.3). In small flocks, often shelter is provided in the form of a building, stable, field shelter or arc. These are all suitable shelter provisions. They also often form the area in which you can gather and hold the sheep for closer inspection, feeding and treatments.

HANDLING SHEEP

Sheep will need to be handled regularly throughout the year for shearing, vaccinations, worming and other treatments or inspections. Having a handling system in place will make these tasks much easier. An area with hard standing underfoot is ideal. This may be a stable or yard area or a farm track or driveway that can be temporarily fenced to hold sheep (Fig. 1.4).

For small numbers of sheep, a stable may be all that is needed but for a larger flock, metal sheep hurdles will be required (see Fig. 1.5). These are used to safely handle sheep and prevent injury to either the sheep or yourself. Agricultural merchants will stock handling systems and fences for sheep. They will also stock weight scales, tip over (turn over) crates and feeding and water trough equipment.

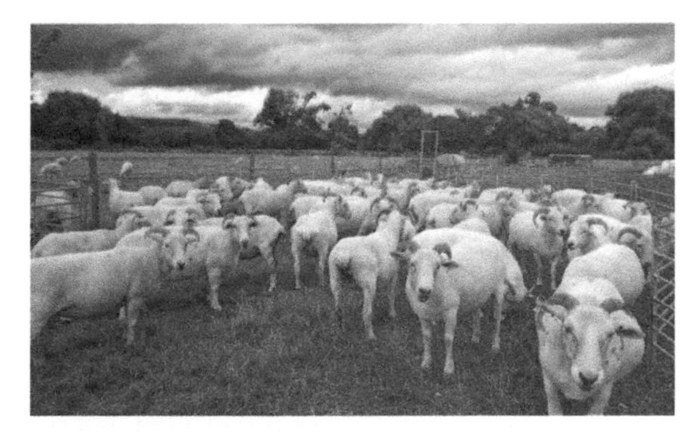

FIGURE 1.4 An example of a handling area.

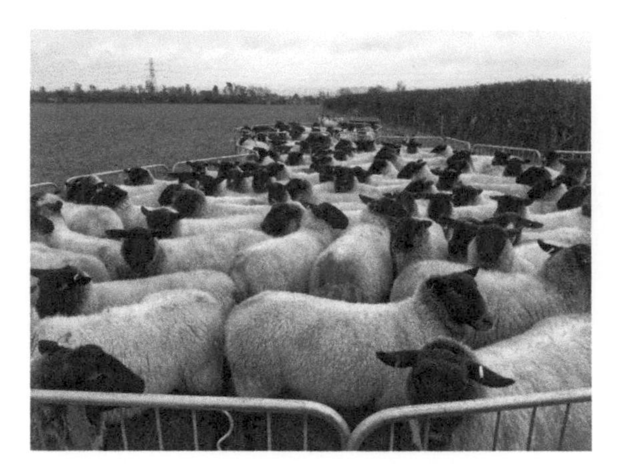

FIGURE 1.5 A mobile sheep handling system.

WATER SUPPLY

Sheep need constant access to fresh, clean water. This is especially important in the drier months of spring and summer due to the lower moisture content of the grazing. In the wetter months, sheep obtain a lot of their moisture from the grass and you may find that if you are supplying water in a bucket, it goes untouched for days. However, if a sheep becomes unwell and dehydrated, it will seek out extra water and often respond to a fever this way. It is therefore essential that the water provision is checked and filled daily. This is also the reason why often ill or dead sheep are found near a water source, that is, a river or stream.

A natural water source such as a river or stream is used as the water supply on many farms. However, this is now becoming a risky practice due to the large increase in infections with the liver fluke parasite. The mud snail *Galba truncata* is required for the life cycle of the liver fluke. The ideal habitat for this snail is wet ground near streams and rivers. Many affected farming systems are now attempting to fence off these areas to control infection.

If there is a history of fluke in your area, then do not use natural streams as a water source. Stagnant water, such as a pond, is not suitable for a water supply. It must be fresh and clean. Field troughs are the best way of supplying water.

Care must be taken with lambs who can playfully jump and fall into water troughs and be at risk of drowning. Placing large stones in the bottom of the trough will help a lamb keep its head above water until it can be rescued. Shallow lamb and ewe troughs are affordable, safer and easier to clean (Fig. 1.6).

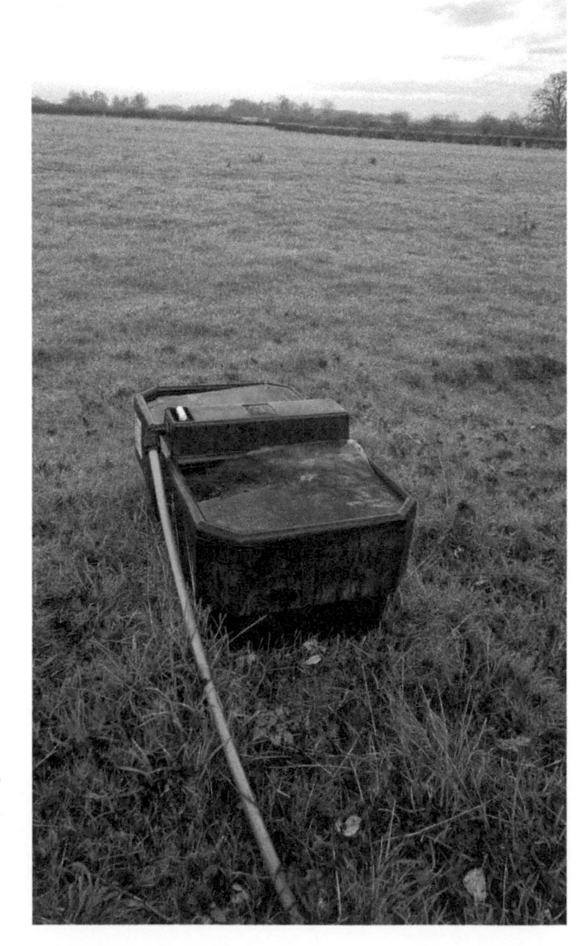

FIGURE 1.6 An ideal water trough for ewes and lambs.

GATHERING SHEEP: DO YOU NEED A DOG?

Moving or gathering sheep is made easier by their instinct to remain as a flock. A good dog can help. Sheep naturally flock together when unsure, alarmed or frightened. The aim of using a dog is not to frighten them each time you move them, but as a cue to the sheep that they are going to be moved or gathered (Fig. 1.7).

A good dog, or shepherd will move sheep using this natural flock instinct. To keep a dog skilled, it will need regular working with sheep and so this may determine whether you decide to use one. An unskilled or untrained dog will cause stress to yourself, stress to the sheep and potential injury; therefore, it needs careful consideration. Not having a dog is far better than using an untrained nuisance dog.

Many small flock keepers will use manpower or feed as a means of enticing sheep to be gathered. Both can be successful if done calmly and with plenty of time to spare in case things don't go to plan (which can be quite often in the sheep keeping world!).

There are health issues associated with feeding too much concentrated feed, which will be discussed later in the book. However, it is appreciated that often this is the only way of being able to gather sheep and so very small amounts of feed may be necessary. Careful monitoring of weight and body condition are essential (see Chapter 4 'Diet and nutrition').

TRANSPORTING SHEEP

There are a variety of sizes of sheep trailers that are used to safely transport sheep. Whether you purchase a mode of transport will depend upon your grazing availability and sheep system set-up and the need for frequent moving, such as to shows, abattoir and markets.

There are certain rules regarding the length and duration of the journey. A comprehensive list of information can be found on the government website regarding the transport of sheep www.gov.uk/guidance/animal-welfare. Before transporting sheep they must be considered fit to travel. Animals that are not considered fit to travel include:

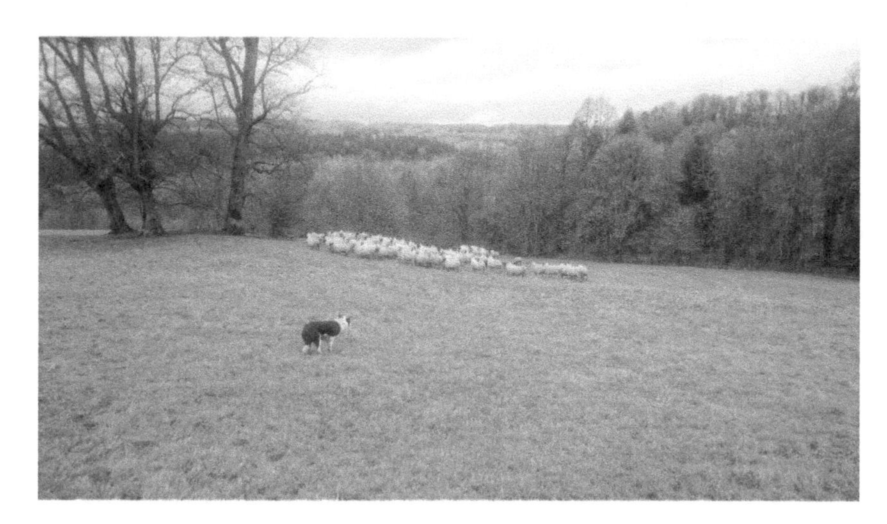

FIGURE 1.7 Using a dog to calmly move sheep.

- Lame sheep that are not weight bearing on all four feet
- Heavily pregnant sheep that are within two weeks of lambing (90% of gestation completed) unless it is for veterinary treatment
- Young animals that are less than a week old
- Sheep that have given birth within the previous seven days
- Sick or injured animals, unless for veterinary treatment

When transporting sheep, they must be accompanied by an animal movement licence, which will state the place of origin, destination, date and duration of the movement. Details of the movement must be recorded and kept in your on-farm records.

LEGAL REQUIREMENTS OF KEEPING SHEEP

Sheep are classed as a farmed species. This is important for many reasons. They are commercially vital to certain areas of the country for the contribution to food production and conservation. Therefore, preventing the spread of disease to animals and the public is crucial.

Whether as pets or in a commercial situation, sheep are vulnerable to the same diseases. Certain diseases such as foot-and-mouth disease can be devastating to the national sheep population. For this reason, a knowledge of the movements and residence of sheep across the UK, whether in large or small flocks, is required. Therefore, before purchasing sheep there are legal requirements that must be followed.

- Before moving sheep onto your land (called a holding) you must apply for a County Parish Holding (CPH) number. To apply for this you must contact the Rural Payments Agency or Rural Inspectorate or Rural Payments and Inspectorate Directorate office
- The place at which your sheep are to be kept must then be registered with your nearest Animal Health Divisional Office. This must be done within a month of becoming a sheep keeper or obtaining a holding
- You will then be given a flock number which will identify your flock and any animals born on your holding. This flock number will be printed onto any future ear tags that are used
- You must keep a holding register which relates to your holding and your sheep. This must be updated regularly to include all sheep moving onto and off the holding, plus births and deaths of sheep on the holding
- If you must replace an ear tag in a sheep on your holding, details of this must also be recorded
- Movements of sheep onto and off the holding must be recorded using the Animal Movement and Reporting Service within 36 hours of the movement

An up-to-date, detailed description of the above information can be found on the government website and it is advised that you read this information fully before purchasing sheep: www.gov.uk/government/collections/guidance-for-keepers-of-sheep-goats-and-pigs

SHEEP IDENTIFICATION

In the UK, sheep are identified by means of ear tags. These tags should display the flock number that relates to where the animal was born and an individual number, if the animal is over 12 months old. Sheep that are less than

12 months and are to be slaughtered for meat do not currently require an individual number. The rules regarding the identification of sheep do change and so to receive up-to-date information it is important to visit the above government website.

Applying the tag

It will be necessary to apply an ear tag to lambs that have been born on your holding or to sheep that lose an ear tag and need a replacement. Figure 1.8 indicates the correct place for the tag application, displayed by the green dot. When tagging young lambs, make sure that you leave a gap between the fold in the tag and the edge of the ear to allow for the ear to grow.

The areas to avoid are the rigid cartilaginous areas and the blood vessel that is enlarged in the position close to the head. Aim to place the tag a third of the way along the ear from the head. The tag can either be placed on the top of the ear or at the bottom (see Figure 1.9).

Ensure that the tags are within the legal specification and that you have the correct matching taggers to apply them. It is also important that you clean the skin surface of the ear with a medicated wipe first. Dipping the tag spike in surgical spirit will also help disinfect the areas of the tag that will pierce the skin.

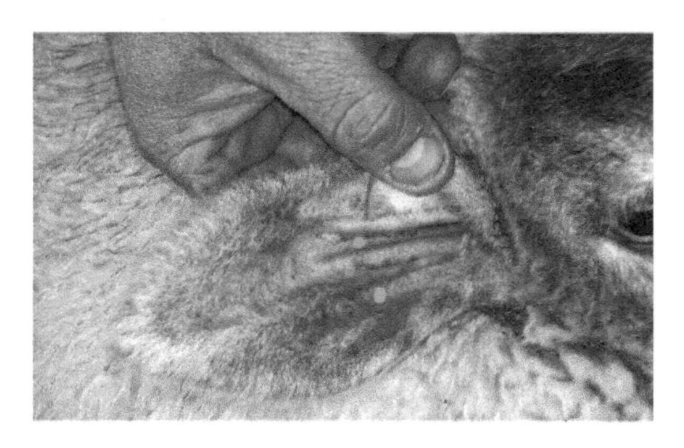

FIGURE 1.8 Correct positions for ear tag placement.

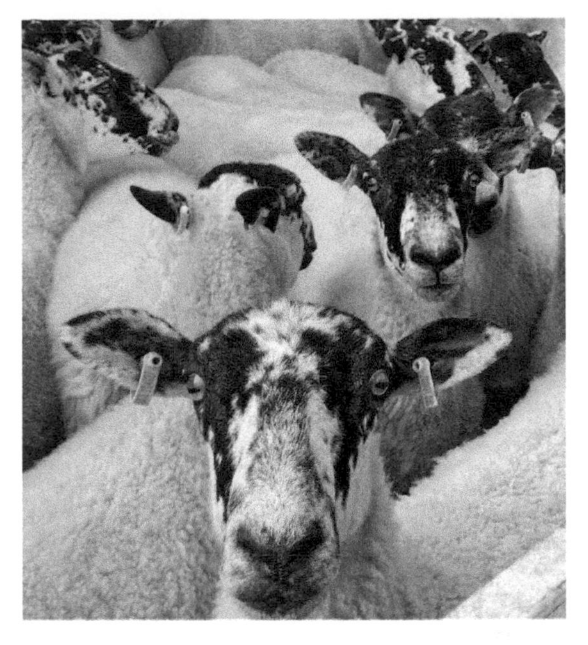

FIGURE 1.9 A good example of ear tag placement.

Tags that have been applied incorrectly can cause infections and severe discomfort to the sheep. If you notice that the skin or hole around where the tag is situated has become smelly, infected and painful, then the tag must be cut out to allow healing. Clean the area thoroughly and be vigilant for fly strike. See Chapter 7 'Sick sheep' for more information on dealing with wounds and fly strike.

BREEDS OF SHEEP

There are many breeds of sheep worldwide, and they have been selectively bred to suit certain environments and production aims. It is therefore important to consider this when selecting a breed for your land. For example, the hill breeds (such as the Swaledale or Herdwick) need a large area of varied grazing over which to roam and will struggle to thrive in small fenced paddocks with permanent pasture. The 'terminal sire' type breeds (such as the Texel or Suffolk) were bred in lowland areas on smaller paddocks and in fenced areas. Always consult breed societies and your vet when considering which breeds to choose.

A FRIENDLY NEIGHBOUR?

If you live in the countryside, it is very likely that you will have some neighbouring sheep farmers. These farmers are a vital source of knowledge and experience and are well worth befriending. It is often wrongly assumed that the motivation of a sheep farmer or any farmer for that matter is primarily financial. Whilst this is a hugely important feature when farming, it is not the true motivation.

These farmers love the stock they work with and the aim of both the large sheep farmer and the smaller flock keeper is to have healthy, happy, productive sheep. Therefore, go and introduce yourself to this valuable resource, who will hopefully provide varying degrees of help and advice in terms of potential breeds to consider for the land and general stockmanship.

WHAT AGE OF SHEEP SHOULD I BUY?

There are some sheep that are not considered suitable for either small- or large-scale sheep systems. In a commercial farming system, when sheep reach the end of their productive life they will often leave the flock as a 'cull' animal. These sheep will either go to slaughter from the farm or they will be bought from a market to be kept for a short period in which they will gain weight before slaughter.

These sheep are therefore often 'aged' or 'old aged'. They are often in poorer condition due to poor dentition or 'lost teeth' (broken mouthed) or due to a chronic disease such as lameness or other diseases.

It often seems unfair that these sheep leave the flock for these reasons and are unable to live out a longer, 'happier' life and there is sometimes the temptation by small flock keepers to purchase these sheep for this reason.

They are not suitable sheep to purchase. Unfortunately, in most cases purchasing or acquiring older 'cull sheep' is not in the best interests of the sheep and they can quickly deteriorate into discomfort and require treatment or euthanasia. Therefore, when selecting the age of sheep to purchase, leave the older sheep alone and look for healthy, young, fit sheep.

CONSIDERATIONS

There are lots of things to consider before purchasing your sheep and becoming a small flock keeper. Think about the points on this checklist before embarking upon your first purchases:

- What land do you have available? Does it include shelter and water and is it 'sheep-proof'?
- How many sheep can you keep on the land? As a guide, use four sheep (not including lambs at foot) to the acre and leave room to be able to rotate fields.
- Are you able to check the sheep every day, 365 days of the year? If not, do you have a suitably trained person to be able to check them?
- Have you done your research into keeping sheep? Why do you want to keep them?
- Are you able to go on a training course/workshop before getting the sheep?

- Do you have a reserve of funds to pay for emergency veterinary care and for routine visits?

REGULATIONS

- Have you registered to keep sheep and obtained a flock number and holding number?
- Do you have a record book ready to record sheep numbers and keep a register?

FLOCK HEALTH PLANNING

As a sheep keeper, you will need a local vet who has an interest in sheep. This may not be the same vet as the one who cares for other pets that you may have. Seek out a local sheep vet ideally via word of mouth and contact them before buying any sheep.

There are many useful forums on the Internet and advice to be found from other sheep keepers, however for the most accurate and up-to-date information it is advisable to seek vet advice. Many of the forums and non-veterinary sources of knowledge can give mixed messages and inaccurate information.

Veterinary advice is often perceived as expensive, but this may only be the case when advice is sought too late into a problem or after incorrect home remedies have been tried. Many mixed and large animal veterinary practices will have a vet with a dedicated interest in sheep. They will often offer training workshops such as for lambing and worm control.

Some practices also offer small holder sheep discussion groups and clubs where knowledge can be shared and discussed. Using your vet in the first instance for accurate advice will prove beneficial for you and your sheep. There is a cost to this but it is a proactive routine cost if used throughout the year, rather than an unexpected cost in an emergency.

Traditionally, there have been routine treatments and practices carried out year-on-year on all sizes of sheep flocks. However, more recently the understanding that every flock is different in terms of health status, treatment requirements and yearly planning is ever more apparent.

The way in which you keep your sheep on your holding will differ, not least due to your land type, available grazing, fodder and sheep enterprise. Farmers and sheep keepers of all sizes of flocks are becoming more aware of the need to discuss the needs of their flock with a sheep veterinary surgeon to create a cost-effective and accurate plan for the year.

The term 'flock health planning' is used for this type of discussion and involves at least one flock visit and discussion with a vet. Usually together the vet–farmer team will decide upon any current concerns with the flock and where to focus attention. They will also draw up a plan for that year based upon routine monitoring, such as worm egg counting, and plan routine treatments, such as vaccinations. This will be discussed further in Chapter 8 'Preventative treatments'.

By engaging with your vet, you will build up a good relationship in which your vet knows your flock, your aims and capabilities. You will then have someone whom you can phone for advice should problems occur. Developing this relationship will be very beneficial for you and your flock.

THE NORMAL SHEEP 2

The normal sheep? This can be a difficult description as sheep can be the masters of disguise, most notably when it comes to pain or discomfort. Their stoical nature means that they will carry on as normal and appear OK until they find themselves in trouble.

Many shepherds understand that sheep can be difficult animals to diagnose and treat. They are aware that subtle signs are often the only signs available when a sheep is sick. Chapter 7 'Sick sheep' will discuss the clinical signs and their causes in detail.

Sheep keepers who have failed to research sheep behaviour or seek help and advice in relation to sheep health can be caught out. An insight into what is normal for a sheep can provide a basis on which to decide whether your sheep are healthy and behaving normally or whether there is an underlying problem.

THE WHOLE FLOCK APPROACH

A daily assessment undertaken by the attending shepherd or sheep keeper involves close observation of the flock. This approach gives an instant indication of any obvious problems and it will also allow you to assess any changes from the previous check the day before. Unbeknown to many of us, shepherds spend each day checking the sheep under their care in this way. This should be carried out once daily and twice daily within the summer months due to the risk of fly strike and during periods of bad weather.

The 'normal' flock will appear settled when you enter the field. Sheep will become very familiar with their keeper's appearance, sounds, accompanying dogs and demeanour. Therefore, on checking the flock they should not be startled or unsettled. This will take a few months of repetition to become established, but over time they will learn that your presence is not a threat.

The flocking behaviour of sheep is a protective one that has remained a strong feature of the domestic breeds. The older, less domesticated breeds such as the Soay and Shetland breeds have a less distinctive flock behaviour and sometimes scatter rather than flock. Learning to work with this can be perfected with practice.

Like many other 'hunted' herd animals, flocking together offers security in numbers. Arranging into a flock means that the target for being attacked is larger and more confusing for the predator (stray dog, unfamiliar person, unusual threat). A flock offers a more efficient 'look out' facility in the direction of danger and hence this enables the safest direction of movement.

When working with different ages of sheep it becomes apparent that the 'flocking' ability improves with age, with older ewes assuming the flock position and being able to be moved far more easily than a group of younger weaned lambs.

By understanding this normal flock instinct, it has become possible to move and control sheep by trained working dogs. This is discussed in Chapter 3 'The organ systems of the sheep'. The main reasons to override this flocking instinct is the maternal instinct or lambing instinct and the sick, unwell sheep.

What do sheep do?

When sheep are awake, most of their time is spent grazing and chewing the cud. Settled sheep will continue to graze once your presence has been noted. They may move away from your position slightly, but usually they should continue with their normal behaviour. Other normal behaviours include drinking, lying on their chest with the head up, lying laterally with their head to the ground (often sleeping and quite startled as you approach), walking to and from the water trough, investigating, assessing your behaviour and interacting with other flock members (Fig. 2.1).

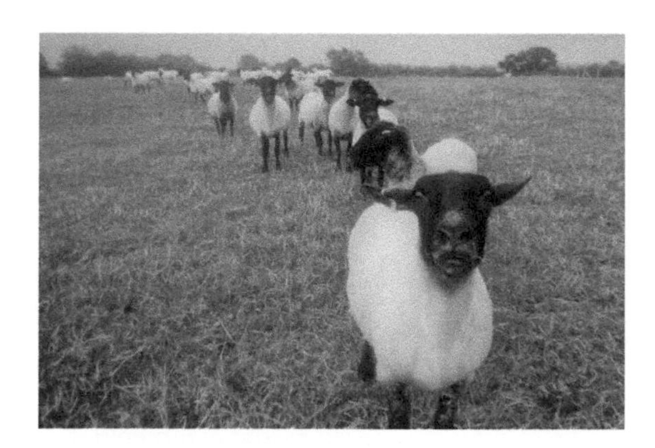

FIGURE 2.1 Inquisitive sheep.

A cause for concern

Sheep that may need further investigation will appear different. These sheep will not look in your direction as you approach or shout or whistle. They may not get up or be able to get up. Often sheep that are unwell will stand with their head bowed and all four feet close together and they will often be found away from the rest of the flock.

When sheep are unwell they are aware of their inability to keep up with the rest of the flock and so will move to a sheltered hideaway, such as in the hedge or under a tree. Unwell sheep often have a pyrexia (high temperature or fever) and so they will seek out a water source to attempt to correct this fever and dehydration. This has contributed to the phrase 'sheep always like to die in the stream or brook' or 'they die in the most difficult place to retrieve them from'!

Following observation of the 'normal' flock, the shepherd will then use the flock behaviour to make a more detailed assessment. By using trained dogs or a simple whistle command, the sheep can then be roused into the flock position and any further abnormalities assessed. For example, a sick sheep will then be identified more easily as either not flocking, moving slowly or lame. The sheep can be counted to identify any missing sheep and the hedgerows and streams checked.

This procedure is followed by shepherds and sheep keepers all over the country as part of their daily routine. By identifying and detecting a sick individual or abnormal behaviour in a flock of sheep early, there is a far greater chance of solving a problem and preventing a deterioration in welfare.

Abnormal flock behaviour

Anything different to previously described could be classed as abnormal and may prompt concern. For example, in a normally well-settled flock, when approached for inspection, a rapid flock together reaction could indicate the presence or recent presence of a 'danger' source. This often involves a stray dog, a dog off the lead, a group of walkers or other perceived danger.

The frequency of stray dogs and uncontrolled dog attacks is becoming significantly more common and so further inspection for evidence of injury, missing or dead sheep would be essential in this scenario. In the absence of physical injury, the stress of frequent disruption by a dog off the lead can cause abortion in pregnant sheep. This has become a frustrating and frequent problem for sheep farmers and requires action in terms of notices on footpaths, reporting to the police and more frequent monitoring where possible (Fig. 2.2).

YOUR
DOG
CAN SCARE
OR HARM
FARM
ANIMALS
PLEASE PUT IT ON A
LEAD NEAR LIVESTOCK

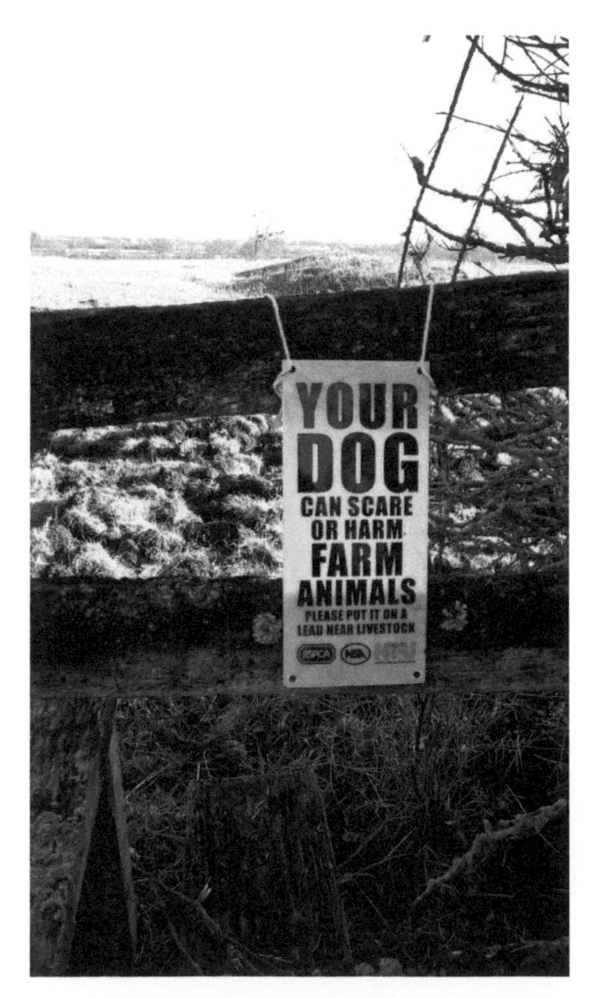

FIGURE 2.2 Educational footpath notices.

Flock assessment

Routine flock assessment will reveal the presence of clinical signs such as:

- Dullness, depressed demeanour
- Lameness
- Excessive itching
- Wool loss
- Scour (diarrhoea)
- Change in body condition. Assessment of body condition also requires the gathering and the handling of sheep for a complete assessment

The detection of any of these issues can then be rapidly dealt with and treated. Successful shepherds and stockpersons are constantly assessing the flock and picking up on subtle signs that will alert them to a problem or a potential problem.

The sudden death of several sheep within the flock can occur when certain diseases are present. These include fluke infection, haemonchosis (blood sucking worm), pasteurella and clostridial infections. These will be discussed in detail in Chapter 7 'Sick sheep'.

The shepherd will also be able to assess the amount of grazing remaining in the field and make supplements or move fields as required.

THE NORMAL SHEEP

As previously mentioned, sheep are very good at disguising symptoms of illness. Sometimes, when the sheep has been noticed and can be examined, the condition is either obvious or the sheep is so ill that it is unable to be treated. Therefore, prompt treatment and investigation is essential. Use your vet to investigate sheep that are unwell and are showing no obvious cause.

CONDUCTING A HEALTH ASSESSMENT

A visual inspection followed by handling can be very informative. Starting at the head:

- *Ears:* They should be pricked and alert (see Fig. 2.3). They should be symmetrical with no enlargements of the ear pinnae (flap) and with no discharges. Always check the skin around the ear tag. An infected tag produces severe discomfort and a foul-smelling discharge. Note that some breeds, such as the Suffolk, have a normal droopy ear position

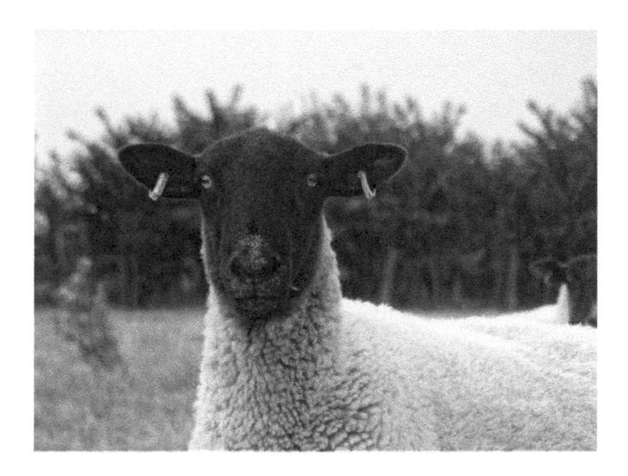

FIGURE 2.3 An alert, responsive sheep.

- *Eyes:* They should be fully open, clear (not cloudy or opaque), the whites (sclera) of the eye should be white and not pink/inflamed or yellow. The area around the eyes should be dry with no excess tears or wetness of the surrounding skin
- *Scent glands:* These are present in the corner of each eye as a darkening in the hair and produce a waxy substance. This is more pronounced in breeds with white or lighter heads and is very normal. Scent glands are also found above the hoof, in between the claws and in the inguinal region (in the groin area)
- *Nose:* The nostrils should be clear from any discharge. Upper respiratory tract infections, pulmonary tumours, parasites and metabolic disease can cause a nasal discharge
- *Skin:* Soft and firm swellings around the cheeks can indicate tooth problems. A submandibular swelling under the jaw, termed 'bottle jaw' is an important clinical sign of several diseases. Swellings below the ear or under the jaw, particularly if they rupture to release an abscess or pus-type material can indicate the presence of caseous lymphadenitis (CLA) disease. This will be discussed in Chapter 7 'Sick sheep'
- *Mouth:* Sheep have teeth on the lower mandible (jaw) with a diastema (gap) separating the front teeth from the rear molar teeth. There is an absence of teeth on the upper area of the jaw at the front. Instead, they have a hard 'dental pad' which is a tough area that enables the grazing of short pasture. This can be seen in Figure 2.4. They do have molars on the upper rear region of the mouth. Observing the condition of the teeth, particularly the front incisors, is important when assessing sheep health

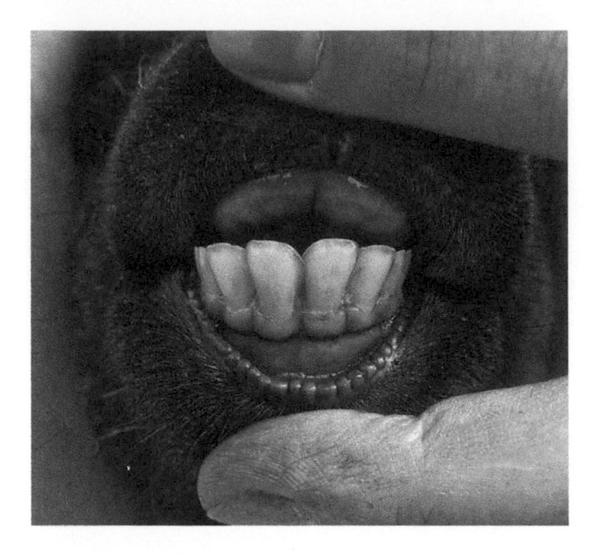

FIGURE 2.4 It is normal that no teeth are present on the upper dental pad.

Use the diastema (gap) in between the teeth on the lower jaw to insert your thumb when opening a mouth for examination. Be extremely careful not to place your fingers to the rear or front of the mouth as they can 'bite', albeit unintentionally.

Ageing sheep

The age of sheep can be determined by their teeth and this is the common method. The fleece can also be useful to determine a lamb from a sheep that has had one shear. The fleece of a lamb is tighter and appears thicker. Lambs can be born with or without teeth. The tooth roots of the lower frontal incisors are visible and in some cases may have already erupted.

By assessing the lower frontal incisors, the age of the sheep can be determined based upon the emergence of adult teeth and the loss of the temporary teeth. Therefore, the age of a sheep after a year old is described by the number of adult teeth, in other words, two-tooth, four-tooth or six-tooth.

Just to confuse matters (if you're not suitably confused already), the age of a sheep is also often related to the numbers of shears it has had. However, this description relies upon knowing the history of the sheep, whereas dental ageing does not.

Table 2.1

AGE	PHOTO/DIAGRAM	REGIONAL/COMMON NAMES
Newborn lamb		
Weaned lamb	1.	Hogg, hogget

12–18 months old

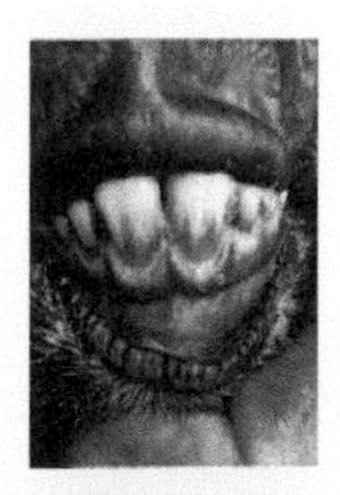

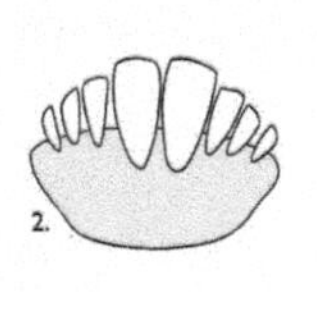

Gimmer, yearling, shearling, two-tooth. Theave (up to first lambing)

18 months to 2 years old

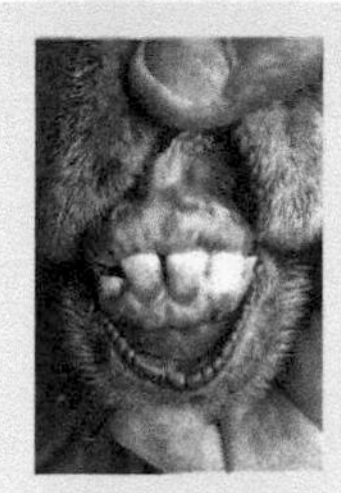

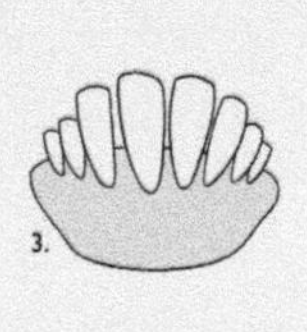

Four-tooth. Double theave (up to two lambings), two shears

2 years 3 months to 3 years old

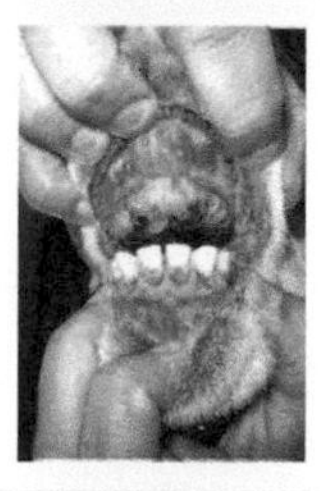

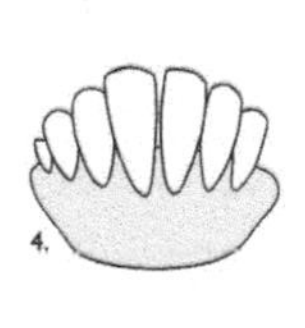

Six-tooth

3–4 years old

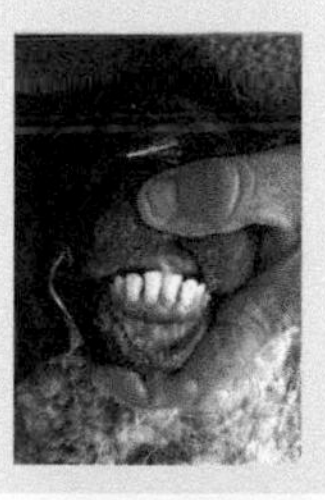

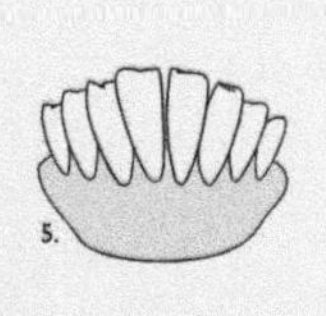

Full mouth

Aged sheep

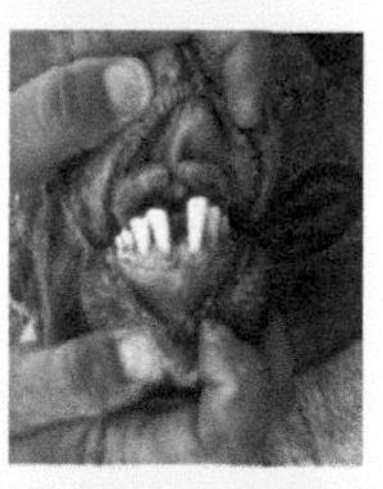

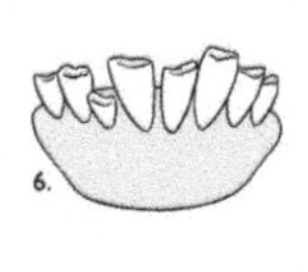

Broken mouth

Old, no teeth

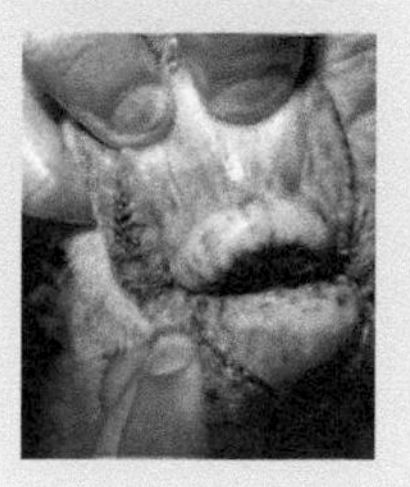

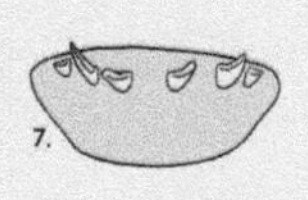

No teeth

(Diagrams: Amanda Aiken)

HEALTH ASSESSMENT: THE BODY

Skin and wool

The fleece of the sheep should be complete and appear full. Sheep use their fleece as an excellent insulator to keep body heat in and also to keep moisture away from the skin layer which would result in cooling. Many breeds of sheep have different wool properties related to the crimp (number of bends along a wool fibre), texture and length. It is these properties that often attract certain sheep keepers to purchasing certain breeds.

- Visually assess the appearance of the fleece – it should appear full and uniform. Darker patches and matted moist areas must be examined further as they can indicate an area of fly strike
- Areas of wool loss – always examine the skin carefully. If crusts and flakes are evident and itching has been observed, then the presence of the sheep scab mite is possible. Lice may also cause this effect. If the skin is normal, wool loss can also be the result of a previous stressful event such as sickness or metabolic disease. This will be discussed later, but you must consult your vet if these signs are present

Body condition score

This is an essential part of any examination and should be carried out every time your sheep are handled. It provides a direct indication of the health of the sheep. Sheep keepers will regularly feel the backs of the sheep as they are handling, moving or doing other routine procedures. They use this to assess their health and performance and as a prompt to adjust feeding or investigate the reasons for poor condition.

It is impossible to visually determine the body condition score of a sheep with a full fleece and therefore it must be handled. Recently shorn sheep can be visually assessed but within a few weeks of regrowth they will need handling again to determine condition.

How to body condition score

1. Either restrain the sheep in a race (metal alleyway) or fill up a pen with sheep so that they are unable to move around too much.
2. Open your hand and place on the spine behind where the ribs finish. This region is the lumbar region (see Fig. 2.5).
3. Roll your hand from side to side using the skin movement to help your hand move and press down firmly.

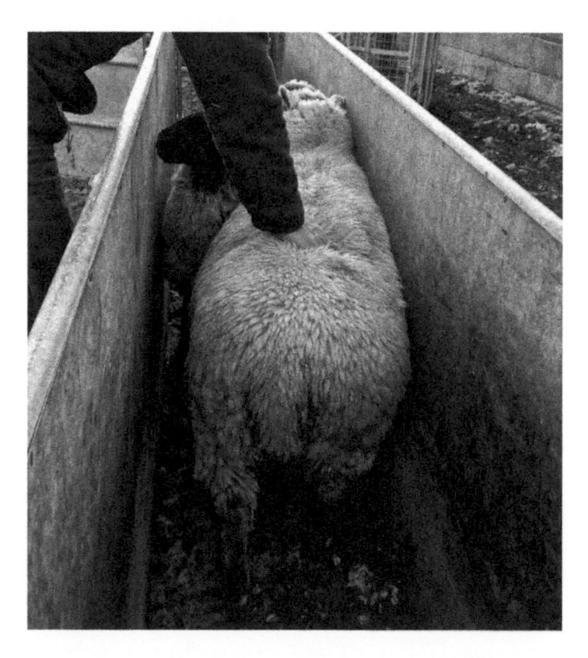

FIGURE 2.5 The lumbar region is felt by placing the hand on the spine, behind the ribs.

4. Use your thumb and palm on one side to roll over and feel the skin covering over the lumbar vertebrae. Use your little finger and palm to feel the lumbar vertebrae on the other side.

The aim is to assess two main areas (see Fig. 2.6: the yellow line demonstrates the spine).

- The area between the spine and the edge of the lumbar vertebrae. This is the green line in Figure 2.6
    - Does this area sink in or dip when you feel it? Score 2 and below
    - Does it feel flat or rounded? Score 2.5 and above
- The area over the edge of the lumbar vertebrae. This is the orange line in Figure 2.6
    - Are the lumbar vertebrae edges easily felt with little pressure? Score 2 or less
    - Do you have to press down to feel the individual vertebrae edges? Score 2.5 or above

Combining these assessments and using the diagram and photographs should help you to assign a condition score. See Diagram 2.8. The body condition scores are numbered 1 to 5. Score 1 demonstrates the thinnest animal and score 5 demonstrates the fattest animal.

The target body condition score will vary depending upon the breed and the time of year or stage of production. However, the aim should be for all sheep to be at least body condition score 2 no matter what stage of the year. Figure 2.7 shows an example of the ewe on the right side of the photo of body condition score 1 and the ewe next to her on the left as body condition score 4.

Try not to worry about assigning a body condition score number and getting it right. The aim should be to regularly handle your sheep and

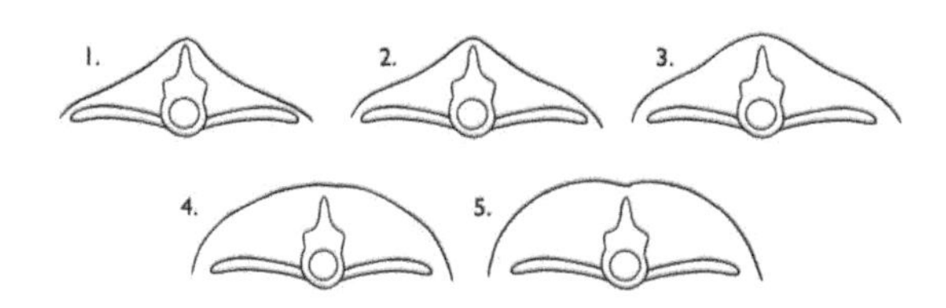

DIAGRAM 2.8

Credit: Amanda Aiken

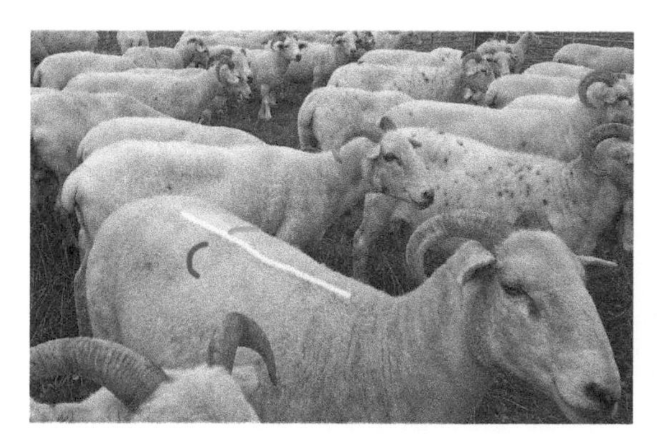

FIGURE 2.6 Areas to feel when body condition scoring (see text for detail).

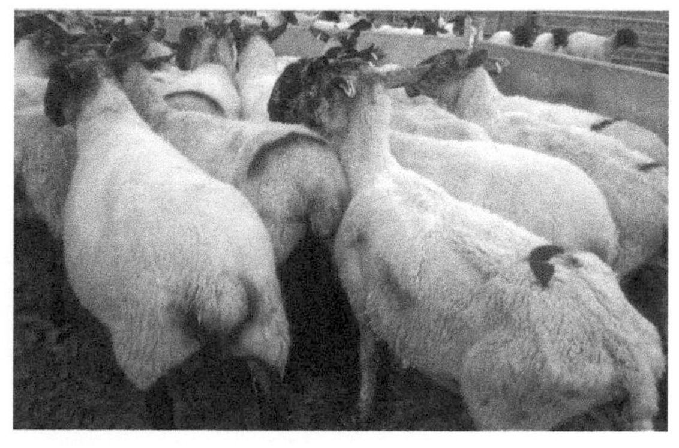

FIGURE 2.7 An example of variations in body condition score.

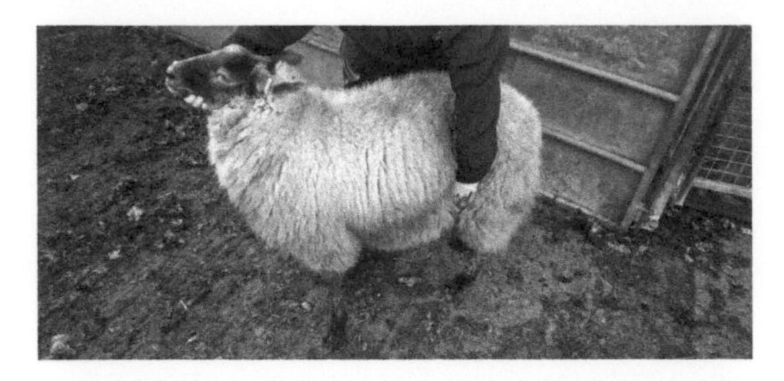

FIGURE 2.8 Position when preparing to turn the sheep.

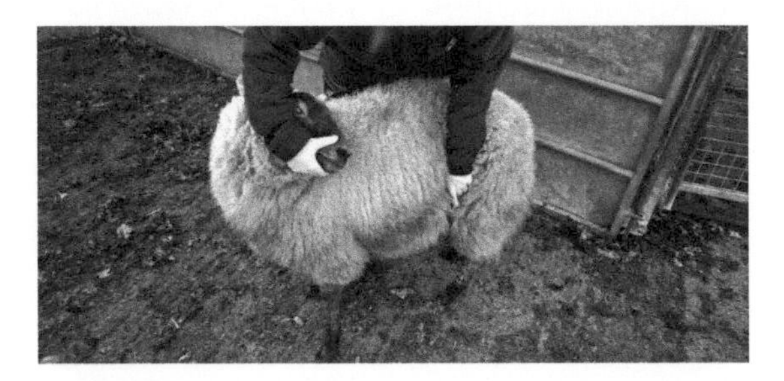

FIGURE 2.9 Turn the head away from your body and aim the nose towards the tail.

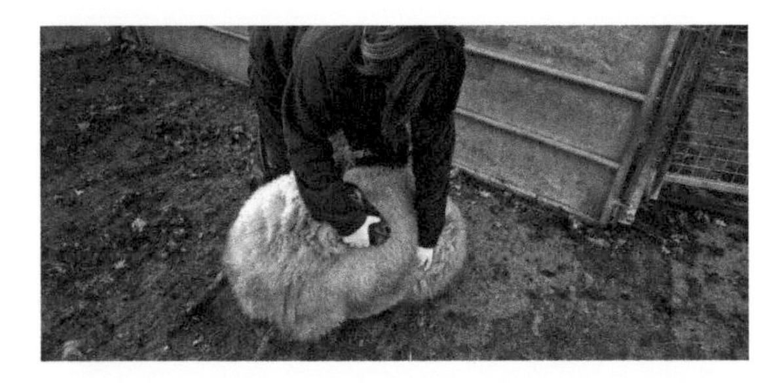

FIGURE 2.10 Press the flank firmly down with your left hand and step back with your left leg.

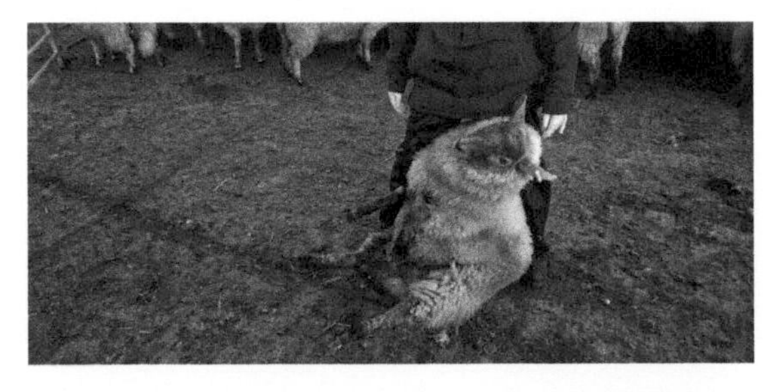

FIGURE 2.11 Securely holding the sheep whilst leaving your hands free.

check that they are in good body condition. It is important to assess the diet and sheep health to determine why they are not holding condition.

Where the flock appears to have lost body condition, reasons often include insufficient nutrition and internal parasites. Individual sheep must be thoroughly checked over including the teeth for any health reasons leading to weight loss. These will be discussed in Chapter 7 'Sick sheep'.

Turning a sheep

To assess the feet and udder, it is important to be able to handle and restrain the sheep confidently and safely for both you and the sheep. Often when you notice problems with one of your sheep, you are on your own and need to investigate. Shepherds have devised a safe and quick technique to assess, treat and shear sheep. This method provides minimal stress and discomfort to the animal and it will allow you to hold the sheep and have your hands free to inspect and treat (after some practice).

This step-by-step guide offers one example of how to turn the ewe. Make sure you have plenty of room around you and no obvious hazards that will result in trapped legs or falls. It can be difficult to turn over a large ewe in a small lambing pen.

Turning a sheep involves using your hands, arms and legs.

1. Stand alongside the sheep with your right hand under her jaw and your left hand in her left flank holding onto the flap of skin (see Fig. 2.8).
2. Using your hand, turn the sheep's head to her left as far as possible. At the same time, step back with your left leg and use your left

hand to push her left flank down (see Figs 2.9 and 2.10).

3. Then grasp her left front leg with your left hand and straighten your back at the same time to an upright position.
4. Her head should then flop over to the right and you can move your right leg over to secure your hold or until you feel in control. You will now be able to let your hands go and she should remain in place (see Fig. 2.1).

This will take a lot of practice! Even with a lot of practice the most accomplished shepherd may still end up on the floor with the sheep looking on, especially after a long night lambing.

For those less agile shepherds, or those with large ewes, or those that would like to prolong the life of their backs, there are turnover crates available from many agricultural merchants. These will still require some effort and practice but provide a very safe restraining method for examination of sheep.

The examination of a ram can be made much harder due to their size. Turning them over often requires two people. When examining feet, many small flock keepers will pick up the feet like a horse, which is fine provided you have help to restrain the ewe at the front.

LOCOMOTION AND MOBILITY

One of the most important health issues affecting sheep in the UK and the global sheep population is lameness. Lameness is an obvious painful affliction that can be observed and recorded by the untrained eye. It is also a condition with which we as humans can associate with. When lame sheep are observed in a field, it will prompt calls from members of the public and it should lead to prompt assessment and treatment by the sheep keeper.

The most common causes of lameness are related to infections caused by bacteria. The extent to which bacteria gain entry to and cause problems within the foot will relate to the challenge present, that is, the level of infection, the number of sheep and the integrity of the normal skin barrier.

The way in which the hoof protects against infection can be affected by underfoot environmental conditions, that is, muddy, warm and wet. It can also be affected by the conformation of the foot, in other words, how the hoof naturally wears down on the ground. If this is uneven, it may cause the entrapment of dirt and stones which will cause further damage. The immune status of the ewe is also important in how the ewe deals with the bacteria which cause foot infections.

The details of these conditions will be discussed in the 'Lameness' section of Chapter 7. The outcome and success of treatment is determined by the speed at which the lameness is diagnosed and treated.

How do you detect a lame sheep?

A very lame sheep is obvious. When at rest, she may hold up the affected foot or only partially bear weight on it. When walking, she may not place the foot down fully or at all, but when running, she may appear sound. It can be more difficult to determine a ewe that is lame on more than one foot and it is difficult to assess a lame ewe that has just started to become lame due to their reluctance to display a disability.

The most effective way to assess lameness is when the sheep are at grass grazing or when walking slowly. With a small number of sheep this should be straightforward and you should be able to identify them as you walk through the flock. With larger numbers it is more difficult and there has yet to be a tried and tested method of identifying them in the field and then once again when gathered.

The only time this can be done is when they have lambs at foot and they have been identified by a number. With larger flocks, it is easier to assess a proportion at a time to have a better chance of finding the lame ones when gathered in the handling pens.

Many shepherds will gather the sheep to catch a lame ewe. They will do this using a very skilful dog and the ability to hold them tightly in the corner of a field, to then catch individuals using a shepherd's crook. Or they may gather into the handling system and try to walk through them to identify lame animals.

These are good indicators that a sheep is lame:

- Grazing on the knees
- Shuffling gait
- Head nod when walking
- At the back of the flock when moving
- Holding the affected leg off the ground or just touching the toe, when at rest (see Fig. 2.12)

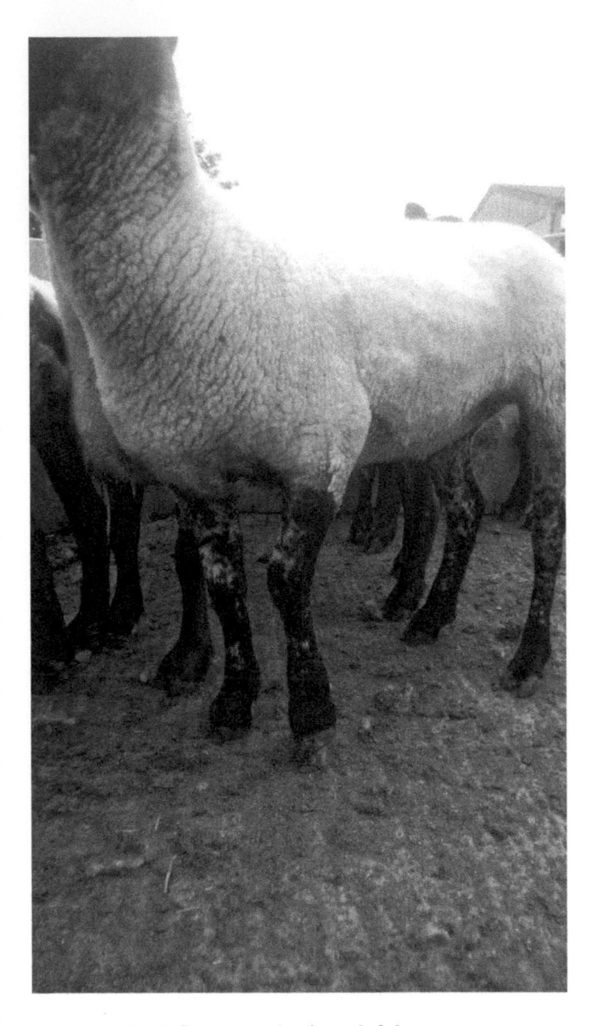

FIGURE 2.12 Lame on the front left leg.

Any sheep showing these symptoms as well as obvious lameness will need examining, starting by looking between the clefts of the hoof and the sole. The area where the haired skin meets the hoof horn (the coronary band) should then be examined and then the examination continued up the leg towards the body.

Seek advice from your vet if you are in any doubt as to the cause of lameness, as the incorrect diagnosis or treatment will delay healing.

It can be useful to measure and record the levels of lameness within your flock and monitor the responses to treatment. Many commercial and pedigree flocks use their vet to assess the levels of lameness within the flock during their flock health visit. They can then decide upon a treatment plan. They will help diagnose the causes of lameness, decide upon an appropriate treatment plan and then evaluate the success and response to treatment measures.

ASSESSMENT OF THE UDDER

The udder of a ewe has two functional teats in contrast to a cow which will milk on four. Examination of the udder is much easier if you have been able to turn the sheep as described above and can be clearly assessed from this position. The udder can also be assessed by observing and approaching from between the hind legs with someone restraining the ewe at the front.

The appearance and feel of the udder varies hugely throughout the year. A lactating udder will be very prominent compared to a ewe that has been weaned for a while, or a ewe that has not had a lamb before. Shepherds will evaluate the udder at significant times within the year.

1. *Before the ewe is mated.* A ewe that has an abnormal udder will not be suitable for mating as the functionality of the udder is likely to be affected. Lumps and bumps and asymmetry suggest that the ewe has had a case of mastitis during the previous lactation. This will affect the amount of milk produced in the next lactation and she will have difficulty rearing twin lambs.
2. *Immediately after lambing if lambing indoors.* This is to assess the presence of colostrum in each side and to ensure that it can be expressed easily in anticipation of the lambs suckling for the first time. The teat canals are often firmly sealed with a protective waxy plug which can sometimes require a firm pull to express it. A normal vigorous lamb will achieve this without help but sometimes a weaker lamb will struggle.
3. *Peak lactation.* At any time, later in lactation or during peak lactation if the lambs appear hungry or are not thriving well.
4. *A sick ewe.* If the ewe appears sick or lame on the hind legs at any time during lactation. This is a common symptom of mastitis.

Normal appearance of the udder

- Symmetrical when observed as the ewe is turned over or from behind
- Smooth and pink skin with no areas of discolouration other than sometimes a darker black pigment
- Warm but not hot to touch
- Pain-free when handled and palpated. A ewe that has mastitis will actively resent you feeling her by kicking your hand away. She will also kick away her lambs to prevent them sucking and causing pain
- The deeper feel to the udder should be symmetrical and soft to firm. This will vary depending upon the stage of lactation and the date of weaning. A ewe that has been weaned up to three weeks ago may still have a very firm and full udder but it should not be painful or hot on palpation

What does an udder with mastitis feel like?

The udder may be hot and painful as described above. It may also feel lumpy and hard to palpate. Both of these can suggest the presence of an acute or chronic mastitis. To assess the udder more thoroughly, milk should be expressed from both sides for comparison. A discharge that is watery, red/brown, contains thick cheesy-type clots or has a strong smell should be examined further and the ewe may need veterinary attention. Mastitis will be discussed further in Chapter 7 'Sick sheep'.

TEMPERATURE

Taking the temperature of a sick sheep is useful to record and add to your list of clinical signs. In many species, it is used as a reliable indicator for the onset of disease. However, as described previously, sheep are very good at masking illness and often the sheep is quite ill before a clinical examination and temperature assessment is performed. In the adult ewe, the normal range for temperature is 38.3–39.9°C.

Temperature readings are very useful in the examination of the newborn lamb. A healthy lamb should have a temperature of 39.0°C . If the lamb appears weak or sick and the temperature is between 37–39°C then it is mildly hypothermic, and less than 37°C the lamb will be severely hypothermic and likely to be collapsed or comatose. This will be discussed further in Chapter 6 'Lambing time'.

RUMINATION ('CUDDING')

This is the process by which the muscular layers of the rumen contract and mix together the contents of the stomach to aid the digestion of grass and other fibrous material such as hay, haylage, straw and silage. These feeds will be referred to as forage throughout the book.

Ruminants can regurgitate their stomach contents and chew them again to break the feed up into smaller pieces. This process is called rumination or 'cudding'. It happens frequently throughout the day and when at rest, sheep can be observed cudding if watched for 30 minutes or so.

It begins with a bolus of food being regurgitated up into the mouth and then the start of chewing. Sometimes saliva will be seen on the floor under the mouth. This is normal. It is abnormal if food is dropped frequently and can indicate a tooth problem or a digestive upset.

The action of cudding is a very good indicator that the animal is well. Disease, a fever, stress, in labour and general reduced health will drastically reduce or stop the action of cudding. Therefore, using the presence of cudding is a reliable way of assessing sheep health.

RESPIRATION OR BREATHING RATE

Sheep have a resting respiration rate of 16–34 breaths per minute. This is rarely observed, as when handling and moving sheep their respiration rate increases. It is important to assess breathing rate along with other signs:

- *Is the sheep breathing with the mouth open or closed?* Breathing with the mouth open can indicated respiratory disease, however it is also seen soon after moving sheep in warm weather or for a long distance. It may also be seen in sheep that have a full fleece in hot weather
- *Rapid, shallow breathing (panting).* This can also be normal in hot weather with or without a full fleece. The respiration rate is increased, even though the sheep are at rest to cool down by the evaporation of saliva and heat. Sheep should not be moved or handled excessively in these conditions and if showing these signs. In hot weather, shepherds will work with sheep either early in the morning or later in the evening when it's much cooler
- *Are there any nasal discharges present?* A clear mucus-type discharge is normal, especially in conjunction with the signs described above. A green or thick yellow-

type mucus discharge can indicate an upper respiratory infection. Copious amounts of nasal discharge can be associated with a more serious respiratory condition called 'jaagsiekte disease'. Speak to your vet for advice

- *Is the breathing noisy?* Particular breeds of sheep such as the Texel and the Beltex can suffer from an inflammation and narrowing of the larynx. This will be heard as a roaring harsh-type sound on breathing. It can be serious and needs veterinary attention immediately
- *Coughing.* Coughing in response to dust inside the shed, for example after bedding down or after moving or after administering a worming treatment, is common and usually will settle down. More persistent coughing in conjunction with other signs such as illness and weight loss can indicate the presence of a parasitic infection or other disease and may need investigating

BEHAVIOURAL RESPONSES TO WEATHER

Sheep can deal with quite severe weather conditions provided they are in good health and can seek out shelter and shade. They are designed to live out in all weathers and have a fleece of varying properties to deal with this.

As described previously, the fleece acts as a water-repellent barrier and also prevents water from seeping down to skin level. If you feel the skin of a sheep in wet weather, the skin would be dry and warm. You will notice that in wet weather, sheep are often seen either sheltering in the hedgerows, against stone walls or stood still in the field. If they move excessively, the wool will part and separate and allow rain and moisture down onto the skin. Therefore, until the rain has passed they often remain standing still with reduced grazing and movement.

Touching fleeces will also cause the repellent layer to be disrupted and water to reach the skin. Therefore, it is advised not to gather, handle or house sheep in wet weather. When left to their own devices they will stand apart from each other and not bunch up when it is wet.

The sebaceous glands of sheep secrete a substance called lanolin. This 'wool grease' acts as an excellent water repellent at the skin and fleece level and so aids their ability to withstand wet weather. As a natural substance, it is extracted from the fleece of sheep and used in the health and beauty industry.

Wool is a great insulator and so the winter months of snow and frost will not pose a problem to a healthy flock of sheep. When assessed with thermal imaging, the visible parts of the sheep are their heads and legs with their bodies remaining well insulated. This is demonstrated in snowfall when snow will remain on top of the fleece without melting, due to the body heat being trapped at skin level.

In hot weather, the fleece can be more problematic and so shearing is required when temperatures increase. The main risk is due to the creation of warm, moist skin under a heavy fleece. These conditions are highly attractive to blowflies and provide an ideal environment in which to lay their eggs.

Sheep will actively seek shade to cool down and escape from the sun. As described earlier, they will also increase their breathing rate or 'pant' to cool down. Sheep are more tolerant of heat stress than cows. Cows begin to suffer heat stress at around 23°C, whereas sheep appear comfortable up to 28°C. Provision of shade is essential in these temperatures and handling, gathering and moving sheep must be avoided in warm weather.

SHEEP SHEARING

Arranging for your sheep to be shorn every year is one of the most important responsibilities that you have as a sheep keeper. Once the temperature starts to rise, which can be as early as April in some years, the risk of sheep suffering from fly strike increases.

The fleece provides a perfect microclimate at the skin level for eggs laid by the blowfly or green bottle fly (*Lucilia Sericata*) to mature and develop into larvae. The warmth of the skin along with moisture from excess sweating and smell from nearby faecal staining will attract blow flies to 'strike' and lay their eggs.

Under these ideal conditions, the eggs hatch and rapidly develop through the larval stages to the visible 'maggot' creating severe skin damage and an open skin wound as they feed from the skin surface. Toxins and further necrotic smells attract more blowflies to the area to lay their eggs.

The eggs hatch after 12–24 hours and within 72 hours under ideal conditions they will have reached the maggot stage and have caused severe damage. Daily flock inspection is essential from March onwards.

Crutching and dagging

Both terms refer to shearing or clipping away the wool from around the tail and over the top of the tail and down the side of either back leg (see Fig. 2.13). This is usually performed early in the spring or summer to clip away faecal-stained wool which would attract flies and gives some extra protection before a full body shear is completed later in the season.

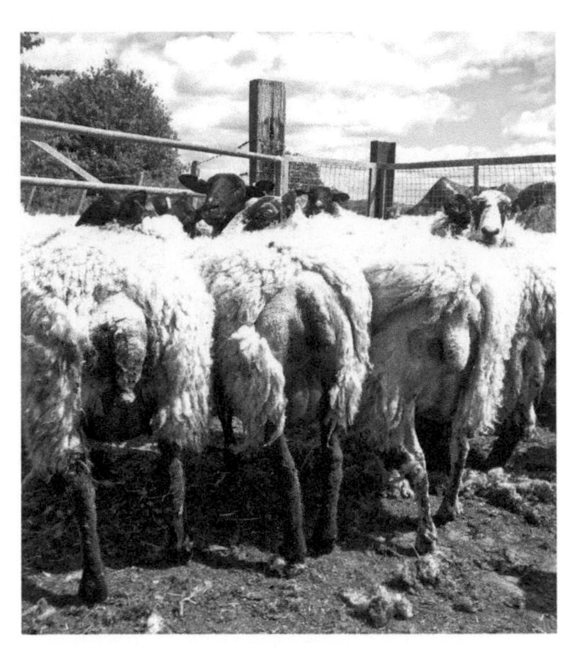

FIGURE 2.13 Ewes that have been recently crutched.

The ewes in the photo are lactating as demonstrated by their full udders. They have been crutched early in the season to remove the occurrence of wool faecal staining from the lush spring grass and hence reduce the risk of fly strike in this area, before the main shearing event. Both ewes and lambs that have started to get some faecal staining will benefit from being crutched. It can be done by yourself using hand shears or by a contract shearer.

Arrange your shearer in good time

Contact your shearer before shearing season. Once the temperatures increase everyone wants the shearer there as soon as possible. Often, smaller flocks are left to the back of the queue if they have not made themselves known beforehand.

It is useful to contact other smaller flocks in your area and ask who they get to shear their

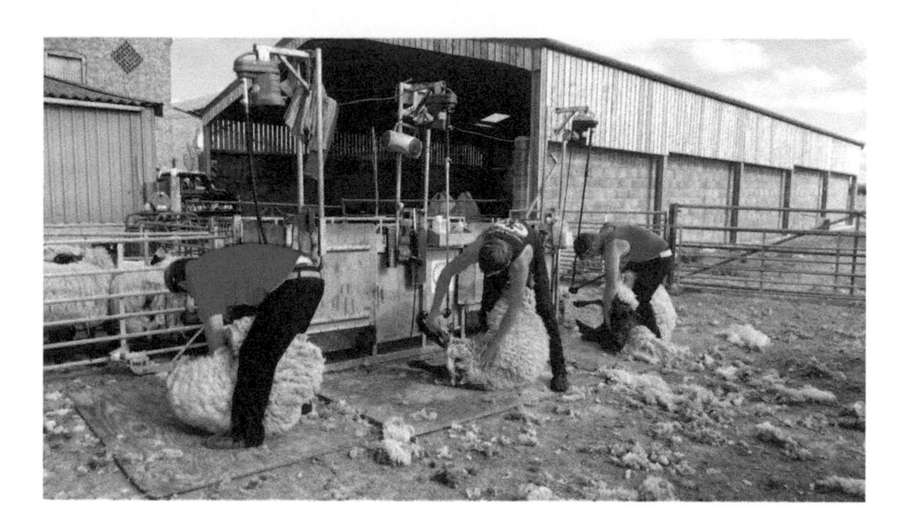

FIGURE 2.14
A shearing gang at work.

sheep. It may then be possible to arrange to shear on the same day to have a better chance of getting your sheep shorn at the correct time.

Alternatively, there are shearing courses run by the British Wool Marketing Board which are very useful. Note, however, that shearing is all about technique and practice and accidents including cuts to the skin or worse can occur if you are not confident or competent.

WHAT CAN YOU TELL FROM LOOKING AT SHEEP MUCK?

Although a strange thing to study, the appearance of the faeces from an adult sheep or lamb can provide an insight into the diet and health of the animal.

Adult sheep

What is normal?

- Firm, dark brown pellets – when on conserved forage, that is, hay and silage, or when grazing in dry conditions
- Softer, greener muck – when grazing in moist, wet conditions or when grazing rapidly growing grass. This can sometimes create staining around the tail region

What is abnormal?

- Very soft/loose dark or almost black watery diarrhoea (scour). This can indicate diseases such as a parasitic worm burden or a toxic response from a sick ewe
- Very loose brown or pasty-type faeces. In sheep that are being fed concentrated hard feed, this can indicate rumen acidosis and a subsequent digestive upset

Newborn lambs, growing lambs and weaned lambs

What is normal?

- Newborn lamb. The very first passage of faeces is the meconium. This consists of the digested amniotic fluid that has been swallowed by the lamb in the uterus. When passed it has a dark green or yellow brown-type appearance. It can be quite firm and often requires the laxative properties of the first milk to aid its passage

It is sometimes passed whilst the lamb is still inside the uterus before birth. When this happens, the lamb becomes a stained-yellow meconium colour (see Fig. 2.15). This can be an indication that the lamb was delayed in being delivered or stressed during the birthing process. It is often seen in lambs that are big or required assistance to be delivered. Sometimes the meconium is seen as soft, dark pellets within the amniotic sac after birth.

- Yellow, soft sticky muck. This is normal muck from a lamb that has started to consume milk from either it's mother or on a bottle

What is abnormal?

- Watery, yellow diarrhoea (scour). This can be seen in lambs that are being artificially milk fed and is often a result of a digestive upset. An assessment of the feeding regime should be assessed or speak to your vet if at all unsure

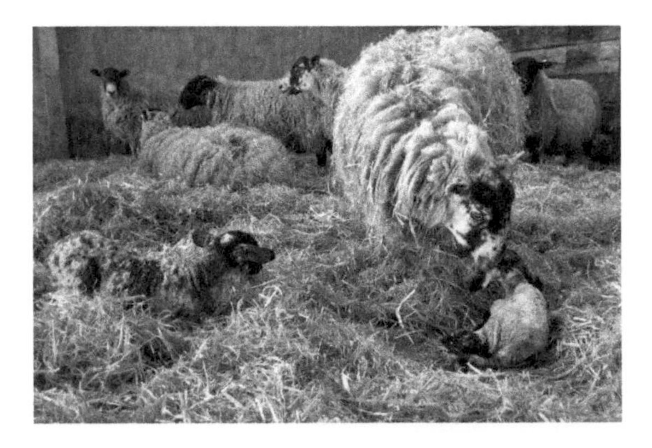

FIGURE 2.15 A meconium-stained lamb on the right.

- Watery dysentery with a darker colour or containing blood. This can indicate the presence of diseases such as lamb dysentery, rotavirus, cryptosporidium infection or *E. coli* and the lamb will require treatment. Lambs can become sick and deteriorate rapidly following the onset of these signs and veterinary advice should be immediately sought

Growing and weaned lambs

What is normal?

- Firm, soft faeces or pellets, darker green in colour. Seen in lambs that are starting to graze and still suckle
- Pelleted dark green faeces or firm but soft and brown consistency. Seen in lambs that are starting to wean and graze effectively and lambs that are starting to eat concentrated hard feed

What is abnormal?

- Loose scour; grey, pasty (some blood staining) faeces causing staining on the tail and perineal region. This is not normal and can indicate disease such as coccidiosis along with other signs
- Loose, watery, green faeces causing staining around the tail as above – may indicate parasitic disease and needs further investigation

The diseases associated with diarrhoea in adult and young sheep will be discussed in Chapter 6 'Lambing time' and Chapter 7 'Sick sheep'.

Internal parasitic disease is one of the most common diseases affecting growing lambs and can cause significant poor growth, death and increased risk of fly strike. All small holdings and small flocks should have a parasite control plan, developed in conjunction with their vet.

Conducting a health assessment of your sheep should be a daily routine. A visual inspection of the flock may be all that is required and it is important to always assess the whole flock. This yields a great deal of information. Then look at any individuals that are not behaving normally and determine if they need further assessment or veterinary attention.

THE ORGAN SYSTEMS OF THE SHEEP

3

Knowledge of some of the specific aspects of sheep biology and physiology are crucial to the successful husbandry and handling of the flock. As previously described, the flock instinct is strong and is very difficult to override. Successful handling comes from working with this instinct. A sheep's sight and vision play a significant role in the expression of flock behaviour and understanding this will improve your success of handling.

UNDERSTANDING SIGHT TO HELP WITH SHEEP HANDLING

Sight is very important to the flock behaviour of sheep. As prey animals and grazing animals, they have a wide monocular angle of vision. They must be able to see other members of the flock to determine the approach of a predator or danger, enabling them to graze whilst being vigilant.

The positioning of their eyes on the side of the head creates a wide angle of vision of 320–340°. This will allow them to graze and scan for 'predators'. They have a blind spot directly behind them and they have a narrow angle of vision at the front (see Figure 3.1). This frontal vision can be restricted further if they are breeds with woolly heads.

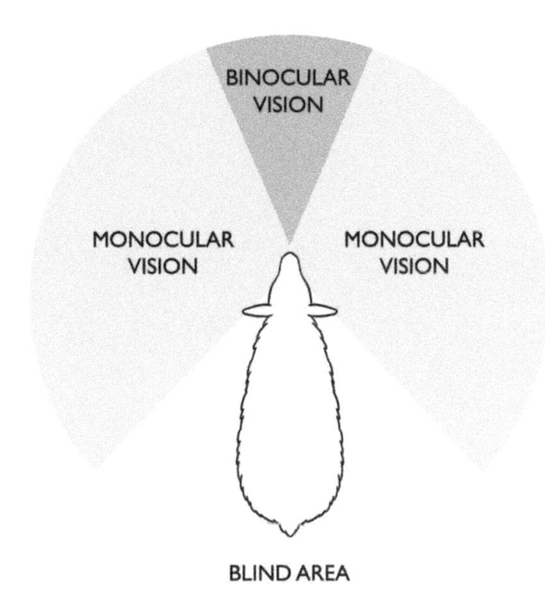

FIGURE 3.1 The visual perspective of sheep.

This type of vision can be used by the shepherd to move them. It is done by working with their point of balance. The point of balance for a sheep is at its shoulder, which can be seen in Figure 3.2 as the red line across both shoulders. By moving your body at a 90° angle to the spine of the sheep behind the point of balance

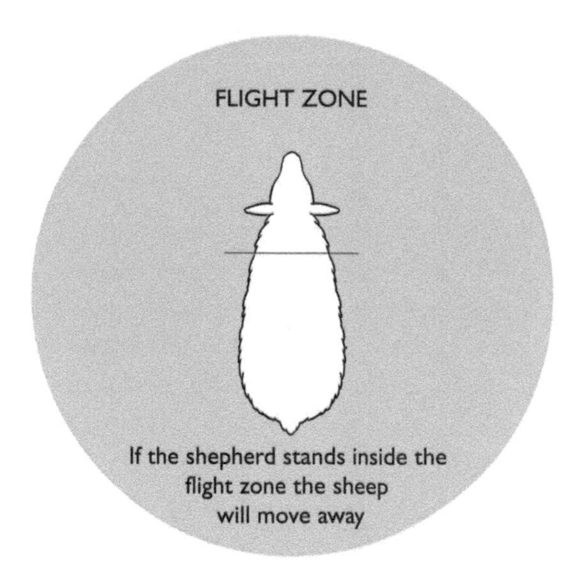

FIGURE 3.2 Diagram representing the flight zone.

(shoulder), the sheep will move forward and away from you. By moving your body in front of their point of balance (shoulder) the sheep will turn away and move backwards. Shepherds use this method instinctively to move sheep and they train their working dogs to work with this behaviour.

The flight zone

Sheep also have a 'flight zone' or an area of personal space (see Fig. 3.2). This is your distance away from a sheep which will not elicit a response to move away. Moving closer to the flock will initiate them to move away when you enter their flight zone and conversely moving out of the zone will stop or slow down their movement.

The flight zone will alter depending upon the type of sheep and the calmness of the shepherd. For example, well-handled sheep will have a reduced flight zone, enabling you to move closer into their personal space. Less-handled sheep or younger sheep may have a larger flight zone and will move away at a longer distance. Increased noise or unfamiliar handlers or dogs will increase the flight zone and sheep will move away sooner.

Sheep use their sight to recognise other members of the flock and research suggests that they can recognise up to 50 individuals within their flock. As described, they use their sight to view other flock members and move together as a flock.

Sheep are followers and there are often dominant leaders within a group. This can be helpful in some situations and unhelpful in others, particularly if the dominant sheep are escape artists or wanderers.

When being moved within a handling system of gates and hurdles sheep will move successfully towards a known exit, for example the gate to the field or towards a perceived 'open' exit. Therefore, it is important to consider this when building or assembling handling systems.

Solid-sided hurdles cast fewer shadows and provide a focussed path of movement with less distraction from outside hazards such as a dog or table/equipment. Creating a funnel effect or a curved effect with minimal right angles will encourage sheep to continue to move and follow the sheep in front.

Sheep can remember and associate good or bad experiences with handling systems. This will reduce the speed at which sheep are willing to move through a system. It is far better (for sheep and farmer) to try and work with a sheep preference for movement rather than trying to move sheep using fear and noise.

Figure 3.3 shows a solid-sided race and sheep visible in the holding pen towards the

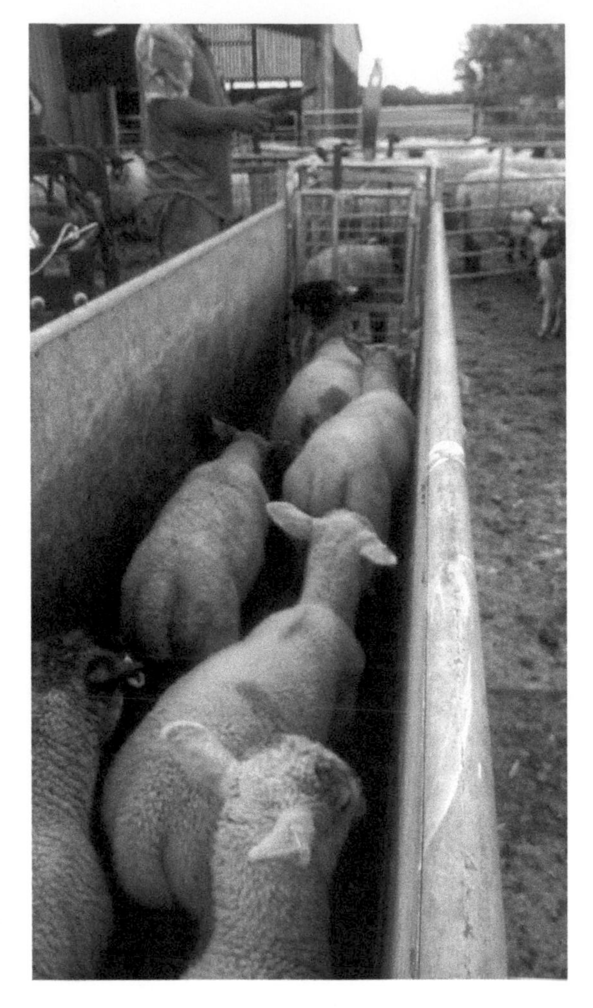

FIGURE 3.3 A sheep race.

exit. Both help with sheep movement through the system.

SMELL AND HEARING

Sheep can use their smell to detect humans and dogs. They also use their sense of smell to identify their young lambs, particularly in the first few weeks of birth. They can detect their own scent from their lambs when the lambs pass faeces produced from the first milk feed.

When fostering on lambs to a foster mother it is important that the lamb sucks the foster ewe's milk. Some methods of adoption involve masking the smell of the strange lamb. See Chapter 6 'Lambing time' for more details on fostering.

Sheep rarely vocalise, which is an adaptation as a prey animal. They vocalise most frequently at lambing time to identify their lambs. Lambs will vocalise vigorously to find their mothers. They also will vocalise to find other members of their flock, particularly if separated. Many sheep have also adapted to vocalise on the sight of a human in anticipation of food, particularly at lambing time.

THE DIGESTIVE SYSTEM

Sheep are ruminants which means, like cattle and goats, they have a unique digestive system to digest forage. A thorough understanding of this system will lead to a thriving and contented flock of sheep. In contrast to humans and other carnivores, ruminants use four chambers of their fore stomach to digest plant fibre. They also have a series of adaptations and mechanisms related to their physiology which makes their system of digestion very efficient and completely suited to a diet of pasture or forage.

A system of chewing and regurgitation enables the breakdown of forage into smaller pieces. The digestive process then progresses with a population of resident microbes which break down the diet further to produce protein and energy.

Breaking down forage

For this system to be successful, sheep must have good oral health to enable grazing and mastication (chewing) and they must also be presented with a suitable diet. Grass or forage enters the mouth using the lower incisor teeth and the hard upper dental pad in a nibbling-type motion. This differs to cattle slightly, who use their tongue more to rip up the grass and pass it into the mouth. Sheep can graze shorter grass than cattle.

On entering the mouth, the food is chewed using the upper and lower molar teeth and a bolus of food is formed. A very important aspect of the sheep's digestive system is the action of chewing.

Fibrous food requires a prolonged time of chewing and during this process copious amounts of saliva are produced and swallowed. Saliva is required to aid digestion by helping the passage of food down the oesophagus and because it contains neutralising properties such as bicarbonate. This helps to maintain the neutral pH environment of the rumen and provide an ideal environment for the rumen microbes or microflora.

The amount of saliva produced by a fibrous diet is almost 60–70% more than a diet that has reduced fibre and increased starch-based carbohydrates.

The swallowed bolus of food travels down the oesophagus and enters the reticulum, a relatively small chamber where microbes can begin to act and where foreign bodies will tend to settle and deposit. The bolus of food then travels into the rumen.

The rumen is the largest digestion chamber of the four stomachs. It has a dorsal (upper) sac and a ventral (lower) sac. Digested food sinks to the bottom of the ventral rumen sac and the most recent swallowed food remains on top as a fibrous mat of food.

Strong rhythmical muscular contractions conducted by the muscular layers of the rumen create a churning effect. These 'churns' happen twice every three to five minutes and it allows the complete mixing of the rumen contents.

This mixing has four main effects:

1. *Rumination or 'cudding'.* The recent bolus of food is regurgitated back into the mouth where it is chewed again to be broken into smaller pieces. The rumen microbes can act more effectively on a larger surface area. Cudding allows more saliva to be added to help maintain rumen pH and aid further digestion.
2. *Eructation.* 'Belching'. The release of fermentation gases. Gases containing methane, hydrogen sulphide and carbon dioxide are produced from the highly fermentative digestion process. These gases are released as a belch (eructation).
3. *Mixing.* The contents of the rumen are mixed to allow further contact with the microbes and for the digested products to sink towards the bottom (ventral) rumen sac.
4. *Movement.* The digested contents are moved towards the exit of the rumen and into the omasal chamber ready for the next stage of digestion.

Figure 3.4 shows the position of the stomachs within the sheep. The reticulum and rumen occupy the left side of the abdomen. If you place your hand behind the last rib on the left side, you should be able to feel the rumen as you apply gentle pressure. You may even feel the rumen contract under your hand.

The omasum and small intestines are on the right side of the abdominal cavity. The abomasum sits mainly on the right side of the abdomen and underneath the rumen.

FIGURE 3.4 The digestive tract.

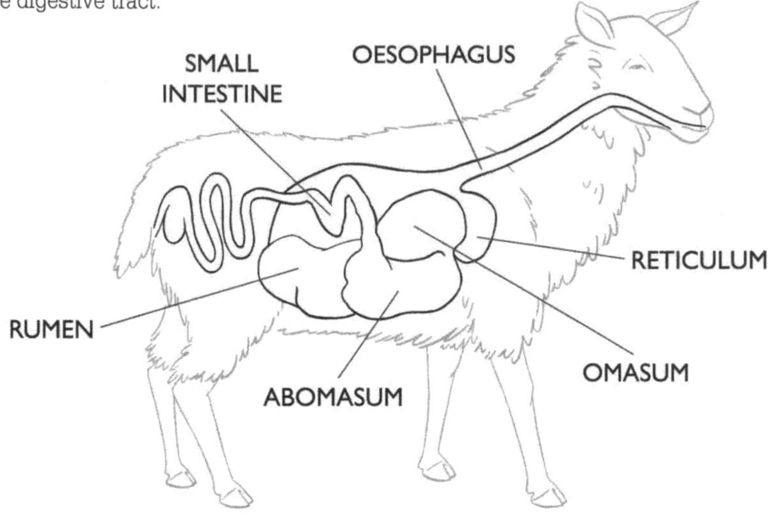

The reticulum

The reticulum lining has the appearance of a honeycomb (see Fig. 3.5). It is separated from the rumen by a ridge of tissue but acts in a very similar way to the rumen. It is of a much smaller size than the rumen and is often the site where foreign bodies such as metalwork, Chinese lantern components and nails become lodged.

The rumen

The rumen is the largest 'fermentation vat' of the ruminant stomachs. The lining of the rumen consists of huge numbers of papillae (leafy projections; see Fig. 3.6). Their function is to increase surface area to improve the absorption of some of the nutrients produced from fermentation.

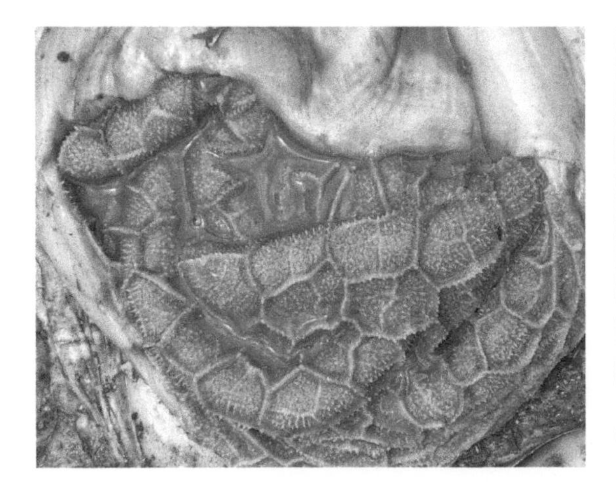

FIGURE 3.5 The reticulum lining.

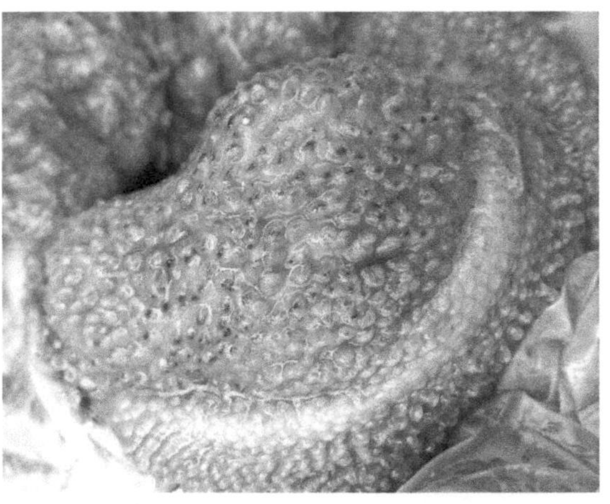

FIGURE 3.6 The rumen lining.

The omasum

The omasum has a surface that is highly folded and almost appears like the pages of a book (see Fig. 3.7). Most of the water absorption occurs here before the digesta moves into the abomasum.

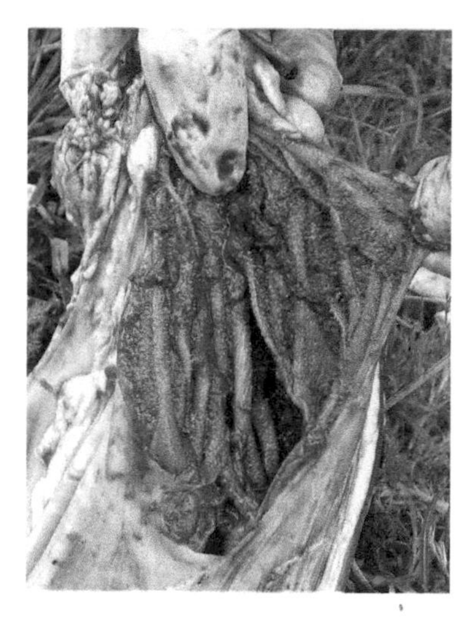

FIGURE 3.7 The omasal lining.

The abomasum

The abomasum is the final stomach compartment before entering the small intestine and is often called the 'true stomach'. This compartment is like that of a non-ruminant and has a glandular secretory lining (see Fig. 3.8). It produces hydrochloric acid and digestive enzymes. It also produces mucus to protect the lining.

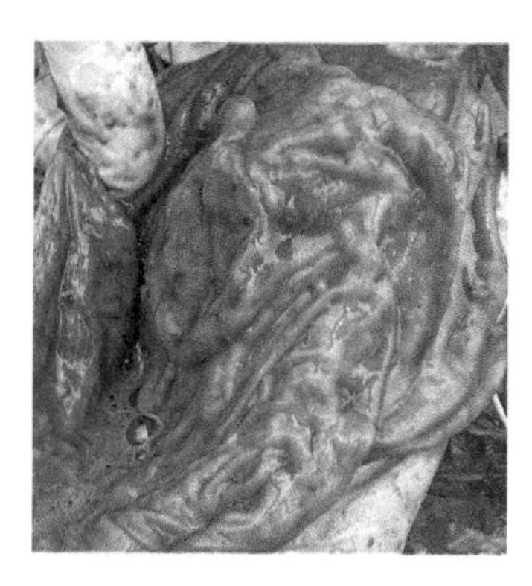

FIGURE 3.8 The abomasal lining.

This acidic environment results in the death of rumen microbes and the production of microbial protein from the dead microbe population. This protein and smaller food particles from the rumen are digested in the abomasum by the action of digestive enzymes rather than fermentation. The contents then move into the small intestine where further digestion and the absorption of protein and nutrients occurs. Finally, it moves further into the large intestine leading to the production of faeces.

The microbe army

Successful digestion is reliant upon a complex population of microbes that live within the reticulum and rumen compartments of the fore stomach. These bacterial, protozoal and fungi-type organisms are responsible for the digestion of food. Without them, or with a reduced population, digestion will be reduced. Therefore, when considering how to feed sheep, you are considering how to feed the rumen microflora.

A diet of grass may appear boring and monotonous; however, it is essential in maintaining a constant feed source upon which these specialised microbes can act. They hate change! These organisms are anaerobic and favour an almost neutral pH 6.5–6.8 environment. They use a specialised fermentation process to digest plant cell walls which consist of cellulose, hemicellulose and pectin. These are carbohydrates that are unable to be digested by species other than ruminants.

Some microorganisms can also digest starch. The population of microbes within the rumen is a mixed population and the amounts of the different species will vary depending upon the type of diet being fed. Therefore, this population is very adaptable if change occurs slowly, for example over a period of two to three weeks. Sudden diet changes are not good news for ruminants.

It is also essential that the products of digestion are constant, to ensure that the working environment for the microbes is kept at a constant pH. This will allow their survival and reproduction.

What do the microbes produce?

The products of bacterial fermentation include microbial protein (from the 'dead' microbes), amino acids, ammonia, B vitamins, volatile fatty acids (used for energy), carbon dioxide and methane. The rumen microbes use carbohydrates, ammonia and amino acids to grow and maintain their population.

The microbes then act to produce volatile fatty acids. The volatile fatty acids are absorbed across the rumen wall into the circulating bloodstream and are used by the liver to produce glucose and other forms of energy available to the sheep.

As the digesta flows through the gastrointestinal tract, the microbial protein and amino acids are digested and absorbed within the small intestine.

Digestive upsets

Whilst the sheep may delight in gaining unsupervised access to the feed store, or being fed extra amounts of concentrated hard feed, their rumen microbe population will not be happy. Large amounts of carbohydrate (hard feed) consumed all at once will create a peak of products, that is, volatile fatty acids.

This peak has the sudden effect of a reduced, more acidic rumen. This, in combination with reduced chewing and saliva production leads to a disrupted, more acidic environment within the rumen, and the effect will be a reduction in population of effective microbes and a digestive upset for the sheep. The clinical signs for this are as follows:

- Sheep appeared subdued and reluctant to feed or graze
- Increased time spent lying down
- Head and ears dropped and appearing restless
- Looking around at their stomach
- Diarrhoea (scour) staining the fleece around the tail and hind legs
- Lying flat or with the chin resting
- Collapse and death

Prompt veterinary attention is required immediately if you are aware that a large amount of grain/hard feed has been consumed or if you find your sheep displaying the above symptoms.

There may just be one greedy sheep affected or the whole group may be affected to varying degrees, depending upon how much grain they could eat. In many cases, when the sheep have started to scour they may then respond well to supportive veterinary care. When collapse has occurred, the prognosis is poor and often the affected sheep won't survive. Details on treating 'grain overload' or 'rumen acidosis' will be discussed in Chapter 7 'Sick sheep'.

The pre-weaned lamb: before life as a ruminant!

A lamb is born without a functioning rumen and without a population of rumen microbes.

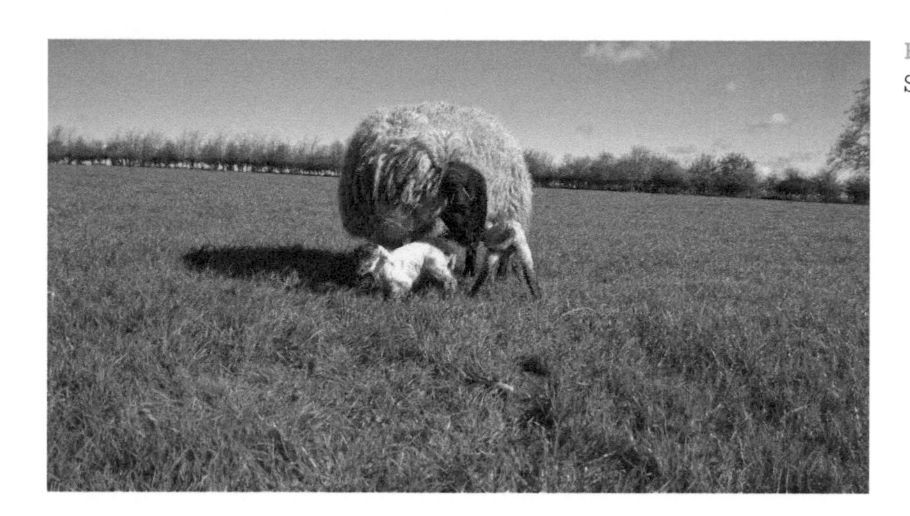

FIGURE 3.9
Successful suckling.

Their diet consists primarily of milk for the first few weeks of life and their digestive system is adapted to accommodate this. The abomasum is the largest stomach compartment in the newborn lamb and milk is digested in this chamber.

The digestive system accepts a milk feed by 'closing' access to the rumen, by the closure of the oesophageal/reticular groove. This groove consists of muscular layers which are stimulated to fold and close. This allows the milk to be directed over the small rumen compartment and through the omasum to the abomasum.

This anticipation of milk is stimulated by the mother nudging her lamb or lambs towards the udder and it occurs when the lambs naturally become hungry.

This amazing adaptation means that the rumen remains free of milk, which would otherwise remain undigested and cause a digestive upset. A lamb suckling with a wagging tail is an outward indication that the 'groove' has closed and the milk is diverting into the correct place (see Fig. 3.9).

Pet and orphan lambs: playing mum!

Lambs that are orphaned or kept without their mothers can often suffer digestive upsets due to too much milk or unusual feeding patterns. If they are fed at set periods throughout the day they will require 'instruction' or a signal that feeding is due. This will stimulate oesophageal groove closure.

This 'signal' could include feeding at regular intervals or mixing up the milk in front of the lambs. This would create enough anticipation to stimulate the oesophageal groove to close. Feeding the milk at the same concentration (as written on the bag) and at the same temperature is also crucial to preventing digestive upsets in lambs. More details on pet lambs can be found in Chapter 6 'Lambing time'.

Developing a rumen

The rumen microbes are introduced into the developing rumen by the lambs exploring their environment with their mouths. The action of their mothers licking their lambs around the head and mouth also helps introduce microbes into the lamb. As they experiment and ingest straw or hay from the environment, the reticulum and rumen compartments are 'scratched' into action and rumen development commences. This development progresses as the diet of the lamb starts to consist of feed and substrates other than milk.

At birth, the reticulorumen chamber accounts for approximately 30% of the total stomach volume. By the time the sheep reaches adulthood, the reticulorumen compartment accounts for approximately 75% of the total stomach compartment.

The ruminant digestive system is such a highly complex system that it is still not fully understood. It provides a fascinating insight into how the selection and adaption of biological systems have evolved to enable the survival of ruminants on pasture-based systems all over the world. The health and success of a ruminant animal is completely dependent upon having a functioning rumen.

THE REPRODUCTIVE SYSTEM

Sheep are seasonal breeders. The onset of their breeding cycle, that is, showing sexual behaviour and the ovulation of an egg for fertilisation, is dependent upon decreasing day length. The breeding season in the UK is typically from late August until late December/early January. The peak breeding season occurs around late October to mid November for most breeds.

The Dorset Horn is a British breed that has a breeding season of around eight months and so can produce lambs over a much longer period throughout the year. The peak breeding period for lowland breeds and crossbreeds such as the Suffolk, Hampshire, South Down and North Country Mules will be slightly earlier and have longer breeding seasons (six to seven cycles) compared to the hill breeds.

The mountain breeds such as the Welsh mountain, Swaledale and Cheviots peak slightly later in their breeding season at around late November to December and have a shorter breeding period of around three to four months (four to five cycles).

This seasonality also affects the rams in terms of the onset of libido and peak fertility. As well as the timing of breeding, there are many other factors that can affect the success of breeding. These relate to nutrition, health status and disease status.

A successful breeding season centred upon optimum fertility is paramount for commercial enterprises to achieve optimum productivity from their flock. The reproductive cycle and breeding will be discussed in more detail in Chapter 5 'Breeding sheep'.

APPROACHING THE END OF LIFE

One thing is certain, that at some point these organ systems will fail and result in the death of the sheep. Domesticated sheep will not usually die due to 'old age'. They are often humanely euthanased to prevent suffering and discomfort.

In large flocks, unhealthy sheep become less productive and they will suffer if they are not either treated or euthanased. As sheep age, they lose or wear down their incisor teeth which means they can no longer graze effectively. The result is a loss of weight and body condition and they can become very thin. Ewes which are very thin due to suspected disease or old age should be euthanased on farm.

Some ewes are healthy but they have lost condition due to lack of teeth, or they have reduced productivity due to poor fertility or poor feet. These ewes can become 'cull ewes'. This means they are either housed or placed on some very good grazing and fed a palatable diet to improve body condition before then entering the cull ewe trade. There is a value to older sheep meat and abattoirs across the country want cull ewes for this purpose.

In many larger flocks, the aim is to maintain a healthy, productive flock and so sheep rarely reach ages above 5 or 6 years old, unless they are in very good condition.

In smaller flocks, where more individual care can be provided, sheep may reach far older ages. However, the rules are the same. If they struggle to eat and maintain condition or they appear to have a chronic disease or are lame due to arthritis or poor foot conformation, then they should be humanely euthanased on welfare grounds.

Euthanasia: what to expect

Euthanasia can be performed by your veterinary surgeon or by a suitable trained operator of a firearm. There are detailed descriptive guidelines for this procedure which can be found on the Red Tractor Farm Assurance website. The document is titled 'On farm humane killing of cattle and sheep'.

A veterinary surgeon will euthanase an animal either by lethal injection of a barbiturate or by using a captive bolt or humane killer. These methods are humane, but it is more common that smallholders request that their sheep are euthanased by lethal injection.

In this procedure, the vet will clip away the wool around the jugular vein and inject barbiturate directly into the vein. The result is an immediate loss of consciousness and then death. This procedure will require someone to hold the sheep securely whilst the vet administers the injection.

It can sometimes be difficult with older sheep or sheep that are sick, to locate and raise the jugular vein. This is often due to poor circulation. Therefore, in some cases it may take time to prepare the vein and several attempts may be required. After death has occurred there may be a final intake of air or sudden movement. This is a normal after-death occurrence and does not mean that the sheep is regaining consciousness.

Can you bury sheep?

Pet sheep, along with other species such as pigs, cattle and horses, can be buried on your land if they were strictly pets, that is, they are kept for purposes other than farming. If you don't have these facilities or if you are breeding sheep to sell, eat or show then you must either take them or arrange collection from a registered fallen stock collector. Vet practices can also arrange for individual sheep to be cremated but this is associated with a significant cost.

DIET AND NUTRITION 4

Given the correct resources, sheep have a fantastic ability to be able to look after themselves. The most important resource required is that of nutrition. As grazing animals, they will actively graze extensive areas in search of new shoots of grass. Hill breeds are adapted to do this in harsh conditions, over large areas and they can successfully maintain good body condition.

Sheep that are housed during lambing and sheep that are grazed on more restricted areas such as a smallholding will rely upon the husbandry skills of the shepherd to monitor their diet and nutrition. This is crucial to the success of a healthy flock. If their body condition is kept optimum and their nutrition adequate, they will be healthy and productive.

GRAZING

'Are sheep suitable lawnmowers?'

Many small flock keepers start their flock with the intentions of maintaining the grass height of a small paddock or lawn. Or land is acquired to accommodate a small flock of sheep. Often the quality of the grazing is not always sufficient to support the number of grazing sheep and either supplementary feed or forage is required.

Sheep keepers are often surprised at how quickly sheep will graze through what appears to be a big area. Sheep are quite fussy animals and will leave grass that is too long and overgrown in favour of tasty new shoots. They can be used as an alternative to a lawnmower but they will be far more selective than a trusty petrol equivalent.

It is very useful to have a basic knowledge of the digestive system and nutritional requirements of sheep and how their performance and suitability of the diet can be assessed. It is also important to regularly handle and assess their body condition. This should be done at least every six to eight weeks to ensure that they are in the correct condition.

Refer to Chapter 2 'The Normal Sheep' for a method of how to assess the body condition of your sheep. Chapter 3 'The Organ Systems of Sheep' describes the unique digestive system of the sheep and how forage is digested.

What can sheep eat?

Sheep can digest forage in the form of fresh grass and conserved grass such as hay and silage or straw. They can also digest leguminous plants such as peas, beans and chicory, and root crops such as kale, turnips and fodder or sugar beet.

Cereals such as wheat, oats and barley are also digestible. Byproducts of oilseeds, that is, soya, and rapeseed and sunflower meal can be digested and are used to make up compound feeds or in home mixes.

Some plant species are poisonous to sheep. These will be discussed in Chapter 7 'Sick sheep'.

HOW TO SUCCESSFULLY FEED YOUR SHEEP

Consider these 'guidelines' when feeding your sheep.

1. *A constant fresh water supply.* A daily supply of water is required in the rumen for fermentation. Sheep will consume around two to four litres of water a day. This will be from drinking and from the water in forage. The amount obtained from the diet will depend on its moisture content.

   The water intake of a ewe will rise significantly during the later stages of pregnancy and in early lactation. A ewe will require four to eight litres of water per day from around lambing and up to six to eight weeks after lambing. Therefore, it is essential to ensure that they have an unlimited supply of fresh water during this time.

   Restricting water supply will also restrict the amount of forage consumed by the ewe and so limit her energy intake. This can also lead to the development of metabolic conditions in the sheep around lambing time (See Chapter 7 'Sick sheep').
2. *Forage.* Most of a ruminant's diet should consist of quality forage. This will be grass throughout most of the year and conserved forages if they are housed over the winter. Many sheep are grazed all year and receive little other changes to their diet other than at lambing time. They will need extra feed sources to maintain condition and prepare for lambing. Extra feed will also be required during adverse weather and when grass quality is poor over the winter months.

   Good forages and grass will have sufficient levels of protein and energy. The quality of the hay or silage depends upon many factors such as grass species, time of harvesting, how dry it is and spoilage during storage.

   Forages are regularly sent away for analysis on larger flocks to assess their feed quality. This analysis can then be used to calculate the amount of extra feed required to meet demand. Poor- to average-quality hay is only useful for feeding to sheep as a maintenance diet.

   Select good forage for pregnant sheep. Increased energy is required when the ewes are in late pregnancy and are preparing to produce milk. Increased protein levels are also required for foetal growth and milk production. Extra protein is also required for growth in young ewes that have not yet reached their mature adult weight.

How do I assess my forage without sending it away for analysis?
It is common for small holders to house their sheep over the winter and during lambing time due to restricted grazing and for easier management. It is also likely that you may need to buy in forage in the form of small hay bales or silage.

To assess the quality, you can smell and feel the hay to detect a good, sweet smell and check for dust levels. Good-quality silage should have very little moisture leakage when squeezed in your hand and should have a nice sweet smell.

This can provide an indication of the quality of the forage but is very subjective and not as accurate as having it analysed. Asking for the history of where and when the forage was made will also help you to assess its likely qualities.

Avoid and do not feed damp, mouldy hay, or hay with lots of soil contamination as the sheep are unlikely to eat it. It may also cause serious disease or abortion from bacteria such as listeria. Mouldy, dusty hay is a sign that it was wet when baled and the forage will be of poor quality.

Forage is best offered ad lib to ensure that all the sheep have a good forage supply available at all times. This will help to maintain a healthy rumen microbe population and help the sheep maintain a good body condition. All sheep including shy feeders will be able to consume the required forage.

The recommended space requirement for feeding ewes is 45 cm feed space per ewe when feeding restricted amounts (once or twice a day) of forage or concentrates in troughs. The space requirement for ad lib feeding is 10–12 cm trough space.

Make sure you regularly (every six to eight weeks) body condition score your sheep by handling them. If their body condition is reducing, then either the diet is insufficient or there are disease problems. Consult your vet as soon as you notice changes.

3. *Grazed grass.* The quality of grass changes throughout the year in relation to climate and growth. Spring grass contains high levels of sugars and so provides high levels of energy and protein. This coincides well with the natural lambing time when the energy demands for milk production are at their greatest. The quality of grazing deteriorates in autumn once the growth rates slow down and the number of sunshine hours reduce.

The height of the grass is important. Sheep favour grazing between 4 and 12 cm in height. Grass will start to go to seed as it increases in height and will then be avoided by the sheep. Grass height less than 2 cm may prove difficult to bite, and older sheep with poorer quality teeth or fewer teeth will struggle to graze and start to lose condition.

Grazing can be improved by reseeding (sowing new seed) with specific grass seeds and the application of fertilisers. The addition of clover to your grazing will increase protein levels and the addition of chicory and mixed herbal leys are useful as an aid to internal worm control.

Red clover. Be aware that pastures containing large amounts of red clover (more than 30 per cent) should not be grazed by ewes for six weeks before, six weeks after and during the mating period. The higher levels of phyto-oestrogens within this plant can cause a reduction in fertility in the ewes.

The importance of teeth. The presence of teeth is often overlooked by novice sheep keepers. As sheep age their incisors become wobbly within the gum and frequently fall out. This is described as a ewe with a 'broken mouth' (see 'Ageing sheep' in Chapter 2). The incisors are essential for nibbling and biting off grass, therefore ewes with a broken mouth are often first seen as losing condition.

It is important to check the cause of weight loss. Unfortunately, ewes with a broken mouth should leave the flock. They will not be able to maintain their health on a grazing diet and will suffer if they are left unchecked. Their diet must be altered to enable them to consume more energy and protein in the form of concentrates and conserved forages.

Rotate your grazing. A way of increasing the amount of grass available is by increasing the rate of regrowth. This can be done by dividing up your available land to create smaller paddocks for grazing (see Fig. 4.1). This will enable you to rotate your grazing and 'rest' your grass. Rotating every three weeks will help improve grass regrowth and reduce the worm burden on the pasture.

In favourable conditions such as during the summer with warm temperatures and some moisture, worm eggs deposited by the sheep onto the pasture will hatch and develop into infective larvae within 5–14 days. Therefore, if there are no sheep to graze and ingest these infective larvae, the larvae will die off and the overall worm burden on the pasture can be reduced (see Chapter 7 in the 'Diarrhoea' section' for more details on the worm life cycle.

4. *Gradual diet change.* If hard sheep feed is required in the form of concentrated carbohydrates, it is essential the process of introducing this food is gradual. The rumen microbes require a constant environment and their functions can be very sensitive to changes. The normal rumen pH is around 6.5–6.8. Despite the products of fermentation consisting of fatty acids, which reduce the pH, the rumen maintains a constant pH by the action of chewing and saliva production. Saliva contains bicarbonate which, when swallowed, can neutralise the acidic conditions in the rumen.

Sudden diet changes affect this process. Compound feeds containing higher levels of carbohydrate are fermented more

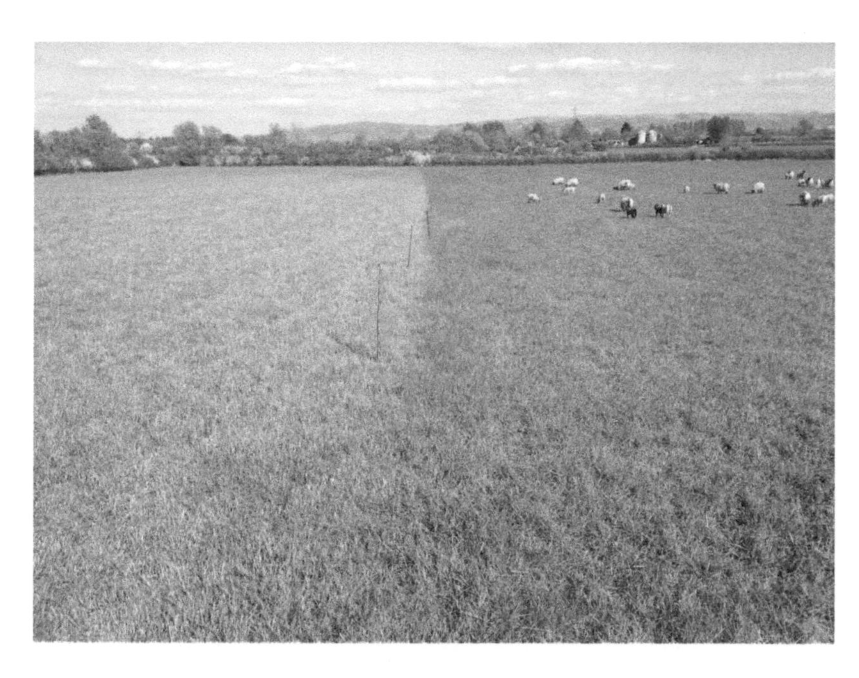

FIGURE 4.1 Using electric fencing to divide up pasture.

quickly and result in an increase in volatile fatty acids. They also require less chewing and reduced cudding. Therefore, less saliva is produced and the buffering capacity is reduced which leads to an overall decrease in rumen pH.

As described in the previous chapter, the result is disruption of the microbe population. This will cause digestive upsets and is discussed in Chapter 7 'Sick sheep'.

TYPES OF COMPOUND SHEEP FEED

Compound hard feeds contain energy in the form of starch (wheat, barley and oats) and sugars (sugar beet and molasses) and a combination of protein sources including soya bean meal, rapeseed, wheat distillers and beans. They also contain formulated vitamins, minerals and trace elements for the target group of sheep, for example lactating ewes, growing lambs and finishing lambs.

Some farmers will make up their own feed each year using home-grown cereals, beans and bought minerals to complement the results of their forage analysis. Most farmers and almost all smallholders will buy and feed a manufactured compound feed. The quality and cost of these feeds varies but they should contain all the requirements needed to maintain a healthy sheep.

Considerations when feeding compound feeds

- *Do not* feed concentrated feed designed for lactating ewes to rams or male lambs – this can cause bladder stones and severe urination difficulties due to the high mineral content
- Make sure the feed can be fed to sheep. Never feed concentrated feed that has been formulated for pigs or cattle only. These contain high levels of copper which can be toxic for sheep
- A good, fresh water supply should always be available
- Regularly monitor body condition to check that your sheep are not getting too fat or too thin and adjust the feed accordingly

How much to feed?

This will depend upon the reason for feeding. If you feed it at housing in the winter period or in the lead-up to lambing, most feeds will be started off at a low rate of feeding, that is, 100–150 g per day or twice per day at approximately six to eight weeks away from lambing. This will be stepped up each week or each fortnight to a maximum of 500 g twice a day in the one to two weeks before lambing.

Sheep should not receive any more than 500 g of concentrate at one feed. A maximum of two feeds per day should be fed. More than this will start to negatively upset the rumen balance and cause effects on the rumen microbes.

These are very approximate amounts and will alter depending upon the body condition, amount of lambs being carried and quality of the forage provided. Therefore, detailed feeding guidelines have been produced which are available online from the levy board or seek advice from your vet or nutritionist.

Many smallholders will feed a small amount of compound feed daily to ensure that they can handle and catch their sheep. This should be around 100–150 g of a general compound sheep feed. They may also need to feed more if grazing and forage quality is restricted or in short supply. This is OK if the correct type of feed is used for the correct group of sheep, for example lambs, rams and ewes, and if the body condition of the sheep is closely monitored. Note that prolonged concentrate feeding can cause issues with excess copper in the diet (see later in this chapter).

FEEDING DURING PREGNANCY

In the first and second trimester of the pregnancy (for the first three-and-a-half months) the ewe will not need much extra feed if her body condition is good (score 3, see Chapter 2 'The normal sheep'). If too much energy is supplied in this period, the ewe may become too fat which will cause lambing difficulties and the increased risk of metabolic disease such as 'twin lamb disease' (see Chapter 6 'Lambing time'). Extra forage should be fed during adverse weather such as flooding and heavy snowfall.

The ewe should not normally need extra feed in terms of concentrates until the final trimester, that is, the last six to eight weeks before lambing. The amount of energy and protein required is based upon the body condition score of the ewe and the number of lambs that she is carrying.

It is always advisable to scan the ewes during pregnancy to identify the number of lambs being carried. See Chapter 5 'Breeding sheep' for more information. Ewes carrying twins and triplets will need more feed than a single bearing ewe.

Most (75%) of the foetal growth occurs during the final six weeks of pregnancy. This growth uses energy consumed by the ewe and her own body reserves. Lean ewes (body condition score 2.5 or less) will need to be fed more energy during pregnancy. It is good practice to separate the lean and multiple bearing ewes from the single bearing ewes and feed them separately.

This is not always possible and so close attention should be paid to the amounts being fed to avoid the problem of oversize lambs that are difficult to deliver at birth. If the single bearing ewes are in good body condition and on a diet of good forage, then they should not need any extra hard feed.

FEEDING AFTER LAMBING

Good-quality nutrition is needed after lambing to enable the ewe to supply a plentiful amount of milk to meet the demands of her growing lambs. Good nutrition is also needed to help her body recover from the demands of pregnancy and prevent further weight loss.

Fresh quality forage should always be available to maintain a healthy rumen. If the ewes were receiving concentrated hard feed before lambing, this should be continued for at least until the ewes and lambs are turned out to grass.

The time of year in which you are lambing and the amount of grass growth will determine how much extra feed you need to provide. If lambing early in February or March, then the ewes will need a daily supply of forage and concentrated feed until the grass starts to grow.

If you are lambing in April or May, in most years the grass growth should be plentiful and of very good quality. Therefore, no further feeding should be required if you do not have too many animals for the amount of available pasture. Make sure you have planned and considered this before you decide when to lamb.

Peak milk production is usually reached at around four to six weeks after birth. During this time, the diet must be able to supply enough energy and protein for the ewe to produce the required milk and maintain her body condition.

If the milk supply is not enough, the lambs will suffer in their health and ability to fight disease and their growth will be reduced. The ewe is also at significant risk of mastitis as the hungry lambs feed more frequently and traumatise the udder. This will be discussed further in Chapter 6 ('Lambing time').

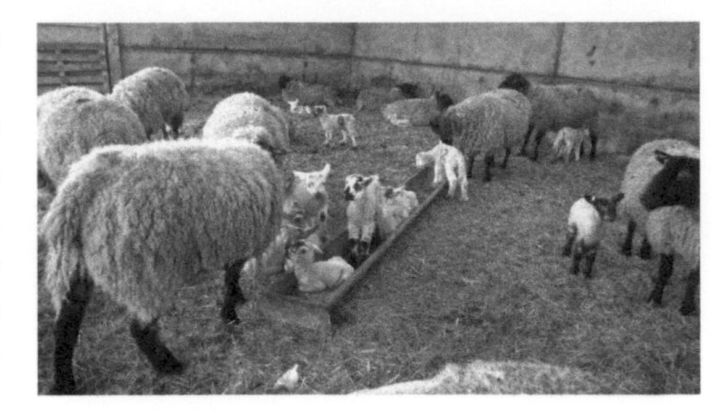

FIGURE 4.2 Well-maintained feed troughs.

FEEDING OPTIONS

Trough feeding

Most small flocks will feed concentrated feed in troughs either out in the field or in the shed. This is a hygienic way of feeding provided the troughs are cleaned and stale feed removed. Make sure these troughs have no sharp edges, that could cause injury (see Fig. 4.2).

Areas around troughs outside can get poached and so make sure they are moved around frequently. This will help to prevent poaching and wet underfoot conditions that can enable the spread of foot infections.

Floor feeding

Feeding on the floor is a common way of administering feed when sheep are housed on straw or out in the field (see Fig. 4.3). Nuts or rolls can be fed on the floor, but not creep sized pellets or home mixes as these may get lost in the straw. Floor feeding can also help exercise the ewes, promote foraging and slow down the intake of carbohydrates. However, make sure the straw is clean and dry and stop floor feeding immediately if an abortion outbreak starts to occur.

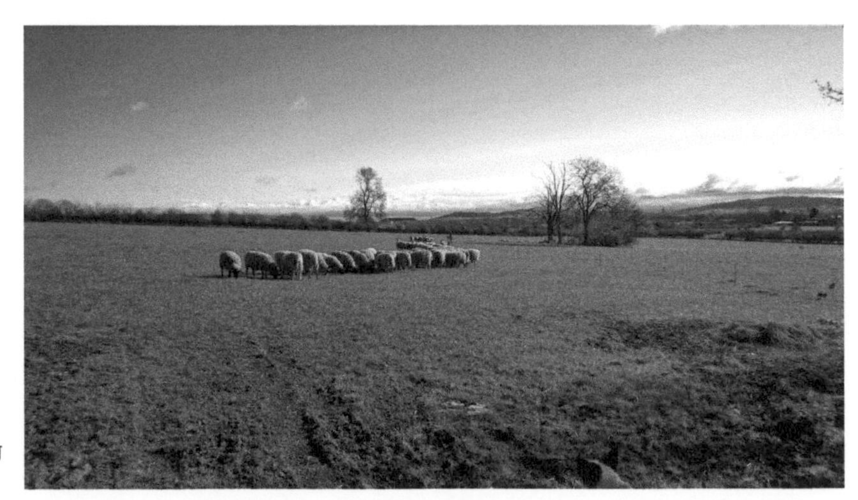

FIGURE 4.3 Floor feeding concentrate feed at grass.

Feed blocks

Feed blocks can be a good way of providing a constant supply of concentrates. Placed out in the paddock they can be useful if outwintering sheep or after lambing time to prevent mis-mothering. However, it is difficult to assess which ewes are feeding and hence detect any sheep that are becoming sick or off colour. They can be expensive and greedy sheep may prevent shy feeders from accessing the feed.

Energy licks

There is a large range of energy licks and buckets available for sheep. If you are feeding a concentrated feed and good forage, then there is little point in adding a lick into the equation.

They can be a way of delivering minerals, vitamins and energy in the form of molasses, but these may not be necessary if the diet being fed is adequate. They can be useful as an extra energy supply where sheep are being outwintered or kept on poor quality grazing.

MINERALS

Minerals such as calcium and magnesium are an essential part of a sheep's diet. Demands for these minerals become pronounced around pregnancy and when the ewe is producing milk. Deficiencies in these minerals can cause serious disease and often death. Low calcium (hypocalcaemia) and low magnesium (hypomagnesaemia) are common problems around lambing time. Most minerals, such as magnesium, are obtained daily from the diet and some are stored and released when required, for example, calcium is stored in the bones.

Forages and grasses are relatively high in calcium and most diets fed to sheep will provide sufficient levels of calcium. Problems with deficiencies in sheep tend to occur in relation to stressful events where feed intakes are disrupted, such as transport, handling, adverse weather and dog attacks.

The demand for magnesium is also highest around lambing time and during milk production. The body is unable to produce or store magnesium and so a daily supply from the diet is required.

Fast-growing, lush pastures during the spring can be deficient in magnesium, along with pastures that have been heavily fertilised, particularly with potassium. Stress and interruptions to feeding will also cause ewes to be at risk. The clinical signs and treatments for these diseases will be discussed in Chapter 7 'Sick sheep'.

Minerals and males!

As discussed earlier, concentrated feeds for ewes contain higher levels of minerals. The mineralisation of these feeds affects the urine mineral composition and can lead to the development of bladder stones. This can cause problems in male sheep. Anatomical differences of their urinary tract, that is, a longer urethra than female sheep, mean that they are unable to pass bladder stones easily.

The result is severe abdominal pain due to urethral blockage followed by bladder rupture and death if untreated or delays with treatment. Your vet must be contacted as soon as possible. It is essential that concentrated feed designed for ewes is *not* fed to male sheep at any time.

TRACE ELEMENTS

These are 'micro' minerals and are required by the sheep for a large range of growth and developmental factors. They are essential for growth, fertility and overall good health of the flock. The most commonly diagnosed deficiencies in the UK include cobalt, selenium, copper and iodine. Clinical signs associated with these diseases include 'white muscle disease' seen with selenium deficiency and poor growth rates seen particularly with cobalt. Poor fertility, reduced lamb vigour and low birth weights can be seen with iodine, selenium and copper deficiency.

Cobalt deficiency

Cobalt is converted to Vitamin B12 by the rumen microbes and this is then used in the production of energy. Deficiency is common in many parts of the UK where soil cobalt levels are low. The main effects are on the growth of weaned lambs. Lambs appear unthrifty with open fleeces due to poor wool growth and with low body weights. Gastrointestinal parasite infections are often present and exaggerate the effects of low pasture cobalt levels.

Copper deficiency

Copper is required for growth, wool growth and fertility. The effects of copper deficiency are seen in young lambs born to mothers who were deficient in copper during mid pregnancy. Inadequate copper affects the nervous system and causes a condition in lambs called 'swayback'. This will be observed as high levels of stillborn lambs or small weak lambs that have difficulty standing and walking, in other words, they appear to sway. This is usually evident at birth but it can be delayed and seen in lambs later in growth.

Grazing and forages normally supply adequate levels of copper, but deficiencies are often seen when the grazing pastures are high in other trace elements such as molybdenum and sulphur. High levels of these elements reduce the amount of copper that can be absorbed from the diet and so higher levels of copper may be required in the diet by means of a supplement.

Copper toxicity

Sheep are susceptible to copper toxicity and if a deficiency has not been diagnosed, sheep should not be given additional copper.

Copper toxicity can occur when sheep have ingested high levels of copper over a prolonged period. It is efficiently stored in the liver but once storage capacity is reached, there can be a sudden release of copper into the blood

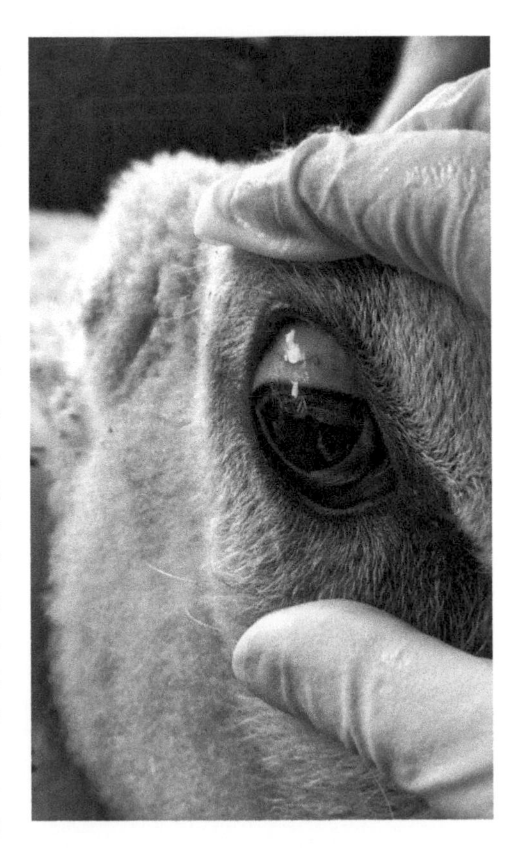

FIGURE 4.4 Copper toxicity in a Texel ewe.

circulation. This results in a 'haemolytic crisis' where the blood and liver cells are damaged and rupture. The result is liver and kidney failure.

This is commonly seen where sheep have been fed cattle or pig feed. Affected sheep will appear depressed, staggering and have rapid breathing. Jaundice (yellowing of the eyes and membranes) will be present (see Fig. 4.4) and collapse and death can occur.

Certain breeds are more susceptible to copper poisoning due to the way in which they store copper. Texels, Suffolks and Longwool breeds are more susceptible to poisoning due to over-supply in the diet.

Acute copper poisoning can result following a trace element or worming drench containing copper. The clinical signs are varied but relate to the development of a 'sick sheep' with increased breathing and heart rate, depression and collapse being common features. Discuss with your vet if you suspect copper poisoning.

Selenium deficiency

Selenium and vitamin E are important for fertility in the adult and for growth and development in the newborn and growing lamb. Deficiencies are common in many areas of the UK.

Low levels of selenium and vitamin E can cause degeneration of the skeletal and heart muscle and so the result is 'stiff' lambs which may collapse when being walked. The effects on the heart muscle can lead to heart failure.

Lambs also require selenium whilst in the uterus to produce good-quality brown fat reserves around the kidney. These reserves are an important supply of energy to the lamb and are required in the first six to twelve hours of life to maintain body heat and help prevent hypothermia. See Chapter 6 'Lambing time'.

If in doubt, consult your vet to determine whether you have a trace element deficiency in your flock. Blood samples from ewes can be tested on a yearly basis by your vet to establish whether supplementation is needed for the next mating period. It is important to discuss any clinical signs that may be related to trace element deficiencies with your vet.

Treatment

The correction of a deficiency should be discussed with your vet and be based upon a diagnosis. This will prevent toxicities being caused and the cost of treating unnecessarily. There are lots of products on the market sold by many different companies. The product chosen will depend upon the length of cover required and the group of sheep being treated, in other words, fat lambs, ewes pre-mating or lambs at weaning.

Free access minerals such as lick buckets are often an expensive and ineffective way of delivering the trace elements. It is impossible to ensure that all your sheep have received the required amounts. Contrary to the myth that sheep will only take the supplements if they 'know' that they have a deficiency, there will be many sheep that avoid the licks altogether and others eat more than is needed.

Individual oral drenches are a more reliable way of delivering trace elements as the whole flock will be treated. However, the effects of oral drenches are short-lived and repeated treatments will be necessary where there is a true deficiency.

Injectable trace elements and boluses will offer longer periods of supplementation, but often only up to between one to five months depending upon the product used. These products are often expensive. Therefore, diagnosing whether supplementation is necessary and discussing with your vet will save your pocket and lead to better outcomes.

WEANING

The lamb starts to explore and chew on bedding, hay, straw and grass from a very young age. The presence of forage entering the stomach starts the development of the rumen. It takes time for the rumen lining to develop and for the microbe population to develop and grow. The rumen starts to become functional as the lamb reaches 3 to 4 weeks of age.

Until around the age of 6 to 8 weeks the lamb will still be receiving much of its protein and energy for growth from its mother's milk. After 8 weeks, a lamb's nutrition will start to be provided by the forage and any concentrated feed it consumes.

During lactation, if the ewe's nutrition is good and her body condition is optimum (score 2.5–3), then the lamb will achieve good growth from milk alone. Otherwise lamb concentrate feed (creep feed) can be offered.

Concentrated lamb pellets, 'creep pellets', have higher levels of protein than ewe feed and they are formulated without the minerals that would otherwise cause bladder stones in male lambs. Hence, male and female lambs can consume lamb concentrates.

They are a smaller pellet than a ewe nut and are best offered from birth ad lib to enable the stomach of the lamb to adapt and consume a constant small supply. Ad lib feeding will require either a specialised feeder for lambs (see Fig. 4.5), or a very secure way of allowing the lambs access to the pellets by means of a small gate, which prevents ewe access.

They should be offered in small amounts over a gradual period if they have not been available from birth. This will allow the rumen microbes to adjust to the change in diet.

At around 10–12 weeks, the lamb will seek comfort in suckling from its mother but will not be gaining much nutrition from her. Therefore, weaning can commence at this age. This will enable the ewe's body condition and udder to recover, which will help improve health and allow her to be ready for the next pregnancy

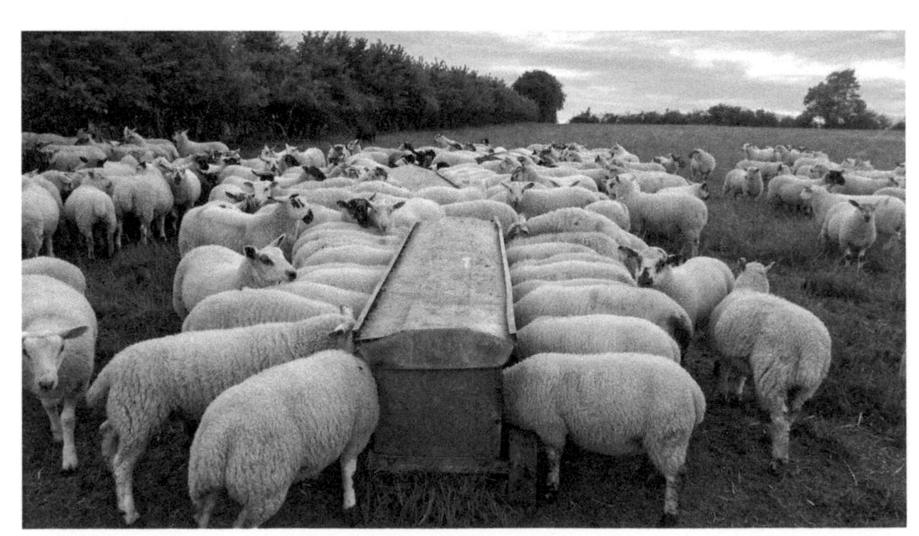

FIGURE 4.5
Lamb creep feeders.

How to wean?

Weaning is best carried out abruptly. Stopping the lamb suckling will stimulate the ewe to cease milk production. Milk is produced in response to suckling and so for weaning to be successful this must be halted abruptly.

Whilst the lambs and ewes will vocalise very loudly for 24–72 hours after weaning, this will soon stop when both parties settle into their lamb and ewe flocks. It is better to remove the ewes from the lambs, so that the lambs remain in a place with which they are familiar and where they know the location of the water supply (Fig. 4.6). The ewes could be housed for a few days or moved to a distant secure paddock.

To help reduce milk supply it is important to reduce the amount and quality of the ewes' feed. Stop feeding concentrates and put the ewes on bare, poor-quality pasture or house them with poorer-quality forage. This will help reduce the milk supply and reduce the risk of mastitis. It is essential, however, that they have constant access to water and clean surroundings. Water does not drive the milk supply and they require fresh water at all times.

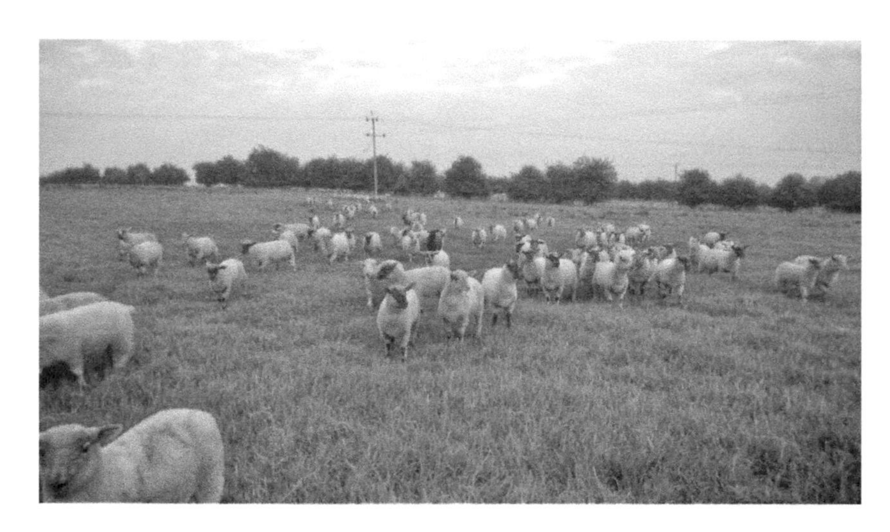

FIGURE 4.6
Weaned lambs.

BREEDING SHEEP 5

Most sheep keepers will breed from their sheep at some point. There are many reasons to breed sheep. Pedigree sheep breeding is very popular for keepers involved in the genetics, showing and sale of their livestock. Others want to produce their own lamb to eat. Many sheep keepers breed from their sheep to experience lambing and the welcoming of new life into the world.

Whatever the reason, it is important to ensure that you have researched and gained some knowledge and skill in sheep health and welfare and have access to an enthusiastic local veterinary surgeon with an interest in sheep. This will ensure good sheep health and welfare.

Many novice sheep keepers will have access to knowledge through pedigree breeders and experienced farmers. This can be extremely useful in times of need. However, be aware that they may not always be contactable in times of need and specialist support in the form of a sheep vet is essential. A veterinary flock health plan can be developed with a vet that includes lambing protocols and practices to suit your flock and your system.

No matter how many times a farmer, smallholder or vet experiences a lamb being born, it is a unique, satisfying and humbling experience. This is the reason why, despite the difficulties, hard work and tiredness, it can be a very rewarding time.

ARE YOU UP TO THE JOB?

Lambing time is the most dangerous time in a ewe's life. Severe risks can occur at the actual time of giving birth in terms of a difficult lambing and afterwards in terms of life-threatening infections such as mastitis, metritis (uterine infection) or metabolic disease (i.e. twin lamb disease). These will be discussed in Chapter 6 'Lambing time'.

It is therefore important to consider the following as the welfare of your sheep is completely your responsibility, particularly at lambing time:

- Have you researched how to manage sheep at lambing time (reading this book is an excellent start)?
- Are you prepared to take time away from work during lambing time? If not, are you prepared to pay an experienced shepherd or do you have experienced help to cover this time?
- Are you able to attend a lambing course beforehand (usually run by your local vet)?

- Are you prepared for the cost of calling out a vet at any time of the day or night to a difficult lambing?
- Does sleep matter? You will be required to stay up and get up during the night over the lambing period
- Are you squeamish and are you prepared to experience the death of animals? Lambs sometimes die during, before or after the birthing process. The ewes may also die. You must be prepared for this and be prepared for immediate euthanasia by calling for the vet or a slaughterman

If you are concerned or unsure about any of the above considerations, discuss these concerns with your vet and do not breed from your sheep until you are ready. Going ahead without careful consideration is irresponsible and not recommended.

The most valuable way to learn, gain experience and build a friendship with an experienced farmer is to offer your services to a local sheep farmer during lambing time. Their experience is priceless and you will rapidly decide whether lambing your ewes is a good idea.

Usually the local farmer will be lambing a lot of sheep in a short space of time. There will be a lot of experience and practice to be gained, which will help when lambing your own sheep for the first time.

Shepherds can rapidly assess newborn lambs and their mothers. He or she is able to determine which ewe and lamb family is fit and well and which needs more attention. To the untrained eye, this process will go unnoticed, so make sure you find a farmer willing to be asked questions and give explanations. Most farmers will be more than happy to do this (provided they have had some breakfast and a little sleep); be considerate with the timing of your questions.

SUCCESSFUL BREEDING

Deciding why you want to breed sheep will help you determine what time of year to breed, the type of breeds to use and where to buy breeding stock. A successful lambing starts with a successful breeding programme. Generally, it is better that the lambing period occurs over a short period. You can then have all your resources together, book time off work, notify your extra help and read up on lambing.

A short lambing period can only be achieved if the breeding period is limited by the removal of the rams a set time after they were introduced to the ewes. However, to ensure that a high proportion of the ewes become pregnant in this time, breeding must take place at the correct time of year for the breed of sheep in question and both the ewes and rams must be healthy and fertile.

The reproductive cycle

Sheep are seasonal breeders. This means that their breeding season starts in response to the season and the length of the light period (daylight). When the day length begins to shorten and the period of darkness increases, the reproductive organs in the ewe and ram are stimulated to become active. This is in response to changes in the reproductive hormones within the body.

A reduction in daylight is recorded by the retina in the sheep's eye which sends a message to the brain. This reduction in light period stimulates an area of the brain called the pineal gland to produce more of a hormone called melatonin. Production of melatonin is therefore suppressed by longer day lengths.

Increased levels of melatonin are detected by another area of the brain called the hypothalamus. When instructed by increased levels of melatonin, the hypothalamus starts to secrete the hormones required for egg development in the ovary and ovulation.

This is gonadotrophic-releasing hormone (GnRH), which acts on the pituitary gland in the brain to release follicle stimulating hormone (FSH) and a luteinising hormone (LH).

Increased levels of FSH start the process of developing a dominant (functional) follicle containing an (egg) in the ovary. LH levels (which are released in pulses) are used to help this dominant follicle rupture, releasing the egg from the ovary (ovulation). The egg travels down the oviduct and can then be fertilised by fertile sperm, if they are present in the ewe's reproductive tract at the correct time.

There are different structures on the ovary that produce hormones. The follicle and then in the space vacated by the follicle, a corpus luteum forms which contains hormone producing tissues.

The hormone oestrogen (produced by the follicle) instructs the ewe to show oestrus (mating) behaviour at an appropriate time for mating to take place in relation to the release of the egg. The hormone progesterone is released from the corpus luteum (from where the egg ovulated) and is responsible for either maintaining a pregnancy if the egg is fertilised or priming the reproductive cycle to start the whole cycle again when blood levels of progesterone start to reduce.

This sudden drop in progesterone will help the next egg (which has been developing over the previous 17 days) to become ripe and ovulate. If the ewe conceived, then this drop in progesterone will not occur and further ovulations will not take place and the pregnancy will be maintained.

How long is each oestrus cycle?

In a non-pregnant ewe, the above cycle happens every 16–17 days during the breeding season.

How long is the breeding season?

The length of the breeding season is influenced by several factors. Some breeds have shorter breeding seasons such as the hill breeds. They tend to start the breeding season later in the year when day length is almost at its shortest. This is an adaptive evolutionary response to delay the start of lambing until the upland climatic conditions in the spring favour better grass growth.

The peak mating season for hill breeds such as the Scottish Blackface, Swaledale, Herdwicks and Cheviots is from mid to late November until January, with lambing aiming to start in late April to late May. These breeds will have approximately four to five cycles within the breeding season.

Lowland breeds such as the Suffolk, Charollais, Texel and the crossbreeds will start cycling earlier with peak mating in late August to late September and they usually have six to seven oestrus cycles. It is therefore important to consider your choice of breed and timing of lambing to achieve the best results in terms of fertility.

When do I put the rams in?

In some flocks, the rams (or tups) will be kept with the ewes all year round, particularly when there is only one ram in the flock. This should be avoided as it can lead to an extended lambing period. Lambing ewes over a long period makes management difficult and often leads to ewes that are over fat and have problems during birth. It is also difficult to administer routine preventative treatments at the correct time. See the 'Vaccines' section of Chapter 8.

It is essential to separate the rams from the ewes when feeding concentrates during lambing time. This can lead to exposure of the ram to ewe feed which can lead to serious urinary tract problems (see Chapter 4 'Diet and nutrition' and Chapter 7 in 'Miscellaneous disease').

Issues can also arise where weaning is delayed and ewe lambs are inadvertently mated by their sire. This can lead to unwanted pregnancies and potentially unhealthy deformed lambs. Rams and uncastrated ram lambs should be separated from ewes and ewe lambs from 5 months of age unless breeding is called for. Puberty will start around this time and unwanted pregnancies can occur. Plan to use your ram or rams specifically for the mating (or tupping) period and then remove them from the flock, keeping them in a separate group.

The length of pregnancy (gestation period) in the ewe is 147–150 days. Ensure that you carefully work this out when planning breeding. For example, if the rams go in with the ewes on bonfire night 5th November, lambing will start on 1st April.

Choosing the correct ewes for mating

Once you have decided upon the breeds to mate and the time of year that you would like to lamb, it is important to have a look at your ewes and decide whether they are suitable or whether you need to buy in more breeding ewes.

When selecting ewes for mating, they must be physically fit and sound. They must be in optimum body condition when going to the ram (2.5–3 for hill breeds and 3–3.5 for lowland breeds); see Chapter 2 'The normal sheep' on how to assess body condition score. It can be difficult and not advisable to try and alter their body condition once they have become pregnant. They can afford to lose a little weight during mid pregnancy, but this should be no more than half a condition score.

When does preparation for mating start?

Selecting your breeding ewes needs to be around weaning time, for example from July or August if your lambing period falls between March and May. Achieving weight gain over the summer when the ewes have stopped milking and rearing lambs is the most successful time to reach the optimum body condition score.

A body condition score is equivalent to approximately 12.5% of a ewe's adult body weight; for example, a 70-kg adult ewe gaining one body condition score is equivalent to gaining about 9 kg in body weight. This can take four to six weeks on very good pasture and six to eight weeks on average pasture. Extra feeding of quality forage and some hard feed can be used where the grazing is poor.

Flushing

Providing improved nutrition for three weeks before mating, during the mating period and in the few weeks after mating, will in some cases improve conception rates. This is called flushing. It will also help the pregnancy to be established and maintained. Ewes that are slightly under body condition will benefit from this far more than ewes that are in optimum condition for mating.

Always aim for optimum body condition scores at mating, particularly if grazing is short or not available. The aim is to graze ewes on the best available grazing for two to three weeks before mating and until at least four weeks after mating.

Why does body condition matter?

The body condition of the ewe in the pre-mating period is crucial to ensuring that the ewe will be fully fertile and ovulate the optimum number of eggs. This improves the chances of conception and implantation in the womb.

A leaner ewe is less likely to conceive and often produces lower birthweight lambs that are not as vigorous. A lean ewe will have poorer quality and quantity of colostrum and milk and hence the growth and health of her offspring will be affected. She is also far more likely to suffer from metabolic diseases (such as twin lamb disease) which endangers the ewe and her unborn lambs.

Over fat ewes can be less fertile and if too fat at mating they may go on to be too fat up until the point of lambing. At this stage, they are at higher risk of vaginal prolapse and having difficulties delivering their lambs due to excess internal fat (see Chapter 6 'Lambing time').

Pre-mating ewe checklist

- *Are they in the correct body condition score for their breed?* Aim for 3–3.5 for lowland ewes and 2.5–3 for hill ewes
- *Examine her teeth:* Ewes must have a good set of functional teeth with no obvious wobbly teeth or lumps around the jaw or molar region. She must be able to chew and digest food to maintain body condition
- *Sound on her feet:* Treat her promptly for lameness (see Chapter 7 'Lameness'). Using most common antibiotics before or during mating will *not* affect fertility, but being lame or having any other type of infection can affect fertility
- *Is she too old?* Ewes that have painful joints or lameness thought to be due to arthritis should not be kept for breeding. They will struggle to keep up with the demands of pregnancy
- *Does she have misshapen feet?* Do not keep ewes that have abnormal feet. They are more likely to pick up infection and become lame
- *Poor body condition:* Sheep that are lean or do not gain weight despite increased feeding may have an underlying chronic disease, a heavy worm burden or both. Seek advice from your vet. A simple worm egg count could be performed in the first instance (see Chapter 8 'Preventative treatments')
- *Mastitis:* If she has had mastitis before then do not breed from her again as she will have a reduced milk supply in the affected quarter
- *Vaginal prolapse:* If she has suffered from a vaginal prolapse, do not keep her for breeding as she is very likely to prolapse again
- *Caesarean:* If she required a caesarean in a previous lambing then she may need one again depending upon the cause of the problem. Your vet may have advised not to breed from her if she has a narrow or misshapen pelvic canal (Fig. 5.1)

Should you worm ewes before mating?

It has been traditional practice to give a worming treatment to all ewes before mating, but recent research suggests that this is not always necessary. This practice has contributed to the development of anthelmintic wormer resistance.

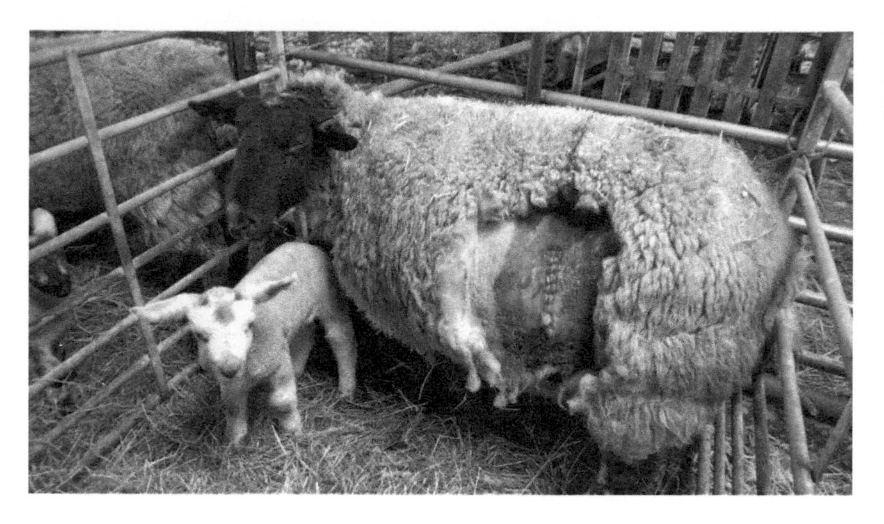

FIGURE 5.1 A successful caesarean section.

Ewes that are in optimum body condition, on a good-quality diet, will have good immunity to worms and will be shedding very few worm eggs. These ewes are unlikely to need worming.

Younger ewes, that is, ewe lambs or yearling ewes, may need a worming treatment. Leaner ewes or ewes that have an underlying chronic disease will have reduced immunity to disease and they may also require worming. See 'Roundworms' in Chapter 8.

It is advisable to collect a muck sample from your ewes and get your vet to perform a worm egg count (see 'How to collect faeces samples' in Chapter 8; Fig. 5.2). This is a cheap test and will give you and your vet information about the worm status of your sheep.

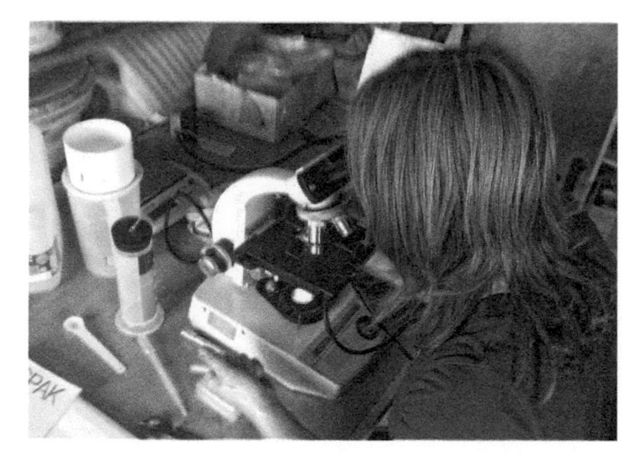

FIGURE 5.2 Using a microscope to perform a worm egg count.

Should I breed from ewe lambs?

Ewe lambs are female lambs kept for breeding from the current year's lamb crop. At the time of mating they will not yet be a year old. Breeding ewe lambs and lambing ewe lambs requires a great deal of experience, skill and confidence and it is not advised if you are a novice at breeding sheep.

Farmers and shepherds sometimes breed ewe lambs to increase the speed of genetic improvement within a flock. Commercially, it will increase the overall lifetime productivity of each ewe by gaining an extra lamb crop. However, for these advantages to work, the ewes must be carefully selected and they are often lambed as a separate group requiring extra vigilance, attention and specific feeding.

When choosing ewe lambs to mate, their body weight and condition is very important. They should have reached at least 65% of their mature adult body weight at the time of mating. A Suffolk cross ewe lamb should be at least 50 kg at the time of mating.

Ewe lambs are not as fertile as yearling or adult ewes. Their oestrus cycle will start later in the season and they will show oestrus for a shorter period than adult ewes. Therefore, the conception rates can be disappointing.

By the time a ewe lamb reaches lambing, she is still growing and her pelvic canal is still not fully developed. Therefore, pregnant ewe lambs are more likely to have difficulties lambing. This is exacerbated if they have been fed incorrectly during the last six weeks of pregnancy. Lambs can become too big to fit through the pelvic canal. Ewe lambs that are too thin will struggle with the demands of pregnancy, produce less milk and poorer quality colostrum. Ewe lambs will struggle to rear twins and so it is advised to remove a lamb and rear as a pet if she has more than one lamb.

Ewe lambs as mothers will also have varying degrees of mothering ability. This can often result in total lamb rejection or mis-mothering, especially if they are disturbed during lambing or need assistance. Think very carefully about your level of experience before putting ewe lambs to the ram.

Choosing the correct ram

Rams can be bought from pedigree shows and sales or direct from farm. Many people buy on appearance and on advice from breeders. Some will base their purchase upon a more detailed analysis of his recorded genetic traits. For example, traits such as growth rates, lambing ease, carcass quality and faecal egg count data are all desirable traits. These are called estimated breeding values (EBVs).

No matter how expensive, a ram's fine appearance or exemplary breeding values are meaningless if he is not healthy and fit for purpose. Performing a basic health check on your new ram is very important. This should be performed every year on existing rams. If a ram is infertile or even subfertile then there will be no or reduced numbers of offspring the following lambing.

You can perform a basic ram health check by assessing the following areas for any problems:

- *Head*

  - Teeth: Does he have good teeth that are not loose or worn?
  - Does he have any obvious lumps, draining abscesses or healed scars below his ears, on the angle of the jaw or under his jaw? This could indicate infection with caseous lymphadenitis (CLA). This is an infectious disease and will be discussed in the 'Lumps and swellings' section of Chapter 7

- *Body*

  - Body condition: He should be well-fleshed and in good body condition of at least score 3
  - Skin: He should not be showing any signs of itching or hair loss or scabs. Make sure you check on his brisket (on the underside between his front legs) to make sure there are no obvious wounds or skin damage from a poorly fitting raddle harness. Also, check the skin on his scrotum for scar tissue, thickened skin or crusting. This could indicate the presence of a previous mite infection or fighting 'foot strike' damage from another ram

- *Legs and feet*
    - Legs: He must have good conformation. Rams spend most of their working time on the hind legs. Therefore, poor hind limb conformation must be avoided
    - Feet: Do not buy a ram that has deformed feet or that is lame. Check carefully that there are no areas of excess tissue or flesh in the space between the clefts of the hoof. These are interdigital granulomas and can be the result of a chronic infection or a hereditary problem. They are very difficult to treat and will result in lameness
    - Lameness: Foot infections such as footrot and CODD are very contagious (see 'Lameness' in Chapter 7). Buying in a ram with these infections will put the rest of your flock at risk. The effects of these infections can be a rise in body temperature, which can have a negative effect on sperm production and quality
- *Testicles:* These are the essential organs for fertility and must be assessed carefully
    - Scrotum: The size of the scrotum has been shown to relate directly to the volume of sperm produced and hence fertility. This can be measured using a tape measure around the widest part of the scrotum with one hand placed at the neck of the scrotum and the other holding the tape measure (see Fig. 5.3).
    - Most rams measure between 30–40 cm with variations in breed and age. They should be at least 30 cm in circumference
    - Symmetry: Feel the contents of the scrotum. Each testicle should be symmetrical and move freely within the scrotum. They should be firm and not hard or soft. Feeling the testicles should not cause pain

A full assessment of the reproductive organs should be carried out by an expert such as your sheep vet. Problems are often very subtle and it takes a trained person to diagnose them. If there

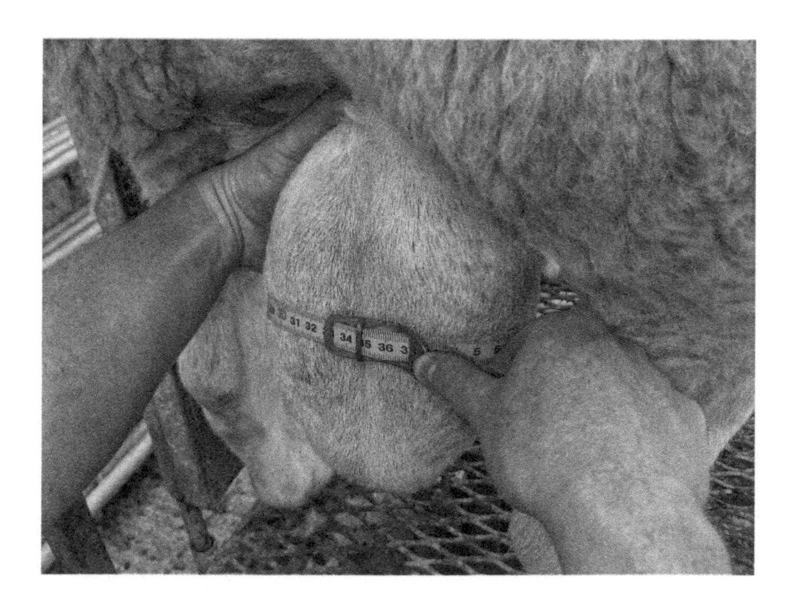

FIGURE 5.3 Measuring scrotal circumference.

are any abnormalities detected or if there are any suspicions around fertility, the vet will be able to extend the examination by performing a full semen evaluation. Your vet will also examine and visualise the penis to check for any abnormalities before breeding.

Rams may fight throughout the year and particularly leading up to the breeding season. A ram kept on his own may be at risk from injury due to trying to escape from his accommodation when ewes are near. In either circumstance, damage to the important area of the testicles, feet and legs can cause significant reductions in fertility.

When should the rams be checked?

The sperm that will be used during mating is produced around seven to nine weeks beforehand. Therefore, the rams need a full health check at least ten weeks before they are due to be used. This requires planning to make sure that new rams are purchased before this time.

It is very important that any diseases including worm or fluke infections, skin infections or lameness are dealt with before this time so that they do not interfere with sperm production. Increases in body temperature caused by infections including lameness will affect the quality of the sperm produced and lead to subfertility if this sperm is used for mating seven to nine weeks later.

Why does body condition matter?

It is common for one ram to be used with 30–80 ewes and even one to 100 ewes in some cases. A fit and fertile ram is capable of successfully mating with this number of ewes over a short period. Rams should be able to achieve a 98% pregnancy rate over a 35-day period and will be very active during this time. He can lose up to one body condition score during this time and so he must be in good body condition at the start of mating. Rams being used for mating should be in 3.5–4 body condition score when going in with the ewes.

In a smaller flock where the number of ewes to be mated will be much smaller, a body condition score of 3.5 would be sufficient. A leaner ram may struggle to have the reserves to mate over the breeding season.

Rams that are too fat when being used for mating, that is, 4.5–5, will potentially suffer from poor libido and lack of energy to work. It is also very likely that rams of this body condition score will have increased fat deposits around the neck of the scrotum. Increased fat in this region will interfere with the thermoregulation of the testicles. The testicles should be cooler than the rest of the body by one or two degrees. Increases in temperature of the testicles will have deleterious effects on sperm quality and fertility.

Rams that are bought from a sale or a show may have been fed intensively to achieve a good body condition. Their appearance may be good but be aware that excess fat deposited around the neck of the scrotum can reduce fertility.

It is important that you monitor your rams and their diet to ensure that they are fit in the two months before mating and not too fat or too thin. A sudden change in diet can also affect fertility, so allowing your new ram to adapt to his new surroundings and diet before he is used for mating is very important.

How can I tell that the rams are ready for mating?

During the pre-breeding check, you may notice the presence of the 'inguinal flush'. This is a dark purple discoloration on the insides of the hind legs extending up to his scrotal region and is best observed when the ram is turned over (see 'Turning a sheep' in Chapter 2). It can look like a bruise but it is an indication that he is 'in season' and ready for breeding. It is not always observed in rams.

Should my ram go straight to work?

Rams are often hired or shared to prevent the problem of keeping rams on their own. This can create new problems in terms of bringing in disease. Any ram brought onto the farm must be isolated and follow a strict quarantine plan.

Any new sheep brought onto the farm, including rams, are a potential source of disease. Quarantine procedures will be discussed later in the book and it is very important to read up on these and have a treatment plan in place. No matter how much you trust the breeder or seller, if you are buying in from a show or sale then you cannot guarantee the health of the animals. They will have been moved through a shed or show ring with many other animals of unknown health status. It is therefore far safer to buy in direct from a farm but still apply the quarantine treatments (see the 'New livestock' section in Chapter 9).

Sharing a ram can be problematic as flocks often want to use him at the same time. Other alternatives to buying or hiring a ram are the use of artificial insemination or buying in ewes that are already in lamb. Artificial insemination is a highly specialised technique and is only performed by expert veterinary surgeons and technicians. It is often performed in pedigree breeding flocks to enhance the generation of offspring from a selected ram. For small numbers of ewes, it is possible to take them to an AI centre, rather than have the technician visit the farm.

Signs of oestrus

Rams use smell and pheromones to detect whether the ewes are on heat. We are unable to detect these subtle signs but you will notice the response of both sexes to the pheromones being in the air!

The rams will show a 'flehmen' response where their top lip will be exposed and curl upwards to detect the maximum amount of smell. When in with the flock they will do this around the tail and vulva region of the ewe. They will also lick and nibble the wool in this region of the ewe and over her rump.

A ewe will respond to this attention by standing still and waiting for the ram to mount. Ewes that have come into oestrus will gravitate towards the rams if they are in the same field or in the field next door and they will present their rear end, holding their tail to one side. The ram will constantly be walking around the ewes and checking for the receptive ewes. Ovulating ewes will display all the above signs and then stand to be mounted. The ram will detect this and mount and then serve the ewe. This happens very quickly and can be easily missed.

Using the rams

To create a compact lambing period, rams are usually put in with the ewes for two oestrus cycles which equates to 35 days. There are different methods available to determine whether a ewe has been mated by a ram. The most common involves the use of coloured paint or wax crayon.

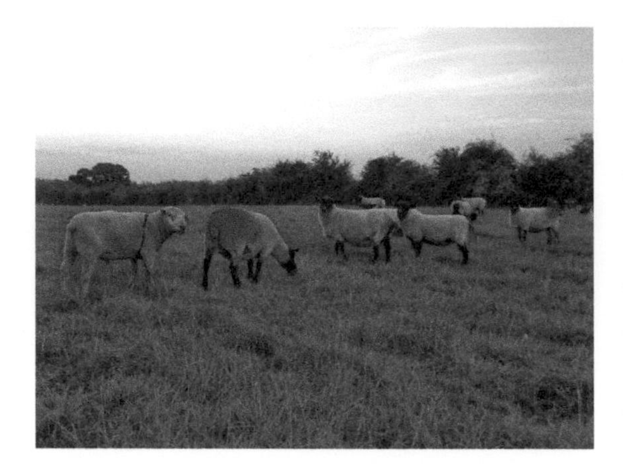

FIGURE 5.4 A raddle harness with wax crayon being put to good use.

An oily-based thick paint can be applied to the brisket or chest region of the ram. Each time he mounts a ewe and creates the forward movement required for service, the paint will rub off and mark the ewe's rump region. This paint needs to be applied daily or at least every other day.

A wax crayon can be used for the same purpose (see Fig. 5.4). The crayon is fitted to a harness and will remain in place and will only need changing when you change the colour. If a harness is being used, it is important that you check it every few days to make sure it is not rubbing the skin and alter the straps as it will become slack as the ram loses weight during the mating period.

If the colour of the paint or crayon is changed after the first week, it is possible to record which ewes are likely to lamb first and how the rams are performing. It will also help you to determine if there is a fertility problem with the rams.

Any ewes that have been marked and then re-marked with a different colour later during the mating period did not become pregnant to the first mating. This can give you an early indication that the ram or ewe is not fertile. If multiple ewes are served multiple times, the ram may need to be changed for a more fertile one. If this has happened, it is wise to consult your vet to determine where the problem may be.

Many smaller flocks do not use paints or raddles but it can be a useful way of telling you when the ewes are going to lamb. This is especially important if your rams live with the ewes. If they have all been marked, you can be more confident that they are pregnant and the ram can stay with them with less risk of any unplanned lambings outside of the lambing period.

Some ewes may lose a pregnancy. This is more common if diseases that cause abortion are present. If the ram is living with the flock, there may be a disrupted lambing period if these ewes are re-mated at a later date.

Ultrasound scanning: is it worth it?

The next stage of management is to ultrasound scan the ewes when they are in mid pregnancy, usually between 50 and 90 days (see Fig. 5.5). This is very useful in terms of managing the correct nutrition and grouping the ewes at housing depending upon how many lambs each ewe is

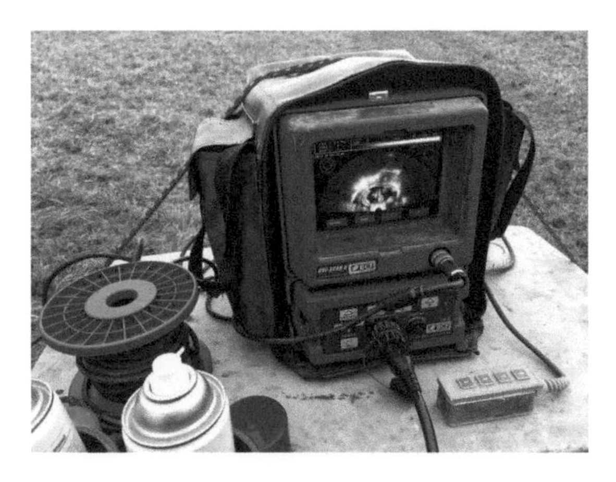

FIGURE 5.5 An ultrasound scanner.

carrying. This will help you to feed the correct amounts of feed to ewes carrying singles, twins or more lambs. It will also help at lambing time to determine how many lambs the ewe should deliver.

Scanning will indicate how many of the ewes are not in lamb (barren or empty). A high barren rate in a flock can be an indication of disease, nutritional deficiencies or infertility in the ram and further investigation by the vet would be required.

It can be difficult in a smaller flock to get a scanning technician to visit and therefore small flocks are often not scanned. If you speak to your neighbouring farmer, fellow small flock keeper or sheep vet, they may be able to recommend someone who will do smaller flocks. A sheep vet may be able to do small numbers as part of a flock visit and flock health plan. This is always an excellent opportunity to gain valuable expert knowledge and for your vet to assess your flock's health during the pregnancy period.

Advancing and synchronising the breeding season

The natural breeding season can be advanced by three to six weeks using hormonal treatment therapies. This involves the use of a melatonin implant to mimic the onset of shorter day length and to initiate the hormonal changes required to start the oestrus cycle.

Another synchronisation method is to insert a progesterone-releasing sponge into the vagina. This creates higher levels of blood progesterone, mimicking an active ovary. This stimulates the release of the other hormones used within the oestrus cycle. The sudden removal of the sponge combined with another hormone injection (pregnant mare serum gonadotrophin) will stimulate ovulation. This method can be used to slightly enhance the breeding season but it is more successful when synchronising a group of treated ewes to ovulate all at the same time (within 24–36 hours). This will help with planning the lambing period. Note that you will need more than one ram for a synchronised flock, if you are mating more than 10–15 ewes.

Vasectomised rams (teaser rams)

Another way to synchronise ewes to ovulate at a similar time is by using a vasectomised (teaser) ram. This uses the pheromones secreted from a vasectomised ram to attract and stimulate the ewes to start cycling. This uses a more natural effect called the 'ram effect' and only works if the rams and the teaser ram are out of sight or smell (such as on another farm) for at least four weeks before the start of the breeding season. If the ewes have already started cycling the ram effect will have little effect. This method will not advance the breeding season but it will synchronise the ewes to cycle very closely together if done properly.

The teasers are introduced into the flock for two to 14 days. The fertile rams must be put with the synchronised ewes no later than 14 days after the teasers were first introduced. Most of the ewes will start cycling immediately. Of these ewes, around 60% will ovulate in 17–18 days after the teaser went in and 40% will have a silent heat on days 4 to 6 and then have an ovulating heat 18 days later. Therefore, there will be two peaks of activity at 18 and 26 days after the teasers go in. Lambing can therefore be planned to occur within a 7–14-day period.

Handling sheep after mating

Once fertilisation has occurred, the formed embryo must implant in the uterus to continue its development. Movement down the oviduct and implantation into the lining of the uterus takes around 30–40 days. It is crucial that the ewes have minimal stresses and handling during this period.

Ideally, ewes should not have to be moved or transported during this time or experience any diet changes. Keep handling and procedures to a minimum. Vaccines should not be given during this time due to the stress of handling and the possible temporary increases in temperature following vaccination.

If any ewes go lame or develop an infection, then they must be treated as soon as possible. Most common antibiotics do not cause any problems relating to fertility. The ewes must be handled quietly and calmly and without dogs.

PREGNANCY

Once mating has occurred and the successful sperm have reached the cervix, there is a period of around 24–36 hours where the sperm are viable. The eggs, once released from the ovary and transported down the oviduct and into the uterus, only have approximately 12–18 hours during which they must be fertilised.

If the ram or rams are fertile and fit, there should be large numbers of successful sperm available for fertilisation. This takes place in the oviduct, the space into which the egg is released from the ovary. For successful fertilisation, only one sperm should penetrate the egg.

Most breeds of sheep will shed more than one egg at peak ovulation and so multiple embryos (fertilised eggs) are common. The embryos will become attached to the wall of the uterus at around 30 days into the pregnancy. The embryo then develops into the foetus.

The length of the pregnancy (gestation period) in sheep is 150 days with a range of 147–150 days. Once implantation in the uterus has occurred, the foetuses can grow and develop via the nourishment of a healthy and developing placenta.

The placenta

The placenta attaches to the lining of the uterus via caruncles on the uterus lining and cotyledons on the placenta. These attachments look like 'buttons'. This type of placenta is also found in other ruminants such as goats and cattle. The transfer of nutrients to the developing foetuses and the removal of waste products occurs via these attachments. The placenta also produces hormones which are required to maintain the pregnancy and stimulate udder development. The umbilical cord is responsible for the transfer of oxygenated blood from the placenta to the foetus.

In contrast to other species such as humans, there is no placental transfer of antibodies and hence immunity from the mother to the unborn lambs. Immunity is transferred from the ewe to her lamb from the colostrum (first milk) that needs to be ingested within the first 24 hours of birth. The first feed of colostrum is needed in the first two hours of life. Further details can be found in 'The impact of colostrum' in Chapter 8.

The placenta develops in relation to the number of foetuses present and the diet of the ewe during mid pregnancy (2 to 3 months). Extreme under- or overfeeding should be avoided during the mid-pregnancy stage.

The foetus undergoes most of its growth in the final trimester which equates to around

75% of their growth in the last six weeks of pregnancy. As described in the earlier chapters, feeding of the ewe around this time must be carefully monitored.

Increasing the quality of feed is important as the space for the rumen is reduced due to the increasing size of the uterus containing the unborn lambs.

Excessive feeding of the ewe at this stage will result in large lambs being born, as excess energy is directed to the unborn lambs and not the ewe. The body condition of the ewe will not alter during the last six weeks of pregnancy but the size of the lambs will increase and potentially cause lambing difficulties.

The later stages of pregnancy and giving birth are the most important and potentially dangerous times of a sheep's life. When deciding upon whether to breed from your ewes, it is important to understand what may go wrong, how to monitor ewe body condition and how to feed the pregnant ewe. Many sheep vet practices will offer lambing courses or workshops before lambing time and it is advised that you attend at least one of these training courses before embarking on the lambing period.

HOW IS PERFORMANCE MEASURED?

In a commercial situation, the profit margin gained from a ewe is important. The only way in which this can be calculated is by recording information. The aim in lowland systems is for each ewe to rear two lambs. In hill and upland areas or native sheep breeds, this is reduced to 1.2 lambs per ewe. For maximum profitability in pedigree systems, two lambs per ewe is desired.

As a smaller flock keeper, you may not have any commercial aims for your flock. However, the other reason for monitoring and measuring performance is that it can highlight areas where disease may be present or where there is a problem with sheep health.

It is a good idea to record the details of your lambing season. In smaller flocks, this should be achievable by means of simple pen and paper recording (see Fig. 5.6). Larger flocks will use electronic individual identification and recording methods to monitor and record the performance of each ewe (see Fig. 5.7).

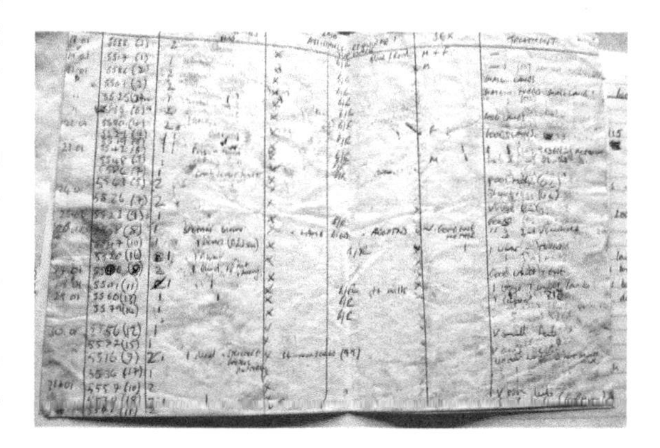

FIGURE 5.6 Pen and paper lambing records.

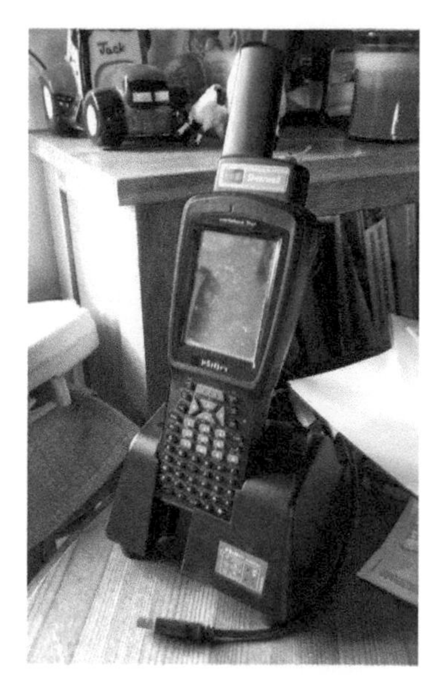

FIGURE 5.7 An electronic stock recorder.

What can you measure?

Scanning percentage

Flocks that ultrasound scan can record how many lambs are to be expected in the upcoming lambing. This is recorded as a percentage over the whole flock.

For example, the number of lambs expected divided by the number of ewes that were put to the ram, multiplied by 100 gives the scanning percentage. Commercial lowland flocks would be aiming for 185–200%.

Barren percentage

Barren or empty (non-pregnant) ewes are calculated by dividing the number of non-pregnant ewes by the total number of ewes put to the ram and multiplying by 100 to get a percentage. Results that are 3% and higher may indicate the presence of an infection.

Lambing percentage

This is the average number of lambs reared per ewes put to the ram. The aim will depend upon how many lambs you expected following scanning. Aim to rear as many lambs as possible. Therefore, the closer the lambing percentage is to your scanning percentage, the better.

Lamb mortality percentage

Recording how many lambs die between scanning and weaning or selling can be a useful exercise to understand and assess flock health. Unfortunately, there are likely to be some lamb deaths during a lambing period. This can be calculated by subtracting the number of lambs that were born, weaned or sold from the total number of lambs that you expected (from your scanning data). This number should then be divided by the total number of lambs that you expected and multiplied by 100 to give you a lamb mortality percentage. A target of 10% or less should be used.

Depending upon the level of your recording, you may be able to break this down further by working out when the lambs died. For example, were they born dead or did they die within the first 48 hours of life or did they die after turnout into the field.

It is important to determine why these losses occurred so that improvements can be made for the following lambing period. Speak to your vet if you appear to have lost too many lambs. Knowing when the losses occurred can give your vet clues as to the reasons for death. The more details that you have recorded, the more information your vet can use to work out the possible causes of death.

The above measurements will be used by your vet as part of your flock health plan. They can be used to compare how successful your lambing has been each year and the impact of any changes that have been made.

Keep it simple

Recording simple numbers of how many ewes you have and how many lambs were born can be very useful. Using a simple chart such as the one below at lambing time can help provide a good insight into your lambing period. It can be recorded and then examined later when lambing has finished and you have regained some sleep. Or, if during lambing a pattern emerges that may indicate that you have a problem in your flock, it can then be used by your vet as part of the investigation into what is causing the problem.

Table 5.1 displays a method of recording individual ewe performance data in the initial lambing period. This can be extended to include the weights of lambs at birth and 8 weeks old and weaning. Measuring daily live weight gains of lambs is a great indication of ewe performance in terms of milk supply and lamb growth rate. Daily live weight gain data can also be used to assess the presence of disease due to parasites or nutritional deficiencies (see 'Diarrhoea' in Chapter 7).

To measure daily live weight gain, weigh the lamb on day 1 and then again on day 7 and then divide the difference in weight by the interval number of days; in other words, 20 kg day 1, then 23 kg day seven. Then divide the difference (3 kg) by the interval (seven days) and the daily live weight gain is 0.42 kg or 428 g.

Table 5.2 is an example of the data that can be collected from a lambing period. This data can be used by your vet to identify areas where losses have occurred and where they are higher than expected. Scanning data can be added to this table in terms of the numbers of singles, twins and triplets expected.

Table 5.1

DATE	EWE ID	NUMBER OF LAMBS EXPECTED	NUMBER OF LAMBS BORN ALIVE	NUMBER OF LAMBS BORN DEAD	LAMB TREATMENTS OR DEATHS BEFORE TURNOUT	COMMENTS
E.g. 03/03/16	2435 'Poppy'	2	2		No	Lambed on her own, good mother

Table 5.2

NUMBER OF EWES TO THE RAM	NUMBER OF EWES LAMBED	TOTAL NUMBER OF LAMBS EXPECTED	TOTAL NUMBER OF LAMBS BORN ALIVE	NUMBER OF LAMBS WEANED OR SOLD	LAMB LOSSES (MORTALITY %)	EWE LOSSES (MORTALITY %)
50	49	93	90	88	5.3	0

LAMBING TIME 6

With newborn lambs running around (Fig. 6.1), lambing is an exciting part of the sheep calendar. However, this is also the period when ewes and lambs are at greatest risk of suffering and death and so commitment and careful attention to detail are needed to protect the health and welfare of these animals:

- Ewes in late pregnancy need to be checked throughout the day and night, to ensure that any having difficulty with lambing receive the assistance that they need

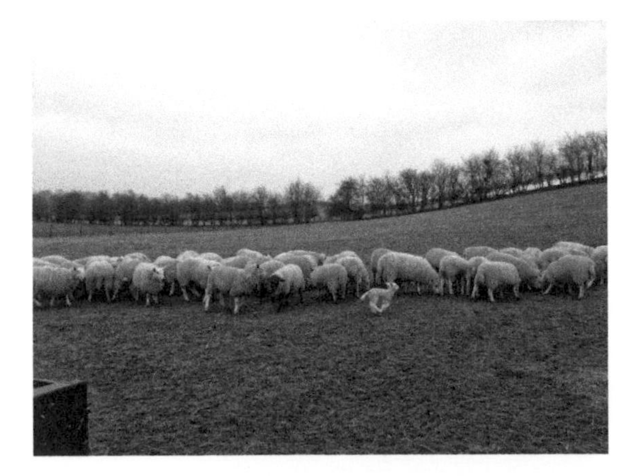

FIGURE 6.1 A young lamb skipping while the ewes are fed.

Photograph courtesy of Miss Kerry Price.

- Young lambs, and ewes that have recently given birth, can deteriorate quickly, therefore regular monitoring for disease and prompt appropriate treatment are essential, as discussed in this chapter

TIME COMMITMENT FOR SUCCESSFUL LAMBING

Ewes that are due to lamb should be checked every two to three hours throughout the day. However, if, during the check between 10 p.m. and midnight, none are showing signs of labour, then it is possible to delay the subsequent check for four to six hours as ewes are less likely to give birth overnight. Where a ewe has started to lamb, monitoring should be increased to every half hour until the lamb is born, or it is apparent that assistance is required (see 'Making the decision to intervene' below).

Young lambs and their mothers also need to be checked several times a day to make sure that they are in the correct place, eating, drinking and alert – rouse them if they are asleep. During these checks, shepherds should look for:

- Drooping ears
- Not eating (Fig. 6.2)

- Excessive sleeping
- Standing or lying away from the rest of the group
- Lounging uncomfortably with eyes half open
- Unresponsiveness or being slow to respond
- Healthy sheep often stretch as they stand up after lying down; animals that are in pain may not do this (Fig. 6.3)

It is also important to keep a watch for hungry lambs. Lambs will get hungry if the ewe does not have enough milk or has mastitis. Signs to look out for include lambs:

- Repeatedly trying to suckle
- Restless when lying down
- Vocalising repeatedly
- A visibly hollow stomach

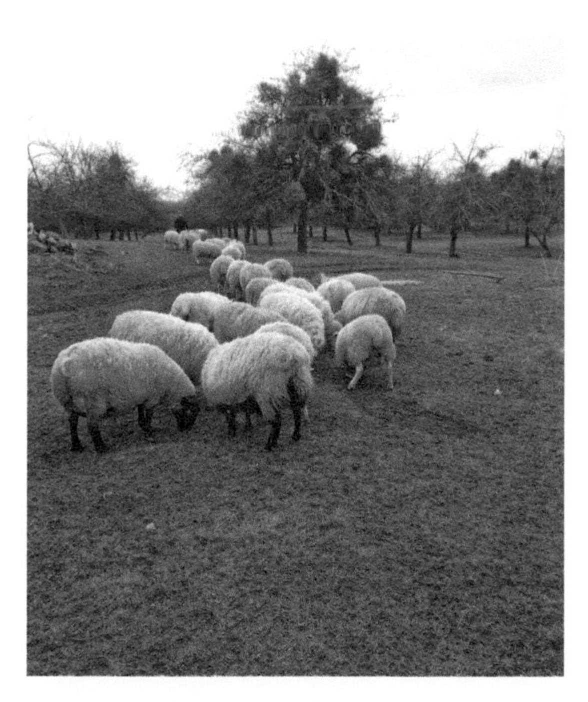

FIGURE 6.2 Feeding time can be a good time to spot ewes that are sick or about to lamb.

Photograph courtesy of Miss Kerry Price.

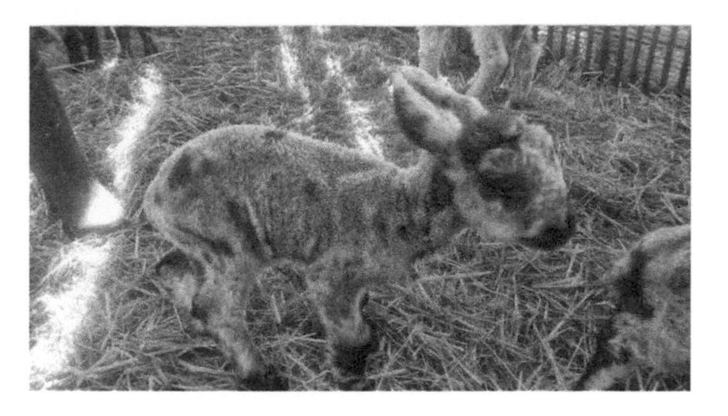

FIGURE 6.3 This hunched lamb is unwell and hungry; it is unlikely to stretch as it stands up.

It is important to watch the normal behaviour of both ewes and lambs as changes to their behaviour can be an early indication of problems; however, it is also important to monitor the general environment to ensure that a change in behaviour is not attributable to another factor, such as:

- The presence of a strange person or dog
- Extreme heat or cold

PREPARING FOR LAMBING

Where to lamb: indoors or outdoors?

Choosing whether to lamb ewes indoors, outdoors, or in at night and out during the day, will depend on several factors, including:

- The time of year and therefore expected weather conditions
- The climate in your geographic location
- Available facilities
- The breed of sheep
- Personal preference

The positive and negative aspects of indoor and outdoor lambing are laid out in Figure 6.4.

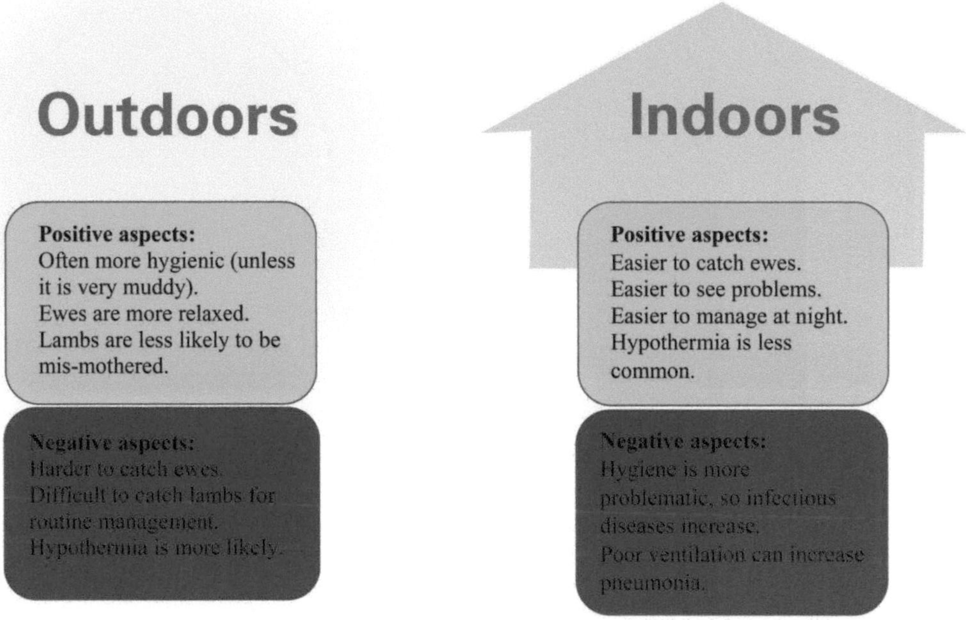

Outdoors

Positive aspects:
Often more hygienic (unless it is very muddy).
Ewes are more relaxed.
Lambs are less likely to be mis-mothered.

Negative aspects:
Harder to catch ewes.
Difficult to catch lambs for routine management.
Hypothermia is more likely.

Indoors

Positive aspects:
Easier to catch ewes.
Easier to see problems.
Easier to manage at night.
Hypothermia is less common.

Negative aspects:
Hygiene is more problematic, so infectious diseases increase.
Poor ventilation can increase pneumonia.

FIGURE 6.4 The pros and cons of lambing ewes outdoors and indoors.

Whichever strategy is selected, contingencies should be considered for switching from one to the other if conditions or circumstances require. For example, in extremely cold weather, are there options for outdoor lambing ewes to be moved indoors? Or, when there is an excessive build-up of infectious disease indoors and sympathetic weather conditions outdoors, can lambing ewes be turned out?

When making a decision to lamb sheep outdoors, consider whether:

- There is adequate shelter to protect ewes and lambs from prevailing winds and rain; in the form of hedges, trees, straw bales, wooden panels or a field shelter
- There are adequate handling facilities; for example, gates, hurdles and a trailer if sheep need to be moved significant distances
- Fields are excessively muddy
- There is a back-up plan in case of severe weather;
    - How can sheep be checked and fed in deep snow?
    - Can sheep be moved to emergency indoor accommodation or sheltered fields during prolonged, severely cold or wet conditions?

For indoor lambing, consider:

- How bedding can be kept clean and dry throughout lambing (Fig. 6.5)
- Whether all sheep have continual access to feed and water, even during hard frosts
- Whether there are low-level drafts that could chill lambs
- The ventilation inside the housing. Things like dusty cobwebs can be an indication of poor airflow
- Indoor lighting and whether this is sufficient to enable work to be carried out

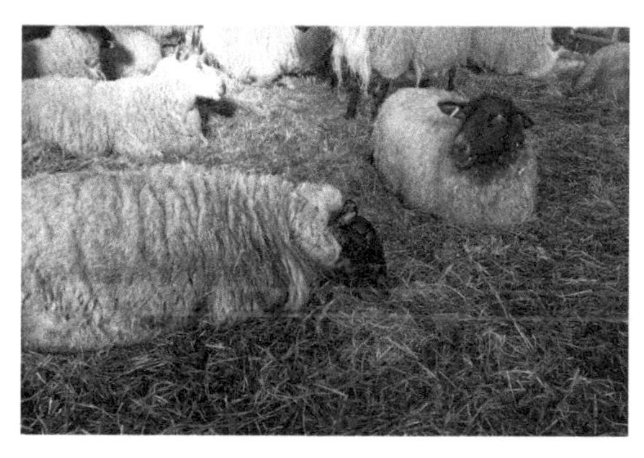

FIGURE 6.5 Ewes laid comfortably in deep clean straw.

Photograph courtesy of Miss Kerry Price.

Lambing equipment

Be prepared a month before the start of lambing: collect all the necessary equipment into clean, well-organised storage containers, close to where ewes will be lambing. Where the flock is small, it may be preferable to share some of the equipment with another local smallholder, however needles, syringes and ear tag applicators must not be shared and all other equipment must be thoroughly disinfected between properties. A lambing equipment list should include:

- The telephone number of your local sheep-friendly veterinary practice
- A ready supply of clean, warm water
- Disinfectant soap
- Clean towel
- Disposable gloves
- Lots of clean buckets
- Lambing lubricant (Fig. 6.6)
- A sheep halter
- A lambing snare (Fig. 6.7) and/or lambing ropes
- Injectable antibiotics. Long-acting amoxicillin and/or long-acting oxytetracycline
- Anti-inflammatory injection
- New needles (19 gauge, 1 inch) and syringes (2 ml, 5 ml, 10 ml and 50 ml; Fig. 6.8)
- A navel dipping cup that does not allow used dip back into the storage well
- 10% iodine solution
- Replacement colostrum – artificial or frozen
- A stomach tube and funnel or dosing syringe without its plunger
- A lamb feeding bottle and teat (Fig. 6.9)

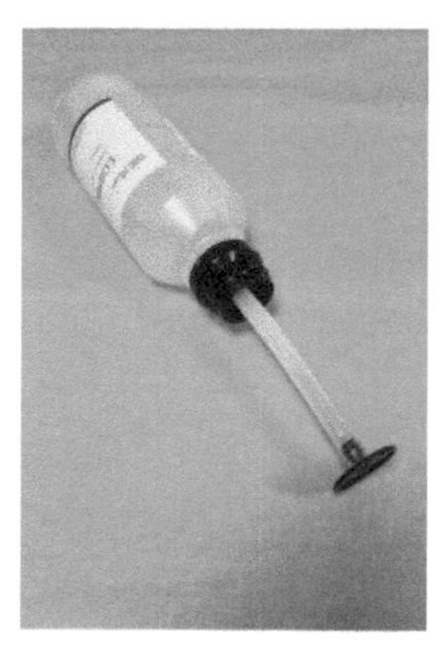

FIGURE 6.6 Generous amounts of obstetric lubricant make lambings much easier.

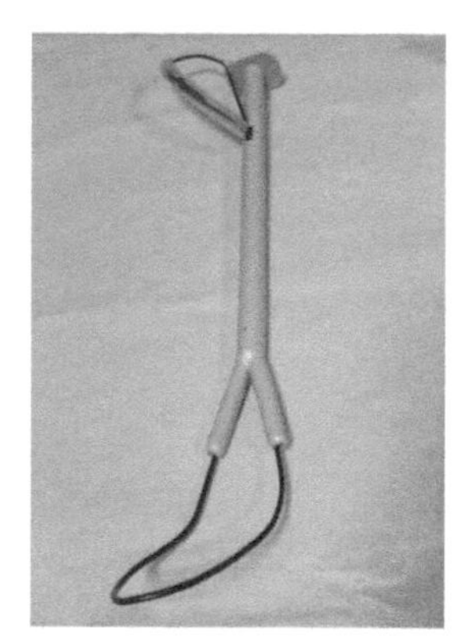

FIGURE 6.7 Lambing snares can be easy to position over a lamb's head, but take care not to tighten them around the neck.

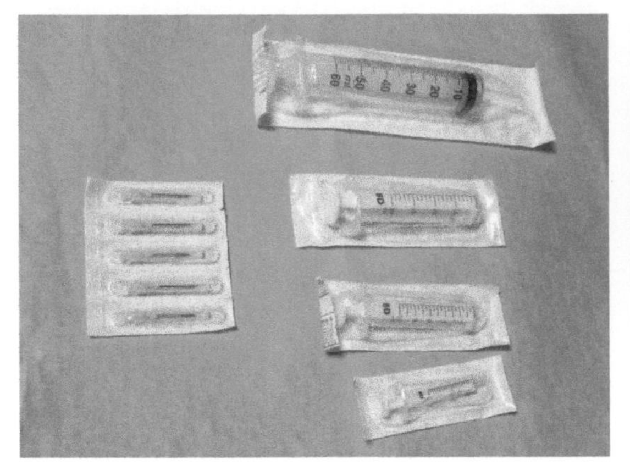

FIGURE 6.8 Have a ready supply of clean needles and syringes.

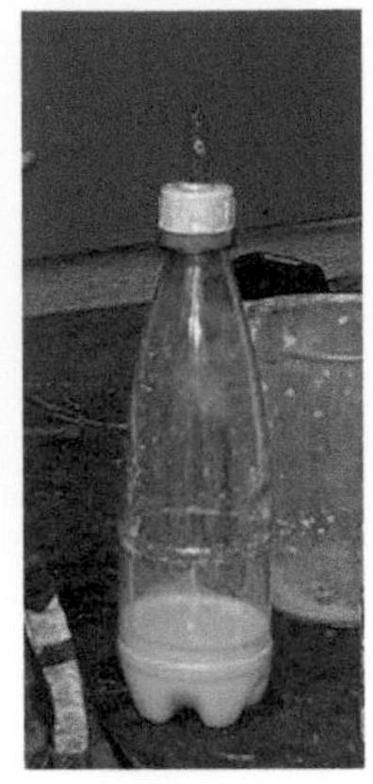

FIGURE 6.9 Lamb's milk in a bottle with a lamb teat.

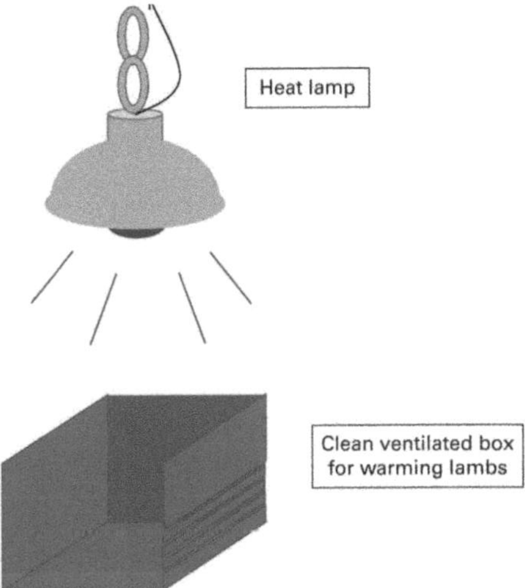

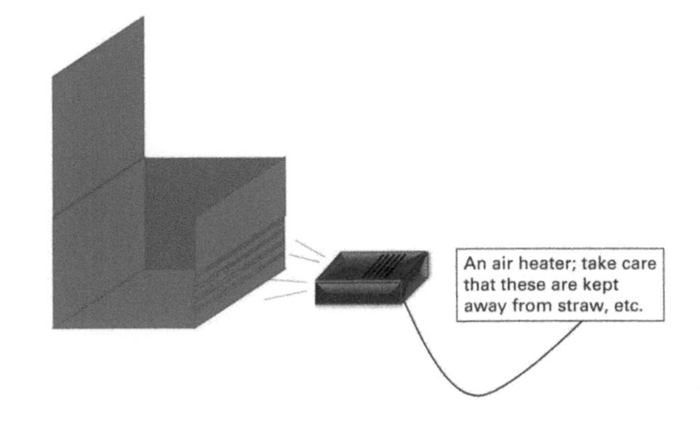

FIGURE 6.10 Warming boxes need to be dry and clean, large enough for a lamb to stand or lie down comfortably, and have a source of heat.

- Twin lamb drench, containing propylene glycol
- Calcium injection
- Injectable glucose
- A warming box or pen for hypothermic lambs (Fig. 6.10)
- Ear tags and tag applicators
- Elastrator and elastrator bands
- Laminated recording sheets and permanent marker pens (see Tables 5.1 and 5.2)

It is also advisable to know where ewe milk powder and prolapse harnesses or retainers may be obtained at short notice.

LAMBING PENS

Pens should be set up before the start of lambing. These are usually constructed from metal or wooden hurdles, pallets or straw bales. Whatever the materials used, they must be securely fastened together at the top and bottom (not just in one place or even in two places close together) and no element should be able to twist or fall onto the occupants. In addition, they must have no gaps through which a lamb could escape (Fig. 6.11).

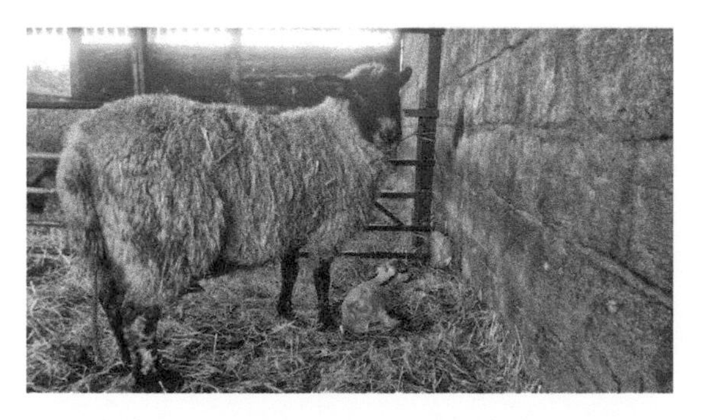

FIGURE 6.11 Lambs can become stuck in, or escape through, small spaces and will starve if they are away from the ewe for too long.

Small pens can be useful for ewes and lambs in the first few hours or days after birth (Fig. 6.12). These pens are normally approximately 3 to 4 square metres in size, but would be larger for ewes with three or more lambs (Fig. 6.13). Pens may be used for every ewe that lambs, which allows the necessary management tasks to be performed in the first 24 to 48 hours

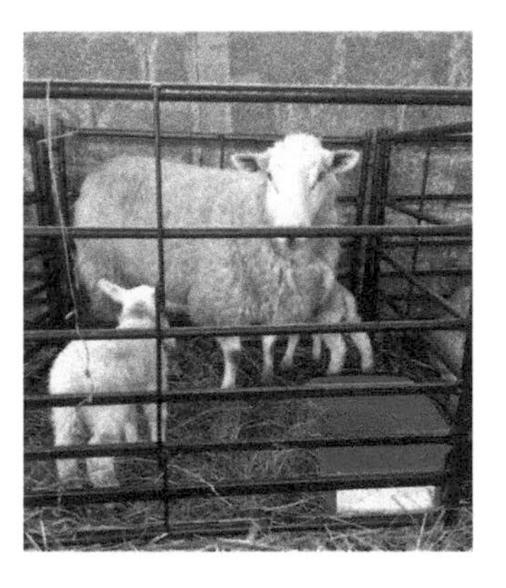

FIGURE 6.12 A ewe and her lambs in a secure, clean lambing pen.

Photograph courtesy of Miss Kerry Price.

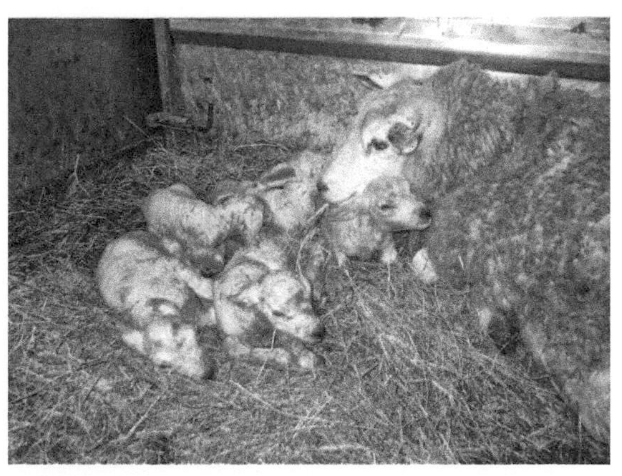

FIGURE 6.13 Ewes with multiple lambs need plenty of space to avoid lying on a lamb. Their lambs also need supplementary colostrum and milk.

Photo by kind permission of Mr John Morgan.

of life; this is often used for lambing indoors to allow close monitoring of ewes and lambs. Alternatively, pens may be used only for specific sets of ewes and lambs, such as:

- Ewes and/or lambs needing treatment or additional feeding
- Ewes with more than two lambs, which need additional milk while a foster mother is found
- Ewes with an adopted lamb, whilst they bond and until the lamb is strong enough to keep up with the ewe

A chalkboard by each lambing pen can be useful to record details about the current occupants, for example the date of birth, treatments given or needed and any specific problems. This information can be recorded before the board is wiped clean between each set of occupants.

Providing feed and water in pens

Ewes should have forage and fresh, clean water available at all times. Water can be provided in:

- Individual small buckets, that are cleaned and refreshed daily. The buckets should be too small for a lamb to fall into and ideally secured to the side of the pen to prevent spillage
- A half pipe that runs the length of a row of pens; either cleaned and topped up regularly (it should never run dry) or with fresh water constantly running through it. The pipe should sit at least 20 cm off the ground to reduce the risk of soiling by ewes. Hygiene is very important as infectious diseases may be able to pass from one animal to all the others drinking from the same pipe

The diet that is provided for the ewes in the pens should be as similar to their previous diet as possible; if ewes are moved straight into the pens from grass, the grass can be replaced by hay, haylage or silage (referred to as 'forage' from now on), but any concentrate feeding should remain the same.

Forage can be offered to the ewes in a number of ways, as long as it is always available, within easy reach of the ewe and none of the equipment can fall onto the occupants of the pen. Sometimes forage is fed on the floor, however it is quickly trodden into the ground and much is wasted. Methods of raising forage off the floor include:

- Hay racks that sit over hurdles (Fig. 6.14)
- Strong plastic feed bags with a hole cut in the side, near the bottom of the bag. When using this method, the hole should not be so large that the ewe could get her head stuck in it
- Hay nets. Whilst these may be used, if tied appropriately and at the correct height, the risk of ewes and lambs getting tangled in them remains problematic, and as such it is not a preferred method of feeding sheep

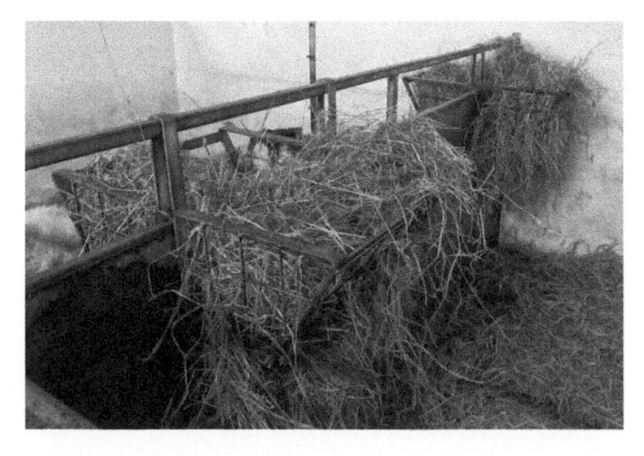

FIGURE 6.14 Small hay racks that hang over gates are useful in lambing pens.

Cleaning and bedding the pens

Various materials can be used as bedding in lambing pens. Straw is most common in the UK, but sawdust, sand and shredded paper have also been tried; whichever substance is used, it should always be:

- Deep enough to give the ewe and lamb comfort and warmth
- Dry and clean
- Topped up at least daily

For the purposes of good hygiene, remove obvious muck, pieces of placenta and dirty bedding. The bedding from each lambing pen should be removed and replaced between each set of occupants. If neighbouring pens are bedded, excessive water should not be used to clean empty pens. Water should only be used to clean concrete floors, it should not be used for cleaning dirt flooring. If possible, after cleaning the pen should sit empty for 24 hours before it is re-bedded with clean material, ready for the next occupants.

Deciding on the number of pens needed

The number of pens required depends on the number of pregnant ewes, how spread out lambing is expected to be and the intended function of the pens. Additional materials for extra pens should be kept close by in case of emergencies, such as busy periods. When setting up the pens, there should be a sufficient number, such that a couple may stand empty at any one time. For indoor lambing, where ewes have been allowed to breed naturally without synchronisation, it should be possible to house 15 to 20% of the ewes in pens at any one time.

If a ewe and her lamb(s) need to be kept in a pen for a prolonged period, the size of the pen should be increased considerably, to allow the occupants to move around.

When should occupants be moved out of their lambing pen?

Do not move ewes and lambs out of their lambing pen until:

- All of the lambs are strong enough to keep up with each other, and their mother at a brisk walk
- The lambs are suckling reliably (Fig. 6.15)
- The ewe is allowing all of her lambs to suckle reliably
- The ewe appears to like all of her lambs, that is, looks for them and calls them when any perceived danger is about, for example dogs, people, and so on

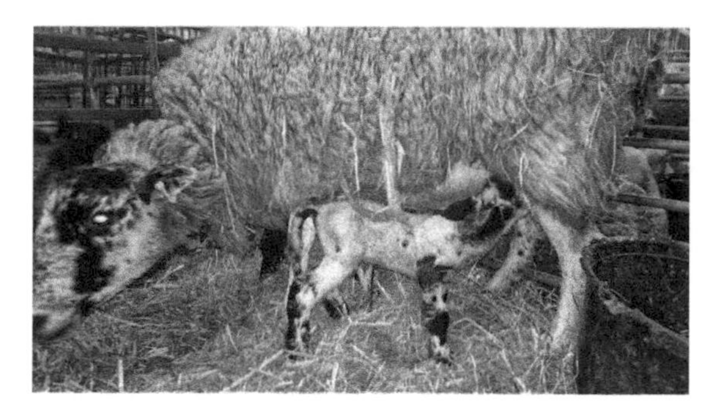

FIGURE 6.15 A newborn lamb needs to be suckling reliably.

An intermediate step: nursery pens or fields

Nursery pens can be set up indoors or in a sheltered area outdoors and used when the weather is bad or the fields are unsuitable for young lambs, for example when the field is too large for a newborn lamb. These nursery pens can be used as an intermediate step between the lambing pens and outdoors. They should be large enough to comfortably house a maximum of ten ewes and their lambs and the size of the pen should be adjusted according to the number of ewes likely to use it. If all is well with a ewe with just one lamb, she could miss the lambing pens altogether and go straight into a nursery pen.

Nursery fields are small fields that can house ewes and lambs if they need close monitoring, for example those that are recovering from disease; ewes that are not reliably allowing lambs to suckle; or ewes that do not have enough milk and their lambs need supplementing from a bottle.

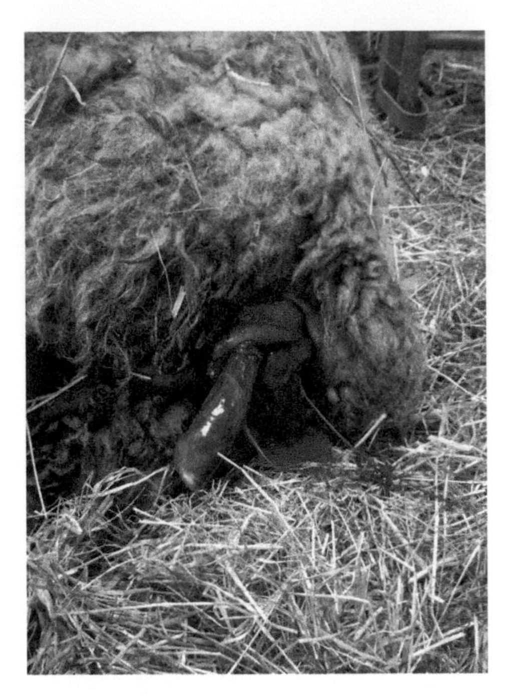

FIGURE 6.16 A ewe aborting a lamb – the membranes are not a healthy colour.

ABORTIONS

There are numerous causes of abortion in sheep. Some are not infectious, including severe stress, rough handling and prolonged lack of food. However, many abortions in sheep are caused by infection (Fig. 6.16), which generally spreads between ewes at the time of the abortion. Spread of infection occurs when healthy ewes come into contact with aborted fluids, foetuses and placenta. The discharge that ewes shed in the weeks after an abortion can also be infectious to other ewes.

All of these substances are potentially dangerous for pregnant women, who should have no contact with sheep for at least a month before or after lambing. Nor should they come into contact with any outer clothing that has been worn by people handling ewes at lambing time or dogs and cats that have been around these ewes. Even people who are not pregnant should be careful when handling aborted material and aborting ewes, as many of the infections can cause other forms of disease in people. Some of the transmittable diseases include *Toxoplasma gondii*, *Salmonella* species, *Campylobacter* species, *Listeria monocytogenes* and Q fever.

It is important to promptly and carefully dispose of aborted material and to isolate aborted ewes to control the spread of infection. The aborted foetus, placenta and associated bedding should be stored in a sealed container, out of reach of animals and children until they are collected for disposal.

Prevention of abortion in pregnant ewes includes:

- Careful handling: wherever possible handle heavily pregnant ewes without dogs
- Ensuring that they are well fed

- Storing feed in a dry place, without access for rodents, birds or cats
- Avoiding contact between pregnant ewes and young cats
- Removing all aborted material and associated bedding as soon as possible
- Isolating aborted ewes from other female breeding sheep for a minimum of a month after the abortion
- Avoiding contact between ticks and ewes that have not had previous exposure to local ticks

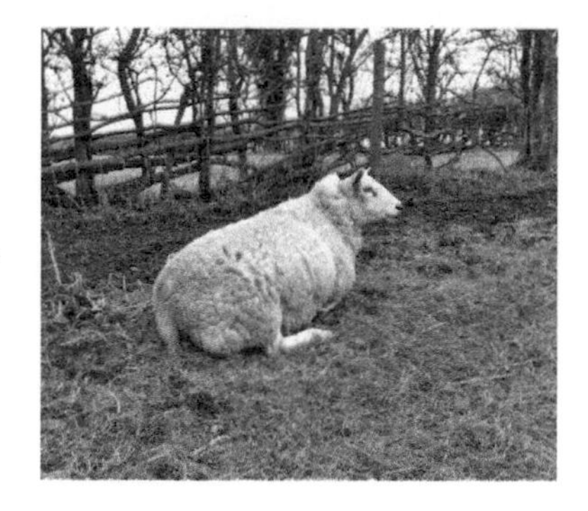

FIGURE 6.17 A ewe lying by herself at the edge of a field, preparing to give birth.

Photograph courtesy of Miss Kerry Price.

LAMBING

A normal lambing

In the few days leading up to lambing, a ewe's udder will begin to fill, her rounded stomach may become 'pear-shaped' as the bulk of the lamb drops closer to the ground and the vulva will become enlarged.

The first stage of lambing can last from several hours to a couple of days. During this time, a ewe's behaviour will change, including:

- Finding a space away from other sheep (Figs 6.17, 6.18)
- Not coming to feed
- Intermittently circling in a small area and stopping to scratch the floor with her front feet
- Lying down and standing up again
- Vocalising
- Trying to steal newborn lambs from other ewes

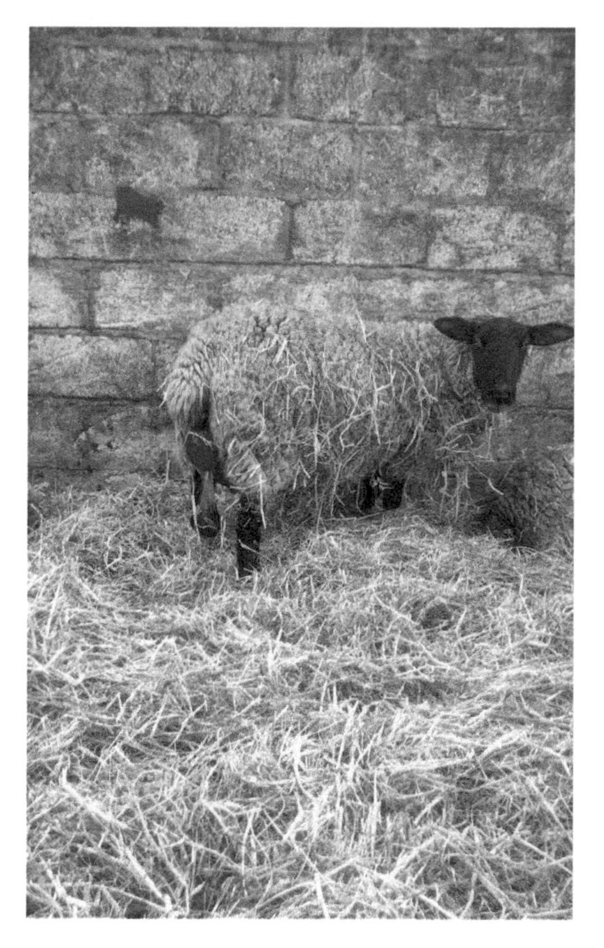

FIGURE 6.18 Ewes often find a spot at the edge of the shed to give birth.

When ewes try to steal lambs it can be difficult to tell which ewe the lamb(s) belong to – check the rear end of the ewes for a bloodstained discharge, which is a sign of recent lambing. It is important to assign the lambs to the correct ewe, as the thieving ewe will reject them once her own lambs are born.

Lambing starts when the water bag is passed from the vulva (Fig. 6.19). You will either see the bulge of the water bag itself or after it has burst the ewe will be wet below the vulva and may have a string of tissue hanging down (Fig. 6.20). The first lamb should be born within two hours of the water bag being passed.

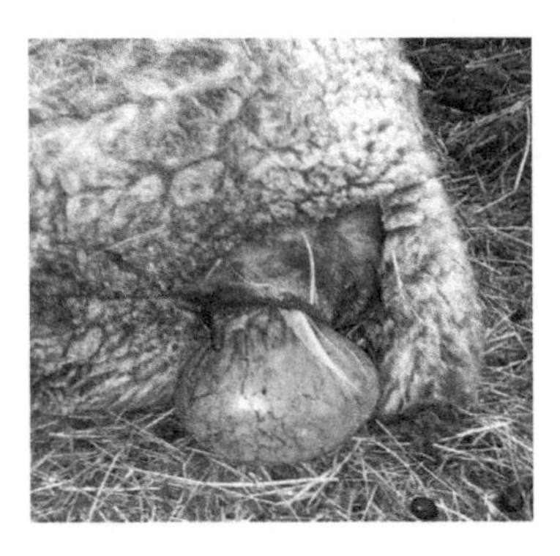

FIGURE 6.19 A water bag coming from the vulva of a ewe at the start of lambing.

Photograph courtesy of Miss Kerry Price.

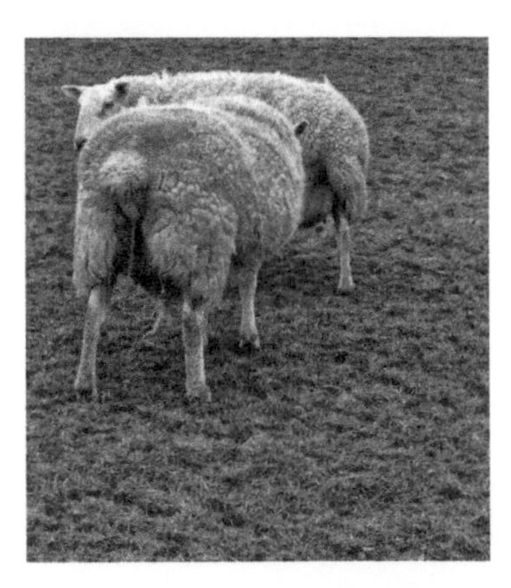

FIGURE 6.20 A burst water bag hanging from a ewe, indicating that she is lambing.

Photograph courtesy of Miss Kerry Price.

During lambing the ewe will be seen straining, either standing with her back legs splayed and head stretched upwards; or lying on her side with her head pointing towards the sky. She may be restless, repeatedly standing up and lying down again. Lambs are normally born head first, lying in the same orientation as the ewe, so that their spine points towards the spine of the ewe and feet towards her feet; the lamb's nose and two front feet all line up together in the birth canal (Figs 6.21, 6.22).

The ewe may pause momentarily with the lamb partly exposed, but then the lamb will drop to the ground (Fig. 6.23) and should start to shake

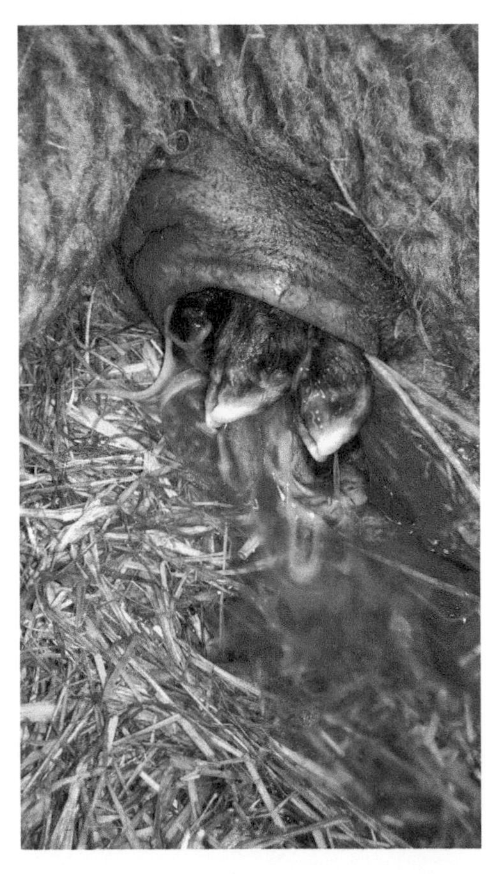

FIGURE 6.21 A lamb being born in normal presentation, with the front feet and nose coming first.

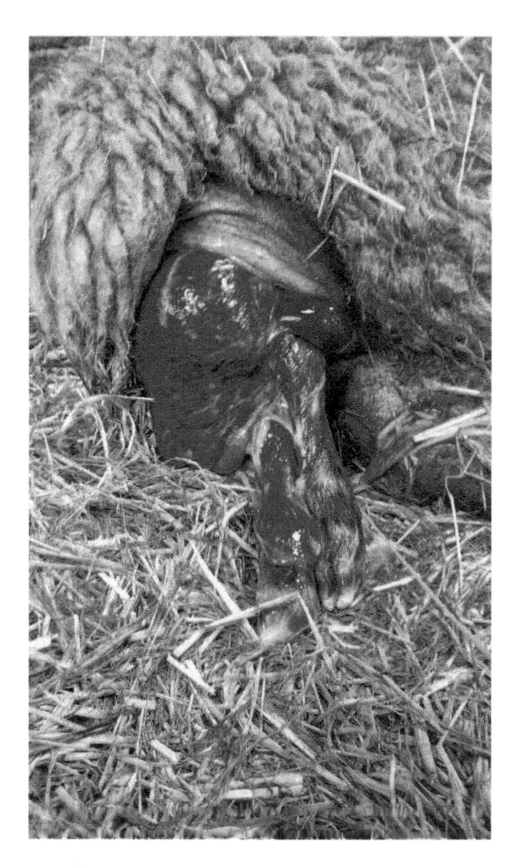

FIGURE 6.22 The head and feet of a lamb during a normal lambing.

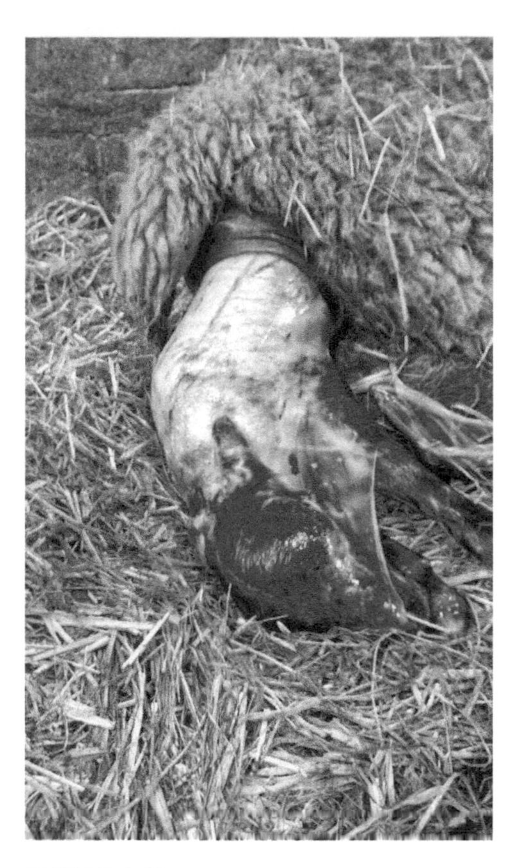

FIGURE 6.23 A lamb reaches the ground, covered in its membranes – these must be removed in order for the lamb to breathe.

vigorously. Occasionally, the water bag does not break open, but covers the lamb's nose; for the lamb to breathe, and so survive, the ewe needs to lick the lamb and break this or the closest person needs to remove the membranes quickly.

Many ewes give birth to multiple lambs; a new water bag will appear for each lamb (Fig. 6.24) and the birth process will be repeated. The placenta should be passed within an hour of the last lamb being born and ewes will often eat this. In order to keep the lambing pens as hygienic as possible, the placenta should be removed from the ground at the first opportunity. If the placenta has not been passed within 24 hours, there may be a problem and the vet should be called.

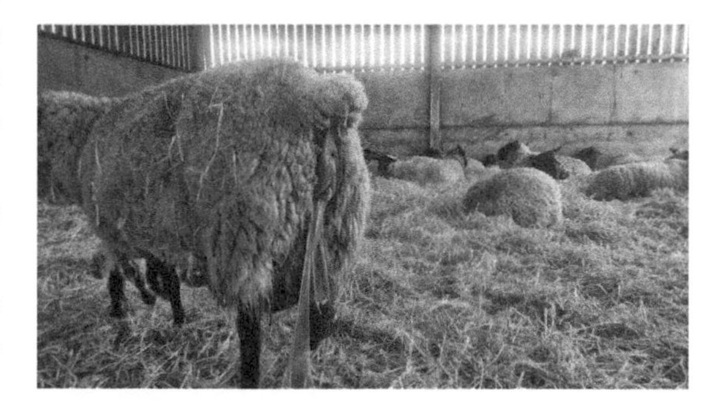

FIGURE 6.24 The second water bag and lamb appearing from a ewe.

Making the decision to intervene

A ewe needs assistance to give birth if:

- She appears to be in discomfort
- She has not managed to give birth in the expected timeframe described in 'A normal lambing'
- She has not given birth after 30 minutes of active straining
- The lamb is not in the expected position; see 'A normal lambing'
- She has a lamb with only its head out (Fig. 6.25) – this requires urgent attention
- The water bag contains meconium (faeces from the lamb; Fig. 6.26). This is an indication of distress in the lamb

Provided a ewe is behaving as expected, it is important to allow enough time for the natural process of giving birth to take place; do not interfere too soon. Make a note of the time when the water bag is first seen and if no lamb has been born:

- One hour later: catch the ewe and introduce a clean, lubricated, gloved hand into the vagina to ascertain the position and posture of the lamb (only do this if your hands are small enough to fit through the vagina, if not call for assistance). If all appears to be progressing normally monitor the ewe for another hour
- Two hours after the water bag appeared: if you have substantial lambing experience, assist the ewe to lamb; otherwise, call for expert assistance

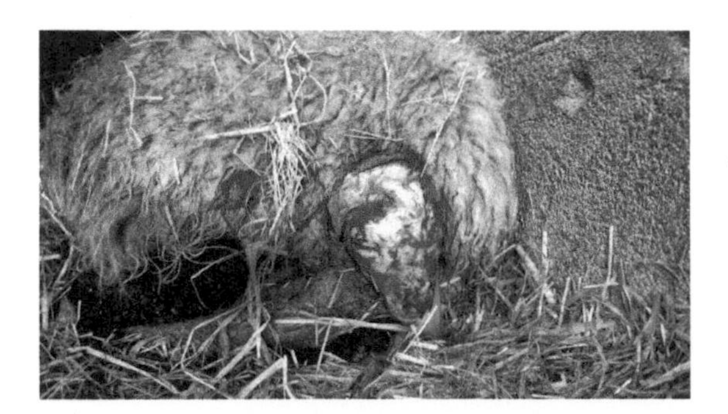

FIGURE 6.25 A ewe cannot give birth to a lamb if the head comes without its legs, this situation requires urgent expert lambing assistance.

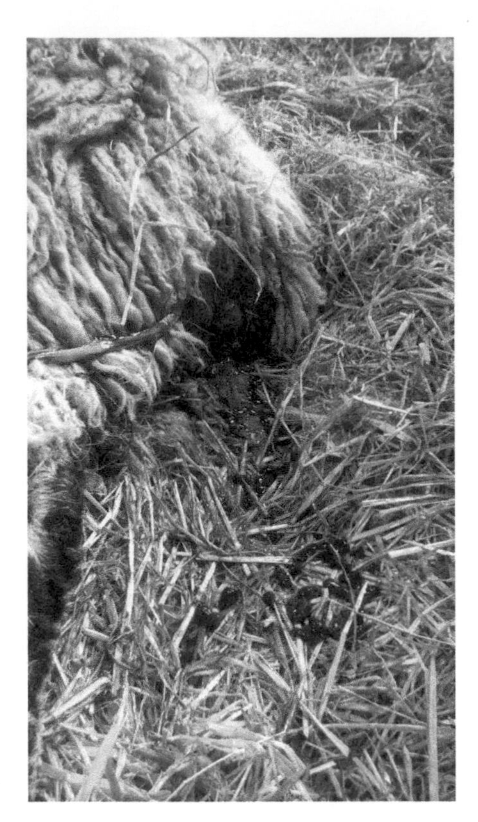

FIGURE 6.26 Meconium passed out of the uterus with fluid from the water bag, indicating that the lamb is in distress.

If you are not sure when the water bag first appeared, the time at which you intervene will depend on how long it has been since the ewes were last checked; if it was:

- One hour: watch the ewe for ten to 15 minutes; if she is behaving normally leave her for 30 minutes before you catch and check her as described above; if not, check her immediately
- Two or more hours: watch the ewe for ten to 15 minutes; if there is no obvious progress in this time, catch and check the ewe immediately; if she is making progress, monitor her until the lamb is born

When a call is made for additional assistance with a lambing, the ewe should be left quietly until assistance arrives.

Assisting a ewe during lambing

There are several reasons that a ewe may require lambing assistance. These include: a lamb in the wrong position for birth; a lamb that is too big; failure of the ewe's cervix to open sufficiently to allow the lamb to be born without damaging the ewe; a small or deformed pelvis in the ewe; a deformed lamb. Distinguishing these causes and assisting a ewe with lambing can be difficult and should only be attempted by those with relevant training and previous supervised experience, otherwise call for experienced help, preferably from the local vet. However, if the ewe is struggling and the lamb is halfway out, it is possible for an inexperienced person to apply gentle pressure to the legs of the lamb and the back of its head to see whether it will come easily.

When assisting a ewe to lamb:

- Restrain the ewe gently but securely: ideally, ask someone to hold the ewe. If no one is available and she is standing, stand her between two hurdles that are securely attached to each other at one end. Allow her to lie down if she tries to do so
- Have a bucket of clean, warm water and dilute disinfectant, containing the clean lambing aids, for example the lambing snare and/or ropes and lubricant (Fig. 6.27)
- Use *lots* of lubricant
- Always have clean, disinfected hands and ideally wear clean disposable gloves
- Be gentle at all times, with the ewe and the lambs
- When repositioning the legs, cover the feet with your hand to prevent them from piercing the wall of the uterus
- Give the ewe an injection of anti-inflammatory after an assisted lambing
- Give the ewe antibiotic treatment after an assisted lambing:

    - If it is a straightforward lambing, give a long-acting antibiotic as prescribed by your vet

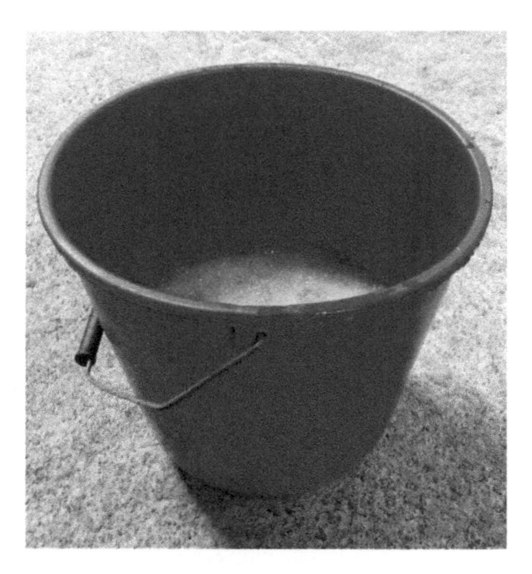

FIGURE 6.27 A clean bucket of clean, soapy water is used for keeping hands clean and holding clean lambing ropes and lubricant.

- If the lambing is difficult or prolonged, or the lamb was dead and starting to decay, speak to the vet about a longer course of antibiotic treatment – start this course on the day of the lambing

- Always check whether there are any more lambs, by reintroducing a clean hand into the uterus; do this even if the ewe has already produced the expected number of lambs
- Mark ewes that have had difficult lambings, and do not breed from them again; also, make a note of their lambs to avoid breeding from these too

There are different approaches to take with assisting a ewe to lamb depending on the position of the lamb being born. If the lamb is in the correct position:

- Slip the lambing rope or snare over each of the lamb's ears and through the mouth (Fig. 6.28)
- Take hold of each foot, or attach a lambing rope to each one above the fetlock (Fig. 6.29) Adult ewes (over 2 years old) can give birth to small- or medium-sized lambs with one front leg back, but if both legs are there, use both
- Ease the lamb out, alternating gentle pressure on each leg and the head
- Once the lamb's shoulders have passed through the vulva, pull it steadily in a diagonal direction down towards a spot behind the back feet
- If the lamb cannot be advanced with gentle traction, call for veterinary assistance

If the lamb is not in the normal position, try to ascertain the following before starting to assist:

- Which legs can be felt in the birth canal (Fig. 6.30)
- The number of legs in the birth canal: if there are more than two, or those two are a front leg and a back leg, the ewe will need veterinary assistance

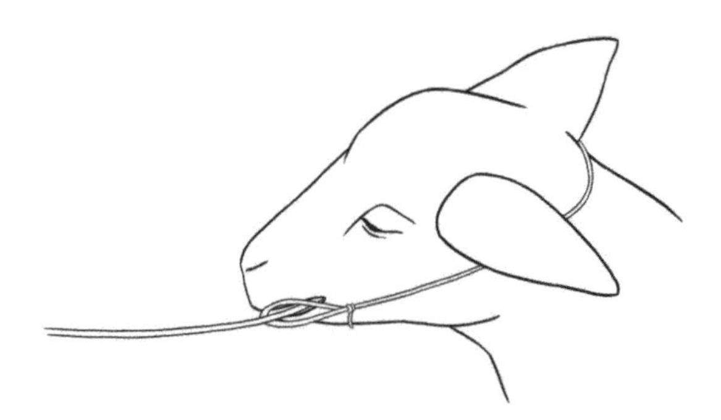

FIGURE 6.28 Position the lambing rope or snare behind the lamb's ears and through its mouth to prevent it from tightening around the neck.

Picture courtesy of Miss Amanda Aiken.

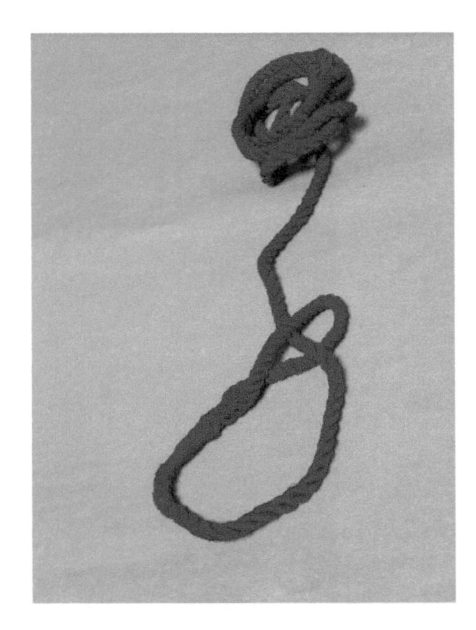

FIGURE 6.29 Loop a lambing rope above the lamb's fetlock and pull it tight to get a secure hold of the leg.

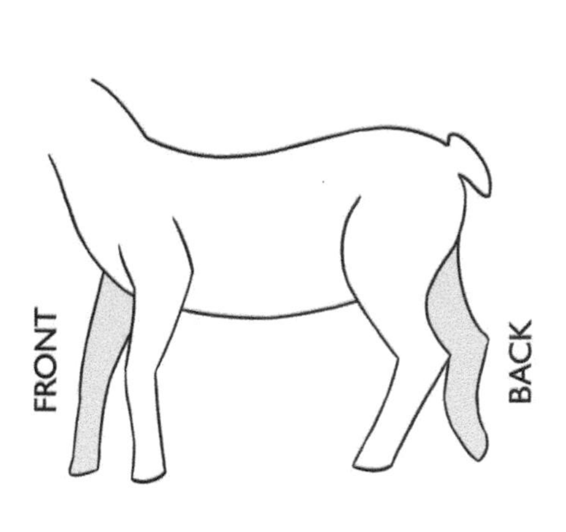

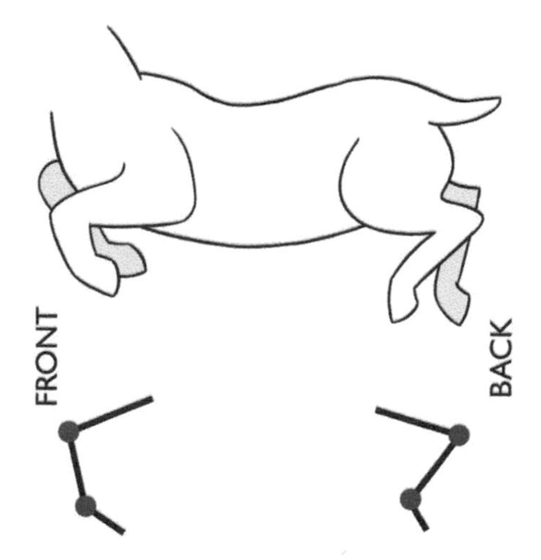

FIGURE 6.30 Knowing that the joints of a lamb's front and back legs bend in different directions allows them to be differentiated by feel during a lambing.

Picture courtesy of Miss Amanda Aiken.

- Find out whether all the legs are attached to the same lamb by gently following them back into the ewe

However, if the intention is to call for expert assistance, do not spend long on checking the position of the lamb as an experienced lamber will soon be able to tell how best to proceed.

When there are further lambs to be born after an assisted birth, a decision needs to be taken as to whether to pull them immediately or allow the ewe to give birth to them naturally if she can. If electing to allow subsequent births to proceed naturally, use the decision-making criteria laid out above in 'Making the decision to intervene', adjusting the maximum time before further intervention to one hour rather than two. Assistance with the birth of additional lambs should be given immediately if:

- The first lamb is stained bright yellow (Fig. 6.31)

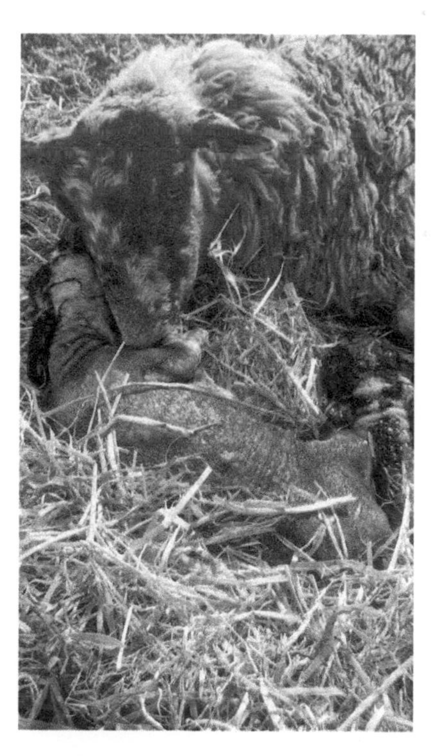

FIGURE 6.31 A newborn lamb stained yellow from meconium, the lamb's first faeces. This is an indication of stress in the lamb during birth.

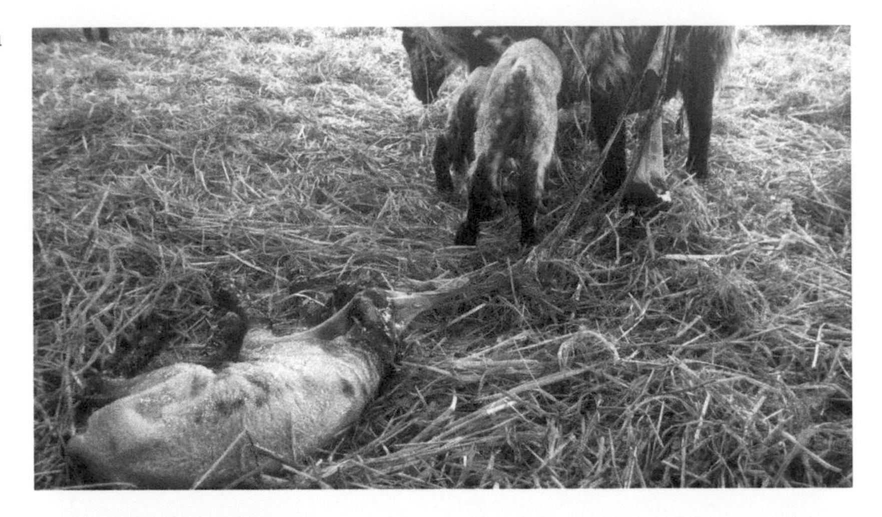

FIGURE 6.32 A newborn lamb still in the placental membranes; ensure these are not covering the lamb's nose so that it can breathe.

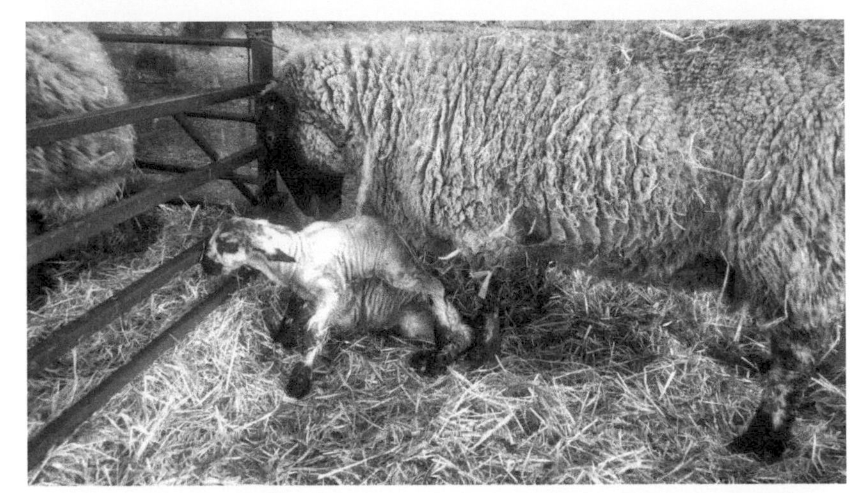

FIGURE 6.33 A ewe licking her newborn lamb; this is essential for the lamb to dry and not become chilled.

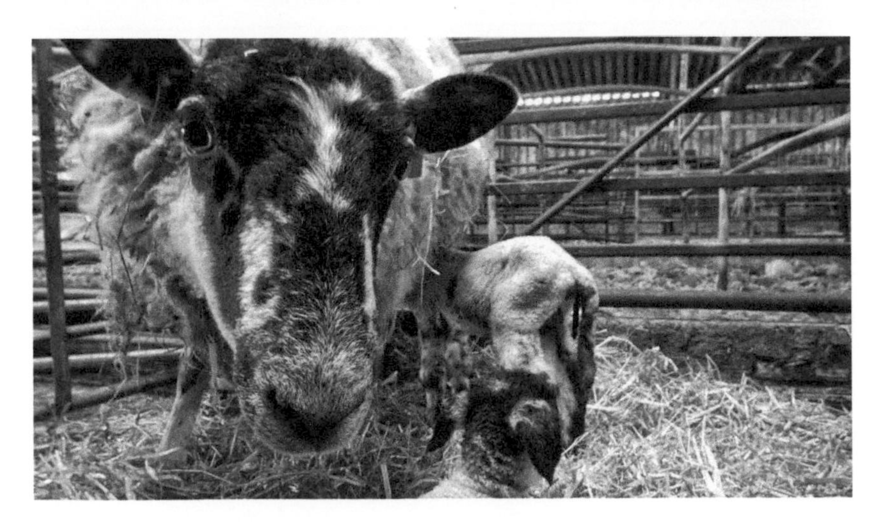

FIGURE 6.34 A newborn lamb passing its first faeces, called the meconium.

- The first lamb was dead or died shortly after birth
- The ewe has been trying to lamb for more than two hours and is exhausted

Immediate actions after lambs are born

- Quickly remove any remaining membranes from the lamb's nose, to allow it to breathe (Figs 6.23, 6.32)
- Check that the lamb is breathing; if not, remove all mucus from its nose and mouth, rub its chest vigorously and prick its nostrils with a piece of straw
- Move the lamb to the front of the ewe for her to lick it (Fig. 6.33)
- Check for additional lambs
- Check that each lamb passes its first faeces – black and sticky meconium (Fig. 6.34) – within a few hours of birth. If not, check that the lamb has an opening at its anus (see 'Atresia ani' below)
- Check that the mother has good milk by expressing a little from each teat

Calling out the vet

If there is any uncertainty during lambing, do not hesitate to seek veterinary advice or assistance. However, there are some specific situations in which veterinary assistance is needed:

- When a ewe requires lambing assistance and people on site have not had relevant training or experience
- For a lamb with only its head out (this requires urgent attention)
- When it is difficult to work out which bit of the lamb is which
- When multiple lambs or the wrong combination of legs are in the birth canal together
- When lambing attempts have been unsuccessful after ten to 15 minutes
- For ewes with a prolapsed vagina (see below in 'Vaginal prolapses') before lambing, which will not stay in
- For ewes that have a vaginal prolapse at the time of lambing (the water bag is not always obvious; if in doubt, call the vet anyway)
- For ewes that have prolapsed their uterus or womb after lambing
- When the lambs are dead and rotten
- For ewes with smelly back ends
- For sick, depressed ewes that are not eating
- For lambs that prolapse their intestines, or guts, through their umbilicus or navel

Lambs that cannot be born naturally, even with veterinary assistance, require birth by caesarean section (see Fig. 5.1). The purpose of this surgical procedure is to save the ewe's life, her lambs' lives or both. These ewes require additional monitoring for signs of sickness or opening of the wound and urgent veterinary assistance is needed in either of these cases.

CARING FOR NEWLY LAMBED EWES

For each ewe that lambs, check her thoroughly and monitor her closely for the following week. Areas to concentrate on include:

- Udder, for milk and signs of mastitis (see 'Mastitis' below)
- Teeth, making sure that she is able to eat the feed and it does not need supplementing
- Feet, for lameness

- Behaviour, make sure that she is allowing all her lambs to suckle and not being aggressive towards any of them
- Smelly vaginal discharges (see 'Metritis' below)
- Signs of ill health, such as dullness, being unresponsive to lambs, not eating, lying down a lot, stiffness or lameness. Seek prompt veterinary attention for sick ewes

CARING FOR NEWBORN LAMBS

Colostrum supplementation

Colostrum is vitally important for the health and well-being of young lambs; they need plenty of good-quality colostrum within two hours of birth. See 'The impact of colostrum' in Chapter 8 for more details about ewe colostrum and supplementary sources. Some lambs will not suckle their mother or a bottle when they are first born (Fig. 6.35) or if they are particularly unwell; in these instances, the lamb will need to be fed by stomach tube until they can suckle – this technique is described in 'Stomach tubing a lamb' below. Details of how to determine whether a lamb has taken a good feed of colostrum from its mother can be found below in 'Checking that lambs are getting enough milk'.

Stomach tubing a lamb

If a lamb is unable to suckle after birth, then it is important that it is fed via a stomach tube until it is able to suckle. In order to safely stomach tube a lamb, the following must be done:

- Make sure there is no damage to the tube
- Warm the colostrum or milk to body temperature
- Clean the tube and funnel, put these within easy reach, with the colostrum or milk (Fig. 6.36)
- Hold the tube against the side of the lamb so that the end reaches the last rib; mark the tube by the lamb's nose to identify how far it needs to be advanced

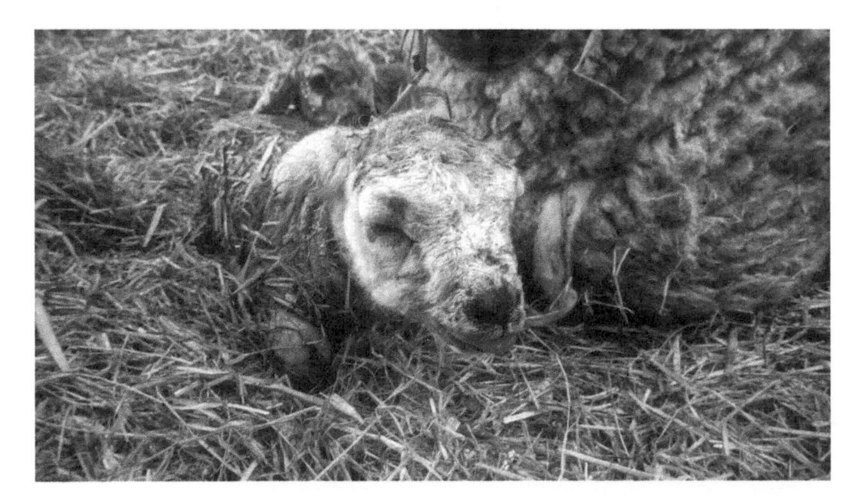

FIGURE 6.35 A lamb with a swollen head and tongue after a difficult lambing needs colostrum by stomach tube until it can suckle.

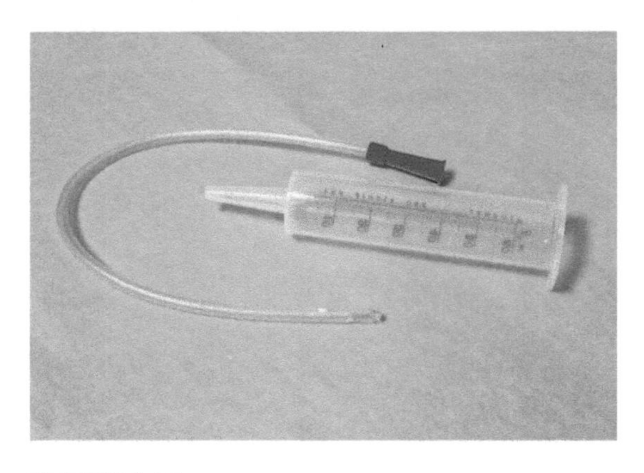

FIGURE 6.36 A dosing syringe without its plunger can be used as a funnel for a lamb stomach tube.

To insert the stomach tube:

- Sit down with your knees approximately horizontal. Hold the lamb gently between your knees so that it is in a vertical position with its head up, tail down and back towards you
- With one hand, hold the lamb's head, with the nose pointing upwards and neck straight but not stretched. Place a finger of this hand in the lamb's mouth to hold it open
- Use the other hand to pass the stomach tube over the tongue and slowly advance it; the lamb should swallow the end of the tube when it reaches the back of the throat
- *Ensure that the tube is in the correct place; see below*

Feeding the lamb using the stomach tube:

- Attach the funnel, holding it above the lamb's head, and pour a small amount of colostrum into it. Check that the colostrum goes down gradually and the lamb does not start to cough. If the lamb coughs, kink and remove the tube immediately and call the vet
- Add small amounts of colostrum to the funnel at a time, allowing most of it to drain before refilling the funnel
- If the funnel stops emptying or starts to refill, wait for 30 seconds; if it is still not emptying, kink the tube tightly between a finger and thumb so that no milk can leak out of it as you remove the tube from the lamb. Try to feed the lamb again later; never force anything into the stomach under pressure, for example never use a syringe with a plunger

The following is a list of checks to help determine that the tube is in the oesophagus, *not* the windpipe/trachea:

- Watch the tip of the tube move down the neck, along the jugular groove (Fig. 6.37), as you advance it
- The tube can be advanced all the way to your mark
- The lamb does not cough
- Air does not move in and out of the end of the tube as the lamb breathes – hold the end of the tube close to sensitive skin or hold something light and wispy over the end

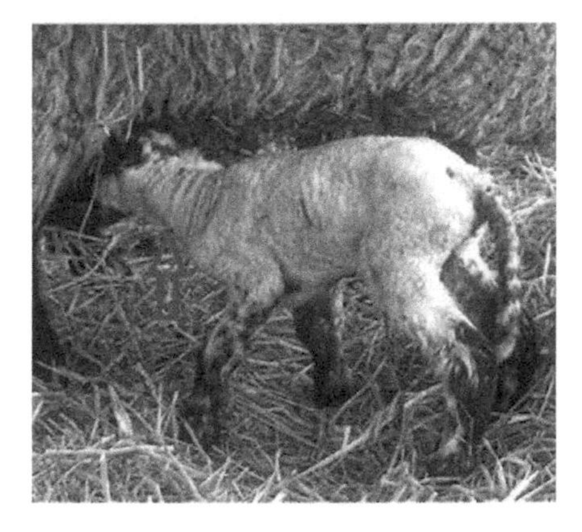

FIGURE 6.37 The red arrow points to the middle of the jugular groove as it makes its way down the neck.

- The tube and windpipe can be felt next to each other in the lower neck; be gentle trying to feel this and be careful not to occlude the windpipe

Navels

The navel, also known as the umbilical cord or vessels, is a common route for infection to get into a lamb. Prevention of these infections is discussed in detail in 'Does navel treatment matter?' in Chapter 8, but it is important that the navel is completely covered with strong (10%) iodine, as soon as possible, and in the cleanest possible manner, after birth.

Checking that lambs are getting enough milk

After lambs are born, it is important to ensure that they are getting enough milk to thrive and grow, as well as fight off disease. Lambs that are getting plenty of milk will:

- Have a bulging stomach after suckling, especially when the lamb is held up by the front legs, when it will look pear-shaped (see Fig. 8.16)
- Suckle continually for a few minutes at a time, then stop and do something else
- After suckling the lambs appear content and no longer vocalise
- Lambs sleep soundly

It is important to be watchful for lambs that are not getting enough milk from their mothers (Fig. 6.38) as early intervention can prevent illness and death. Signs of underfed lambs can include:

- Hollow bellies, even when the lamb is held up by the front legs

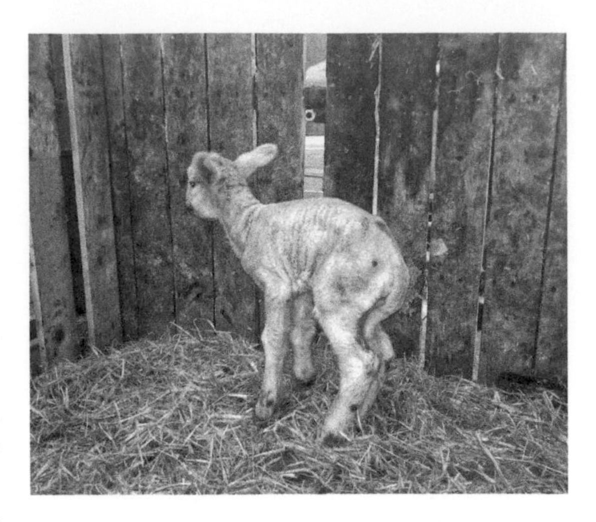

FIGURE 6.38 A thin, hollow lamb.

- Repeated vocalisation
- Repeated attempts to suckle, including releasing the teat and looking for it again
- Ewes moving away every time a lamb tries to suckle
- A discontented appearance
- Depression; this is an advanced sign of starvation and these lambs will need a lot of care, including rehydration; seek veterinary advice

When hungry lambs are identified, their mother's udder should be checked for signs of mastitis: pain, heat, cold and a change of colour to red, purple and/or black. Also check the udder for milk, by squeezing the teats in a downwards motion from top to bottom, but do not forget that if a lamb has a full stomach there may not be much milk left in the ewe's udder! This is especially important where a ewe has birthed more than one lamb, as the others could be suckling well and only one be underfed.

If there is no sign of mastitis, but the ewe has no milk, all of the nutrition for the lambs will need to be provided by milk replacer and/or milk pellets, depending on the age of the lamb(s). See the 'Pet lambs' section below for more details. If the ewe has insufficient milk and the lamb(s) will take some milk from a bottle, they can be given ewe milk replacer two to three times daily. The amount of additional milk that is needed can be judged by how hungry the lambs are and how well they are growing. If the ewe's milk remains insufficient, these lambs will need concentrate feed as well; but if she starts to produce enough milk, they will refuse the artificial milk.

Some ewes will have little or no milk at lambing time, but will then produce a normal milk supply two to three days later. In these cases, leave the lambs with the ewe, giving them all the colostrum and milk that they need for these first few days and keep checking the ewe's udder.

Carrying lambs

Young lambs are relatively tender, and as such can be unintentionally injured if handled incorrectly. However, it is often necessary to carry them close to the ground, so that their mothers can see them and will follow you with them. A common way to carry lambs for this purpose, is to hold both front legs above the fetlock in one hand, with a finger placed between the two legs; the back legs are allowed to hang downwards, but should be kept off the ground (Fig. 6.39).

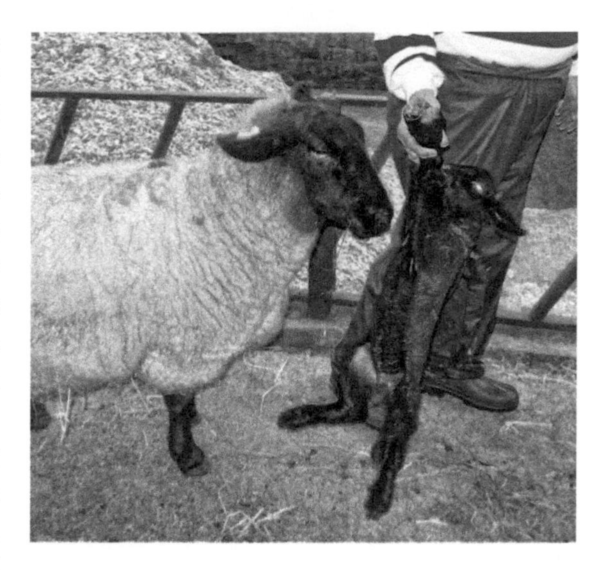

FIGURE 6.39 Lambs should be carried by holding a minimum of two legs.

Triplets

Ewes that give birth to three or more lambs will need extra care and feeding. In most cases, the ewe will not have enough milk to rear more than two lambs, although occasionally a ewe with lots of milk will be able to rear three. However, in this situation she will need to be kept with a small group of sheep for close monitoring. Ewes that rear triplets (or more) need good grass and/or forage, with additional concentrate feed, for six to eight weeks after lambing. Often triplet lambs will also need extra milk from a bottle.

In the majority of cases of triplets, the best course of action is actually to allow the ewe to rear two lambs and either rear the additional lamb(s) artificially or foster it/them onto other ewes with a single lamb. It is recommended, when taking lambs for artificial rearing or fostering, that the strongest lamb(s) are selected as these lambs are the ones most likely to survive the change. However, if any of the lambs are small and weak, it is best to leave equally matched lambs with their mother and give the smaller ones additional care and attention.

After the birth of triplets, ensure that all the lambs get some colostrum from their mother, then give each of them some supplementary colostrum; the ewe's colostrum should be better quality than any supplementary colostrum but she will not have enough for them all.

Tail docking

Lamb's tails are docked by the application of a tight rubber ring (Figs 6.40, 6.41) and by law this must be performed within the first seven days of life. Rubber rings are used because they cut off the circulation of the tail, causing it to die back and the bleeding to stop before the tail drops off. The tails of docked sheep must be long enough to cover the anus and vulva of female lambs and the tail should be left an equivalent length in male lambs. Always put the rings on as cleanly as possible to prevent infection from tracking up the spine from the tail and ensure that nothing is trapped in the ring with the tail.

Lambs and sheep with docked tails are less susceptible to blowfly strike later in life because soft faeces are less likely to become trapped by short tails. For sheep breeds that are prone to diarrhoea, tail docking is recommended. However, for some native UK hill breeds this is less of a problem and their tails protect them against the weather; tails are not normally docked in these breeds (Fig. 6.42).

Owners should find out what is standard practice for tail docking in their breed of sheep. This can be done through the breed society. Sheep should also be monitored over several years to see whether they get mucky back ends. If this does not appear to be a problem, it is possible to consider not docking lambs' tails, but this should be discussed with the local vet before any changes are made because undocked sheep must be monitored more carefully than docked sheep, particularly for blowfly strike, and vaginal and rectal prolapses, as these can be hidden by the tail.

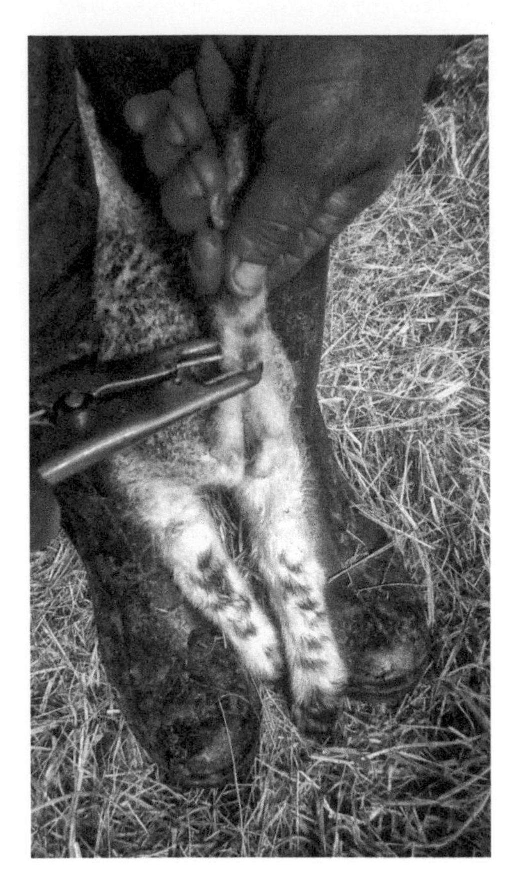

FIGURE 6.41 A lamb's tail being docked using a rubber ring.

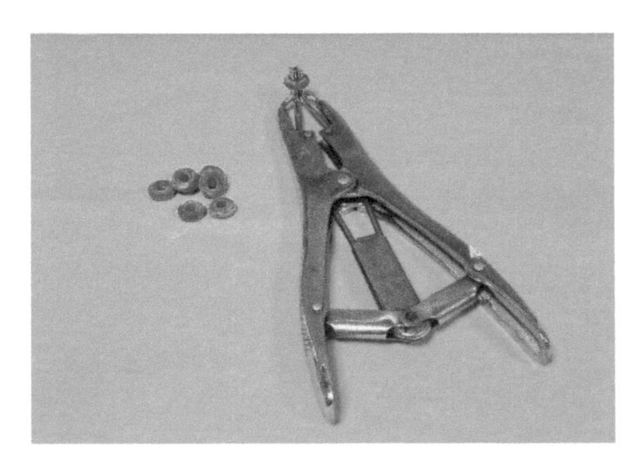

FIGURE 6.40 Rubber rings used for tailing and castrating lambs.

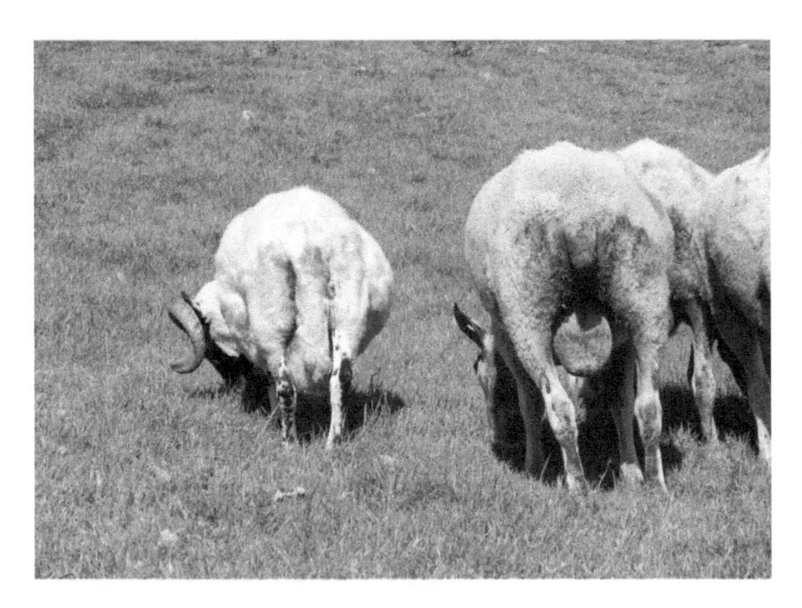

FIGURE 6.42 Susceptibility to diarrhoea varies between breeds of sheep and affects whether their tails are routinely docked.

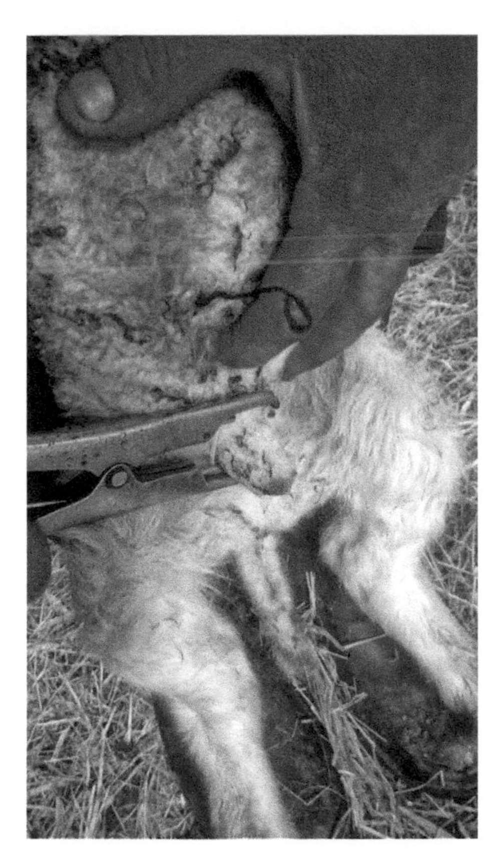

FIGURE 6.43 Male lambs can be castrated using rubber rings; this is a specialist procedure requiring training.

Castration

Male lambs can be castrated using the same tight rubber rings that are used for docking tails (Fig. 6.43); however, this is a specialist procedure and as such should only be performed by a suitably trained individual. Speak to the local sheep vet to find out about relevant training.

Castration is not necessary if male and female sheep over 4 months old can be successfully kept apart; speak to your local vet if this may be possible. If it is not possible to separate male and female lambs then castration should be performed to prevent unwanted, and potentially harmful, pregnancies in young ewe lambs. By law, castration must be performed within the first seven days of a lamb's life.

Pet lambs

Rearing pet lambs is time-consuming but very rewarding. Newborn lambs need colostrum (at least 50 ml per kilogram of their bodyweight) every two to three hours for the first 24 hours, then ewe milk replacer – do not try to substitute cow's milk as it does not have the correct constituents to provide the lambs with the nutrients that they require. The manufacturer's instructions for the replacement ewe milk will give the correct guidelines for mixing the milk and the total volume required at each point from birth to weaning. Table 6.1 gives an overview of pet lamb milk requirements.

Most smallholder pet lambs will be reared on milk from a bottle; once the milk is finished the bottle should be removed as suckling an empty bottle can cause digestive problems. Milk buckets (Fig. 6.44), with multiple teats, can be used to feed several lambs at once; and some farms with a large number of pet or orphaned lambs use milk feeding machines. These feeders automatically mix the milk and send it to several teats; these are convenient and provide lambs with a constant supply of milk. All milk feeding equipment, whether individual bottles or feeding machines, must be kept clean to prevent the build-up of infections.

Lamb starter or milk pellets need to be introduced in small amounts until all the lambs are eating their share. This prevents individual lambs from overeating the pellets and making themselves unwell; gorging on concentrate feed can be fatal for sheep and immediate veterinary attention is needed where gorging is suspected. The manufacturer's instructions for the pellets will give guidance on how much to feed.

Lambs should be fed at roughly the same time each day, with approximately even gaps

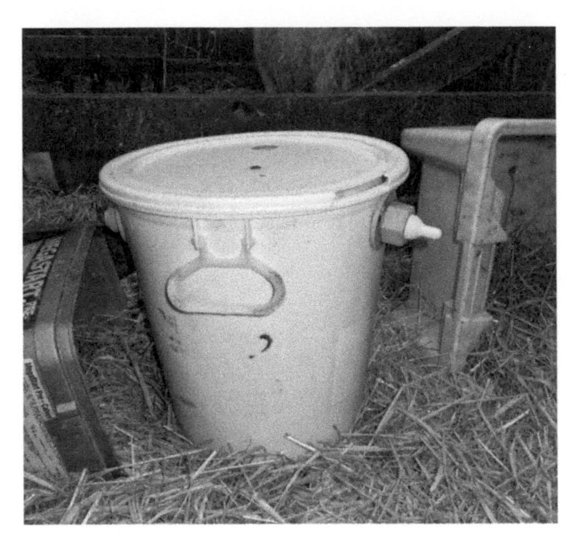

FIGURE 6.44 A milk bucket with a teat can allow lambs to take milk little and often, reducing the risk of digestive problems.

Table 6.1 An overview of pet lamb feeding until weaning.

TIME SINCE BIRTH	FEED REQUIREMENTS
Day 1	Colostrum every two to three hours; see 'The impact of colostrum' in Chapter 8.
Days 2 to 5	Warm ewe milk replacer every four hours (overnight as well).
Days 5 to 7	Gradually cool the milk replacer until they are taking it at room temperature by day 7; feed milk every six hours.
Days 8 to 14	Cold milk replacer every eight hours. Give a small amount of lamb milk pellets or starter pellets to introduce the taste.
Days 15 to weaning	Cold milk replacer every eight hours, gradually increasing in volume; with an increasing amount of lamb pellets.
Weeks 5 to 6	Wean: stop feeding milk suddenly once the lambs are over 10 kg in weight.

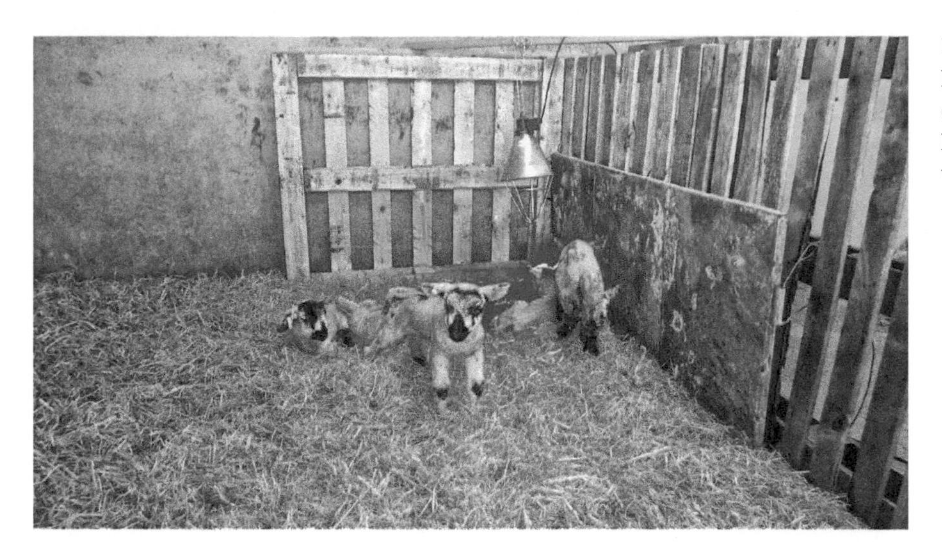

FIGURE 6.45
Pet lambs in a clean, dry pen, with a heat lamp to keep them warm.

between feeds as they learn when to expect their milk; disruption to this routine can interfere with digestion. Lambs should also have a source of fibre to chew on, either as clean straw or hay, and as always, bedding should be kept clean and dry (Fig. 6.45).

Adopting lambs

Young lambs that cannot be supported by their own mother can sometimes be 'adopted onto' another ewe that has just given birth and has only one lamb of her own. During or immediately after the ewe has given birth, the orphan is put with the ewe's own lamb and covered in the birth fluids so that they smell the same. It is best if the orphan lamb is no more than a few days old and the lambs are similar in size. Only attempt to adopt one orphan lamb onto a ewe, do not try to give her two even if she has none of her own.

If a ewe loses her only lamb, but has plenty of milk, she can sometimes be persuaded to adopt an orphan lamb. Some farmers will skin the dead lamb and use the skin to make a jacket for the new lamb, so that it smells right to the ewe. This should only be attempted by people with a lot of experience of sheep rearing as, in the case that the dead lamb was carrying infection, this could be passed on to the orphan.

When adoption is attempted, the ewe and her lamb(s) must be kept in a lambing pen and monitored carefully for the first week. Make sure that the ewe is standing to allow the lamb to suckle, and that she is not pushing the adopted lamb around, or worse still, being aggressive towards it.

If the ewe does not immediately accept a lamb, she may need to be tied up for a couple of days using a sheep halter. Tie the rope no higher than 15 cm off the ground to something secure that will not move and give the ewe just enough slack rope to access food and water, but not enough to get tangled in. A length of approximately 20 cm is usually sufficient. Food and water should be placed immediately in front of the ewe for easy and obvious access. Keep a close eye on the ewe and lamb throughout this period, checking that the ewe can reach food and water and that the lamb is suckling.

Do not attempt to adopt lambs onto ewes when the lamb is over a week old because the ewe is unlikely to accept an older lamb as her own, due to a difference in the smell and behaviour of the older lamb. If the ewe has not accepted the lamb after two days, return it to artificial milk and 'pet lamb' status.

DISEASES OF EWES AROUND LAMBING TIME

Ewes are more susceptible to disease around lambing time than at any other time of year; therefore, they must be kept well fed, with clean surroundings and monitored closely for changes of behaviour and feed consumption. The common diseases associated with lambing are described below; however, other conditions may also become more obvious during this time of increased metabolic strain, such as those described in Chapter 7.

Twin lamb disease and hypocalcaemia

Twin lamb disease and hypocalcaemia occur in the weeks leading up to lambing; and, in the case of hypocalcaemia, after lambing as well. The symptoms for these diseases are similar (see Table 6.2) and the conditions have similar predisposing factors, so they will often both affect a ewe at the same time. For this reason, it is best to always treat affected ewes for both conditions. Veterinary samples can be taken to confirm the diagnosis, allowing preventative measures to be put in place for the rest of the group.

Ewes are most at risk of twin lamb disease and hypocalcaemia if they are either excessively fat or excessively thin. In addition, anything that interferes with access to feed, or sudden changes in diet or management can precipitate these conditions.

Veterinary assessment of affected ewes is necessary to confirm the diagnosis (see 'Listeriosis' in the 'Behavioural changes' section of Chapter 7 for another similar disease seen at this time of year), but it is possible to treat suspected cases prior to veterinary diagnosis. As such, it is prudent to have the basic treatments for these diseases on the farm from a month before lambing and to give the initial doses of these treatments while waiting for the vet. These treatments can be beneficial for sick ewes, so if the vet gives a different diagnosis, they are unlikely to have been wasted or harmful. Once the vet has made the diagnosis, it is important to continue treatment for the advised length of time and to follow advice for prevention in the rest of the group.

Treatments and care that are required for animals with these conditions include:

- Propylene glycol given by mouth; first dose 120 ml, then 60 ml twice daily for 3 days
- Calcium: 60 to 80 ml injected under the skin, spread over three different sites, twice daily for 3 days
- These ewes will often need anti-inflammatory and antibiotic injections as well, speak to the vet about these
- Provide palatable feed and clean water within easy reach of the ewe
- Check these ewes twice a day for lambing; they may not show obvious signs and are unlikely to give birth without assistance
- If the ewe is not responding to treatment within 24 hours, seek more veterinary advice

Twin lamb disease can be difficult to treat; some ewes will not survive despite your best

Table 6.2 Symptoms of twin lamb disease and hypocalcaemia (milk fever).

BOTH CONDITIONS	TWIN LAMB DISEASE	HYPOCALCAEMIA
A ewe does not come to feed	Blindness	Mild bloat
Unresponsiveness	Head pressing	Green discharge from the nostrils
Weakness of legs	Seizures or fits in the late stages	
Lying down and unable to rise later in the disease (Fig. 6.46)		
Die within a few days if untreated		

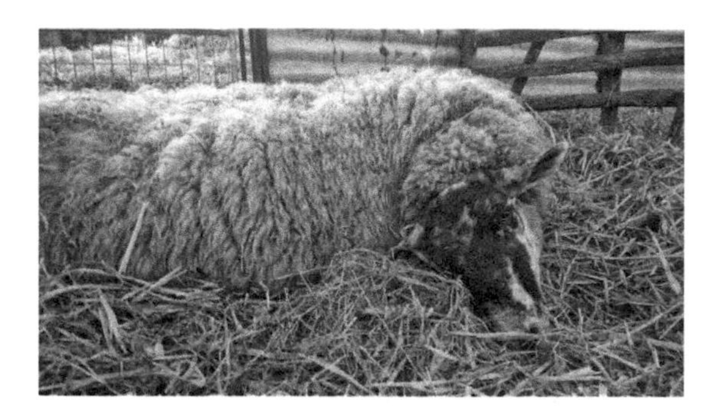

FIGURE 6.46 A depressed, sick ewe that is unable to stand up.

efforts, but starting treatment early increases the chances of survival of both the ewe and her lambs. Affected ewes are unlikely to be able to rear their lambs, therefore, although it may be beneficial to the ewe to keep her lambs close by, all their nutrition must be provided as described in the 'Pet lamb' section above.

Prevention for both these diseases includes:

- Avoidance of stressful movements and handling in late pregnancy
- Keeping ewes in good body condition, not too fat nor too thin (see 'Body condition score' Chapter 2)
- Maintaining a constant supply of feed
- Avoiding sudden dietary changes – apply changes gradually, for example, ewes that are to be lambed indoors should be fed the lambing diet (forage and concentrates) for at least a week before housing
- Provide mineral supplementation, including calcium, magnesium and phosphorus, when feed is cereal-based – seek specialist advice from a nutritionist

Vaginal prolapses

Before lambing, the pressure in a ewe's abdomen builds up, which can cause her to push before she is ready to give birth. Sometimes the vagina will be forced through the vulva, causing a pink bulge to appear under the tail (Fig. 6.47); this is a delicate structure that is easily damaged (Fig. 6.48). Prompt treatment by a person with previous training and supervised experience is necessary; a veterinary surgeon is the best person to treat these animals (Fig. 6.49).

For those who are suitably qualified, the stages of prolapse treatment are outlined below; however, if the prolapse cannot be replaced without excessive force or it re-prolapses, it is important to seek veterinary attention as soon as possible. Excessive handling of the prolapse is likely to damage it, so care must be taken at each stage.

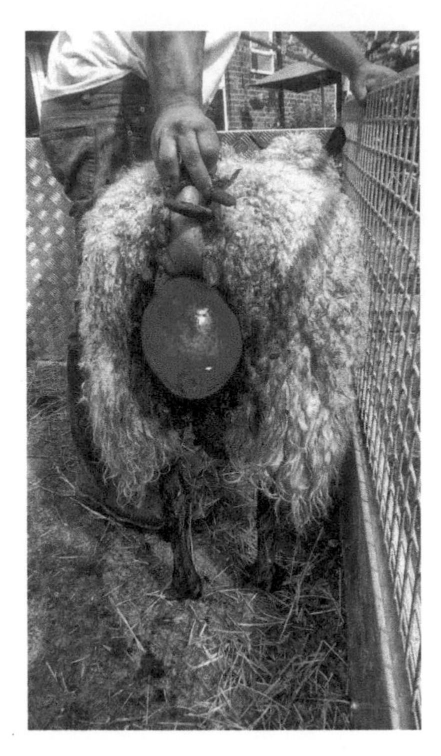

FIGURE 6.47 A ewe that has prolapsed her vagina before lambing.

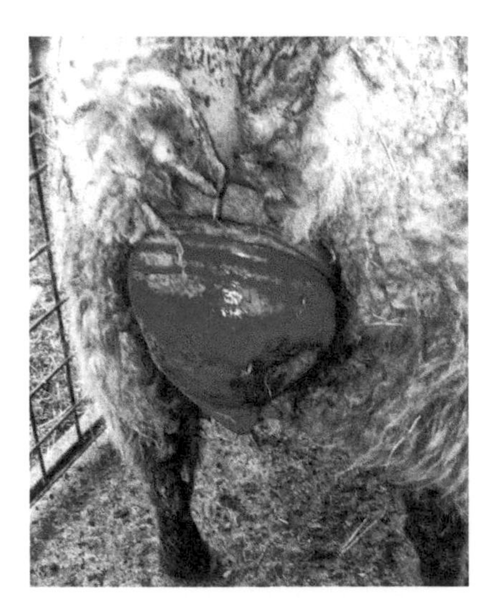

FIGURE 6.48 Vaginal/cervical prolapse with some early signs of damage.

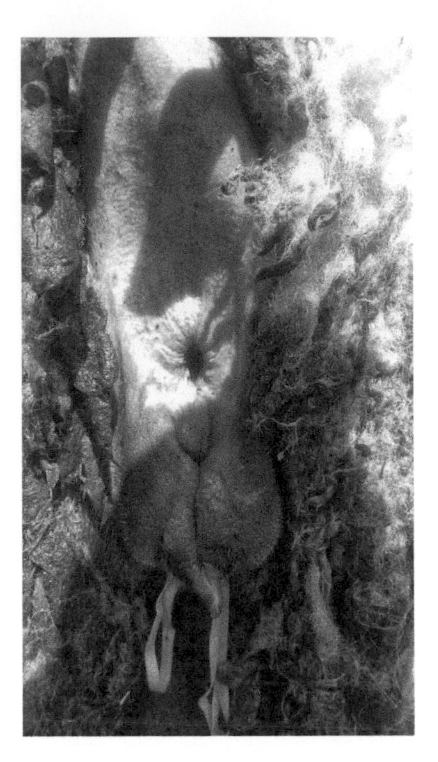

FIGURE 6.49 Vets will stitch the vulva of a prolapsing ewe, so that she can urinate but not prolapse. This stitch must be removed for the ewe to give birth.

Stages for prolapse replacement (only to be attempted with suitable training and supervised experience):

- Wash the prolapse with dilute disinfectant (Fig. 6.50)
- If any fluid or membranes come out from the cervix call the vet immediately, as the ewe is trying to lamb but will not be able to do so through the prolapse
- Apply obstetric lubricant to the prolapse
- Replace the prolapse gently with the flat parts of the hands; avoid using fingers which can puncture the tissue
- Small prolapses may stay in place, but most need to be held by a retainer; several products are available to buy for this purpose,

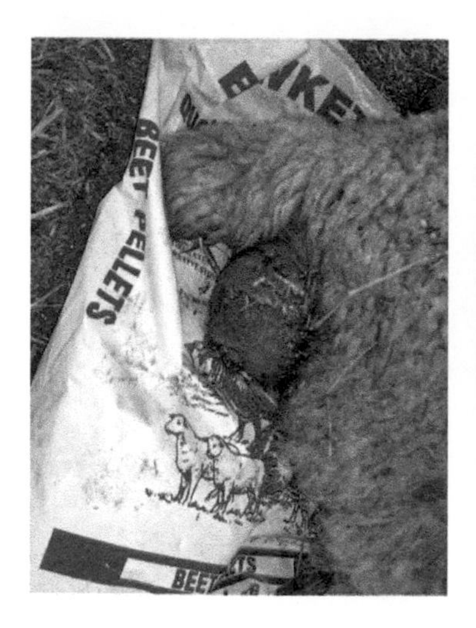

FIGURE 6.50 The dirt and straw on this prolapse needs to be gently washed off before it is put back into the ewe.

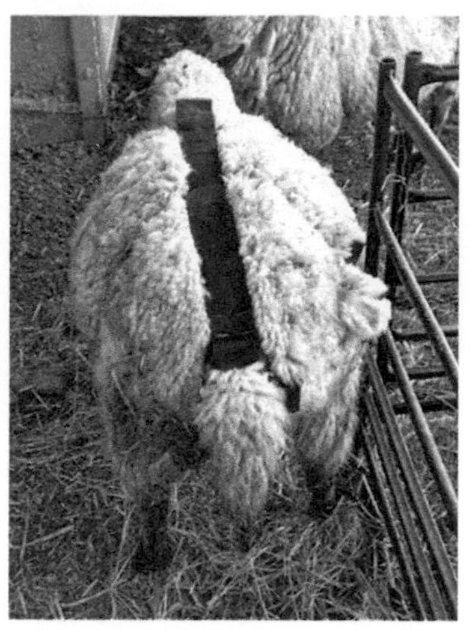

FIGURE 6.51 Well-fitted harnesses can be good for retaining vaginal prolapses.

Photograph courtesy of Miss Kerry Price.

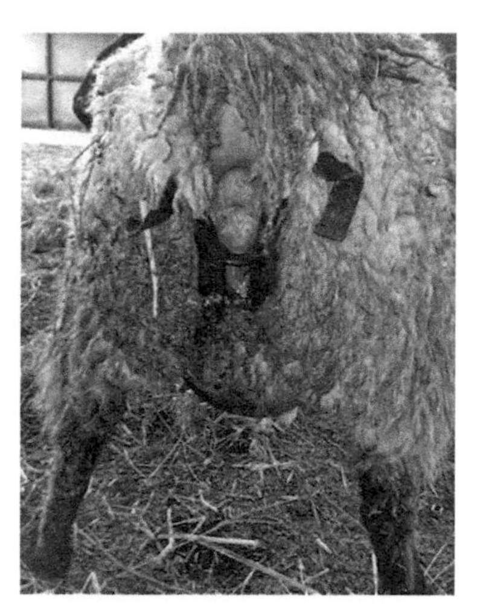

FIGURE 6.52 Harnesses have the potential to rub, so should be monitored carefully.

Photograph courtesy of Miss Kerry Price.

including harnesses (Fig. 6.51) and 'spoons'. These devices must be used according to the manufacturer's instructions and closely monitored, for example harnesses can rub the skin and make a ewe uncomfortable (Fig. 6.52)

- Give long-acting antibiotic and anti-inflammatory injections, according to veterinary advice
- Keep the ewe where she can be monitored closely
- As soon as the ewe shows signs of lambing, the prolapse retainer must be removed
- If the ewe prolapses while lambing, or is having any other difficulties, call the vet immediately

Ewes are more likely to suffer from vaginal prolapses if they are excessively thin or fat, carrying multiple lambs or kept on moderately to steeply sloping fields. Some breeds and some individual sheep are more prone to this condition. Therefore, prevention of the condition involves careful feeding and monitoring of ewe body condition during pregnancy; and not breeding from ewes that have prolapsed in the past or their daughters.

Hypomagnesaemia ('staggers')

Lactating ewes are at most risk of 'staggers', a disease which, as its name suggests, causes the ewe to stagger and become twitchy. However, affected ewes are often found lying on the ground fitting or already dead. This condition is due to insufficient daily magnesium consumption, particularly when sheep are eating fast-growing, lush, fertilised grass in spring and producing milk for their lambs.

If this is a known problem in your flock, prevention can include providing hay for ewes on lush spring pasture or magnesium supplements

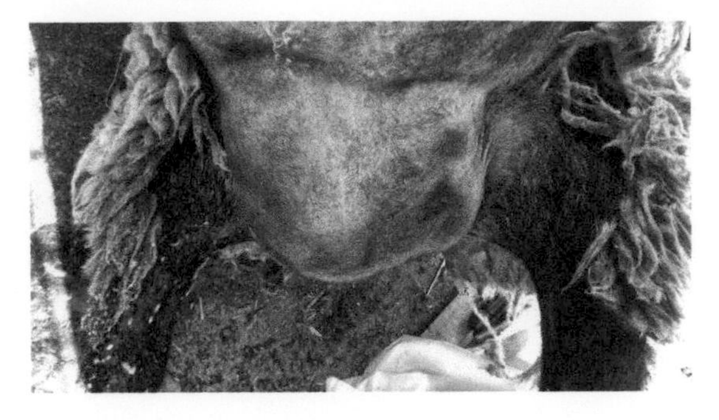

FIGURE 6.53 An enlarged mammary gland in a ewe with mastitis.

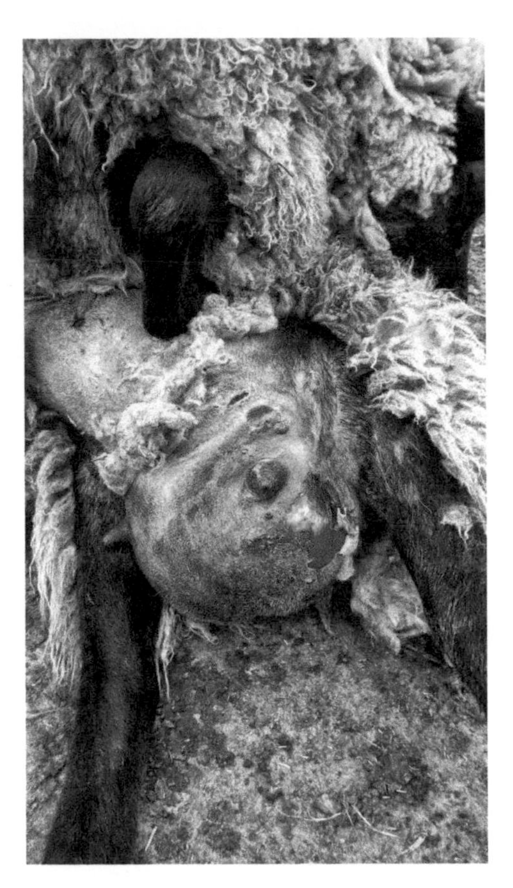

FIGURE 6.54 An enlarged, erupting udder in a ewe with severe mastitis.

added to drinking water, in 'licks' or as a powder. Some people also think that rock salt supplements are useful.

Mastitis

Mastitis is an infection of the mammary gland or udder, which results in very painful swelling and hardening of one (Figs 6.53, 6.54) or both glands. Mastitis in ewes has been linked to the following predisposing factors:

- Poor milk production, which may be due to a low-protein diet during late pregnancy and early lactation
- Cold winds
- Orf infection
- Flies
- Dirty surroundings
- High milk production without suckling lambs
- An asymmetrical udder
- Lumps in the udder
- Watery, lumpy or discoloured milk, with or without a pungent smell

Early signs of mastitis can include:

- Hungry, discontented lambs
- A ewe refusing to let her lambs suckle
- Hind limb lameness or stiffness
- Depression
- A ewe that is not eating
- An udder that is either hot or cold; painful; hard; and red, purple and/or black

Mastitis normally prevents an affected gland from ever producing milk again, therefore a ewe that has mastitis in one side of her udder is only likely to be able to raise one lamb in the future. However, a ewe that has been affected in both glands will not be able to produce milk for any lambs, so should not be bred from again. Some udders may slough off and these ewes need a lot of care, including fly prevention treatments to stop the flies from spreading infection to exposed flesh and laying their eggs in the udder.

The local sheep vet will be able to advise you about treatment for simple mastitis cases, however cases that are unresponsive to treatment, or ewes that appear particularly unwell with mastitis, should be examined by a veterinary surgeon. General good practices for mastitis treatment include:

- Cleaning the affected teat and milking out as much of the milk as possible
- Anti-inflammatory and antibiotic treatment, according to your vet's advice
- Feeding the lamb(s) if the ewe is no longer producing enough milk to do so (it can be difficult to persuade older lambs to drink from a false teat; these lambs will need lamb starter or milk pellets)
- If the ewe does not improve within 24 hours seek further veterinary advice

Mastitis prevention includes feeding ewes sufficient levels of quality protein, providing shelter from prevailing winds, fly control and good environmental hygiene.

Uterine prolapses

After lambing, occasionally a ewe might push all of her uterus or womb out through her vulva (Fig. 6.55); this is red with a knobbly surface (these knobbles are normal). If this is observed in a ewe, the vet should be called immediately.

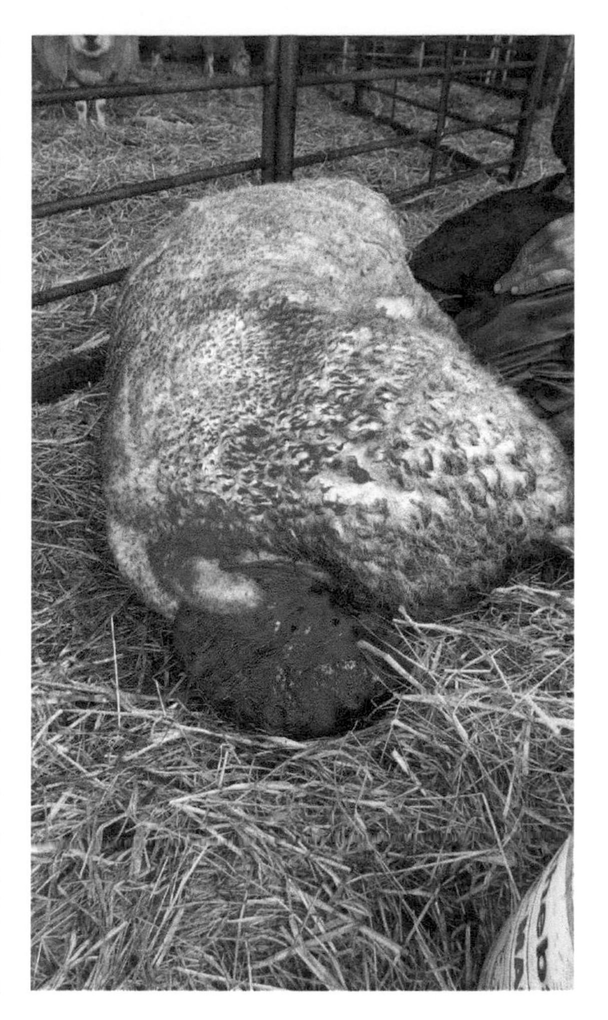

FIGURE 6.55 A ewe that has pushed her uterus out after giving birth.

Metritis

A ewe's womb can become infected during the days after lambing and these ewes become depressed, anorexic and unresponsive, with an unpleasant vaginal discharge; they must be seen by a vet promptly. This is known as metritis. In addition, any unwell ewe should be examined by a vet at lambing time, as during the strain of late pregnancy and lambing, it is possible for other, less serious diseases to become worse.

LAMB DISEASES AND TREATMENTS

Weak/hypothermic lambs

Lambs are small and if they do not get enough milk, are susceptible to the cold, particularly in wet conditions. Therefore, smaller, weaker lambs are more prone to hypothermia, which will normally result from a combination of cold conditions and starvation. Always check the mother of hypothermic lambs to make sure that she does not have mastitis, has enough milk and is allowing the lamb(s) to suckle. Hypothermic or starved lambs are unresponsive, stand with their heads drooped, take no interest in their surroundings and have a hollow stomach. Work through Figure 6.56 when deciding what these lambs need. Glucose is not needed for lambs under 5 hours old because of the fat reserves that they are born with, called 'brown fat'. Lambs that are in a warming box should be checked every 30 minutes at least and should be fed after the first 30 minutes of warming.

Injecting glucose (Fig. 6.57) into the abdomen of a hypothermic, starving lamb, provides life-saving energy without the lamb having to digest milk. If the decision-making tree in Figure 6.57 suggests that a glucose injection is needed, follow the instructions below:

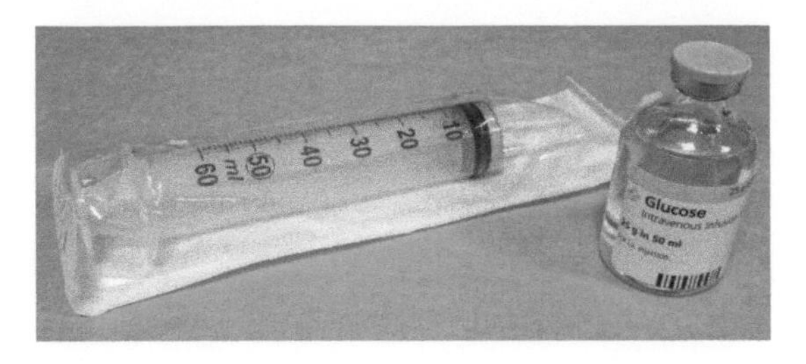

FIGURE 6.57 Glucose should be mixed with boiling water, so that by the time it reaches the lamb it is at body temperature.

- Use a *new* needle (19 gauge, 1 inch) and *new* syringe (50 ml)
- Mix together:
  - 4 ml/kg of 50% glucose (20 ml for an average 5 kg lamb)
  - 6 ml/kg boiling water (30 ml in 5 kg lamb)
- Hold the lamb by the front legs
- Spray a spot of oxytetracycline spray 2 cm (1 inch) below and 1 cm (½ inch) to the side of the navel

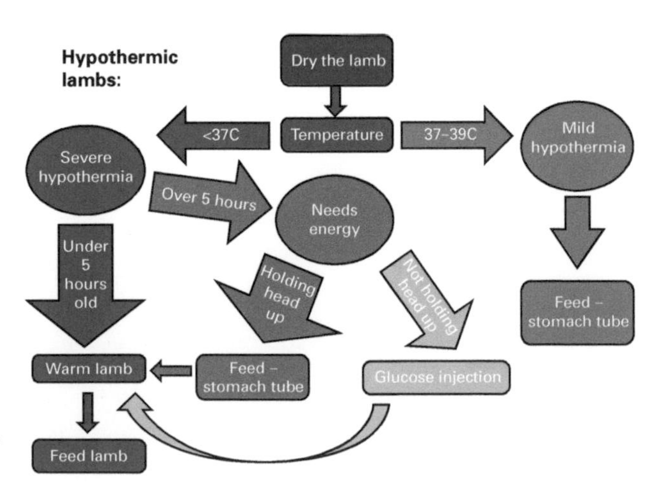

FIGURE 6.56 Decision tree for hypothermic, starving lambs.

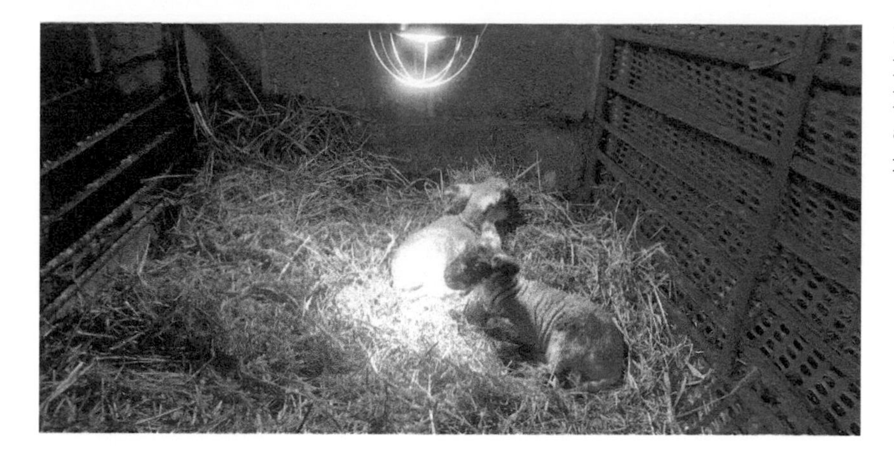

FIGURE 6.58 Lambs being warmed under a heat lamp, looking bright and alert, indicating recovery.

- Insert the needle here, directing it towards the top of the tail
- Inject the solution slowly

If a lamb still appears to be unwell once it is warm (Fig. 6.58) and fed, have it examined by a vet.

Watery mouth

Watery mouth disease is an infection of the stomach in lambs that are typically 1 to 3 days old and causes depression and weakness. Affected lambs usually have cold mouths and drool excessively; in severe cases, their stomachs are enlarged with gas and fluid, which has spawned the name 'rattle-belly'. This empty belly can, at first glance, replicate the look of a full stomach of milk, but is in fact an enlarged abdomen. If there is any doubt as to the condition of the lamb, it should be examined by a vet.

Lambs that do not get enough quality colostrum within the first few hours of life are at greatest risk of watery mouth. The incidence of cases often increases towards the end of lambing as infection builds up in lambing sheds. All lambs in pens should have the temperature and wetness of their mouths checked at least once a day, for example in the evening as part of the final daily check.

Watery mouth is difficult to treat unless it is detected early. Treatment includes:

- Warm rehydration fluids (see 'Fluids' in Chapter 7); give 50 ml twice, three hours apart by stomach tube
- Leave the lamb with the ewe, if possible with a safe heat source
- Antibiotics and anti-inflammatories as prescribed by your veterinary surgeon
- If the lamb is not suckling after six hours, give 50 ml per kg of milk from the ewe, by stomach tube or bottle

If a lamb is deteriorating despite treatment, the kindest course of action is to have the lamb euthanased to prevent unnecessary suffering.

Good colostrum is the best preventative for watery mouth. This requires ewes to be fed sufficient quality protein during pregnancy and lambs to receive at least 50 ml/kg of colostrum within the first two hours of life. Clean, dry surroundings for newborn lambs also help. If more than one case is seen within one week, the lambing shed should be cleaned out or lambing ewes moved onto clean fields and veterinary advice should be sought.

Atresia ani

Lambs are sometimes born without an opening at their anus (Fig. 6.59), this prevents them from passing any faeces and is eventually fatal. Check that every lamb is passing faeces in the first few days of life. Affected lambs will appear normal, suckling and behaving like any other lamb; but after a few days their stomachs get very large and eventually they become depressed and anorexic.

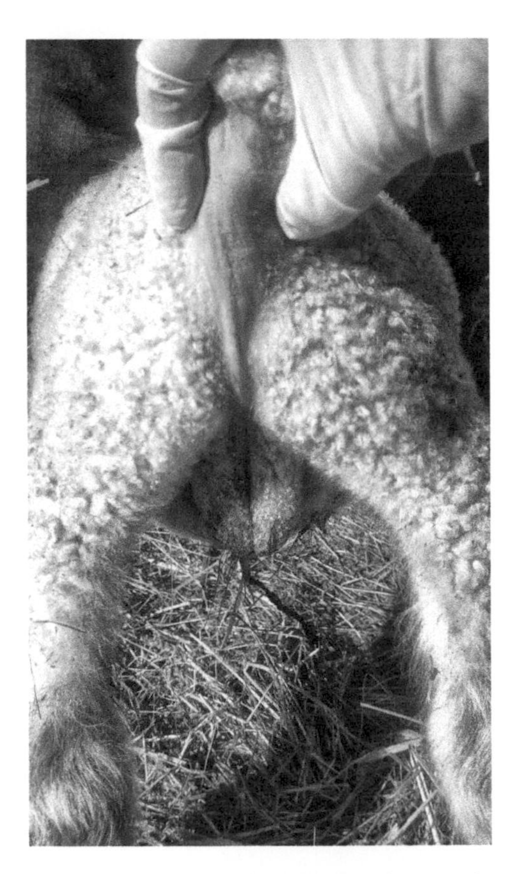

FIGURE 6.59 A newborn lamb with no anal opening to allow faeces to be passed needs veterinary attention as soon as possible. Some can be corrected surgically, others cannot.

Diarrhoea

Diarrhoea in young lambs has a variety of causes, including sudden changes of diet, poor nutrition and infectious diseases. However, the most important consideration when a lamb has diarrhoea is that they are very susceptible to dehydration. If a lamb has diarrhoea, it will excrete watery faeces that either form a steady stream or dribble down the lamb's hind legs. Colour can vary from yellow to brown, green or even bloodstained red.

Young lambs often have paste-like faeces, especially if they are receiving a good milk supply; but if faeces become runny, the lambs need to be monitored for other signs of disease; watery faeces need immediate action.

The mainstay of treatment for diarrhoea is oral rehydration fluids; lambs should be given at least 50 ml per kg at a time by stomach tube, see 'Fluids' in Chapter 7. If the lamb is not suckling milk from its mother, alternate fluid and milk feeds, with up to one feed every two hours. If a lamb is dull, has blood in the diarrhoea or is not improving within 24 hours, seek veterinary attention. When several lambs are affected, seek veterinary help to find out the cause of the outbreak.

Prevention of diarrhoea is similar to watery mouth, including good colostrum and hygiene management.

Lamb dysentery

If pregnant ewes are not vaccinated for clostridial diseases, or their lambs do not receive enough colostrum, lamb dysentery can cause many lambs to die. This disease causes severe stomach pain, with or without bloody diarrhoea, and affected lambs die very quickly. Treatment is rarely successful and the disease is very painful; so, these lambs should be seen by a vet to confirm the diagnosis and euthanased immediately.

Navel ill

Navel ill is an infection of the umbilicus in which the navel is slightly enlarged, warm and painful, and the lamb becomes depressed. Prompt antibiotic treatment is required, according to veterinary recommendations. Navel disinfection at birth is the best prevention for this condition, as described in Chapter 8 'Does navel treatment matter?'.

Joint ill

Joint ill occurs after infection gets into a lamb's bloodstream from the navel, mouth or a wound. The infection then settles out in the lamb's joints. Lambs are more likely to suffer from this condition when navel treatment is ineffective or late, colostrum is insufficient, wounds are common or surroundings are dirty. Lambs normally show signs of joint ill at 2 to 3 weeks of age; walking stiffly, lying down a lot, struggling to keep up with other lambs or their mother – so they are often hungry and hollow. The joints are normally, but not always, enlarged and warm to the touch.

Treatment of joint ill requires anti-inflammatory and antibiotic therapy, according to the local sheep vet's advice. Many lambs will relapse if the course of antibiotics is too short; therefore, keep affected lambs in a small paddock or pen with the rest of their family unit, so that they are easy to catch for repeated treatments when they start to feel better. Most lambs need seven to ten days of treatment for a complete cure.

Severe joint ill in multiple joints can be associated with tick pyaemia, which is caused by tick-borne fever, a bacterium that is transmitted by ticks. This infection results in poor immunity in the lamb, allowing other infections to run rampant and severe joint ill is one of the potential outcomes. Seek veterinary attention for affected lambs as this is a difficult condition to treat.

Joint ill prevention is similar to the other bacterial diseases discussed above; including good colostrum, navel treatment and hygiene. Occasionally, outbreaks of joint ill are encountered in spite of these precautions. Where this occurs, new cases can be reduced by disinfecting navels a second time, four hours after birth.

Entropion

An abnormality in the eyelids of some newborn lambs causes them to turn inwards so that the hair on the eyelids meets and rubs against the surface of the eye (Fig. 6.60). This causes pain and ulceration of the cornea (the outer surface of the eye). In extreme cases, the scarring can cause permanent blindness. This is thought to be an inherited condition that can be passed down to lambs through the ewe, ram or both. Affected lambs are normally only a few days old, they hold their eyes partially closed (Fig. 6.61) and tear staining (Fig. 6.62) can be seen below the eye(s). In one lamb, each eye could be affected in the upper, lower or both eyelids.

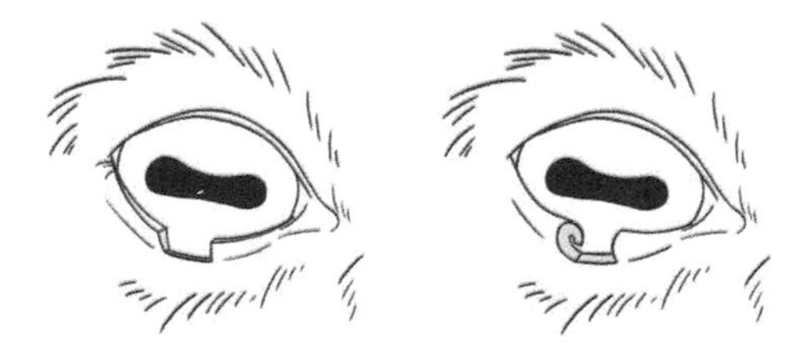

FIGURE 6.60 In lambs with entropion, the eyelids are turned in, with hair and eyelashes rubbing against the eye.

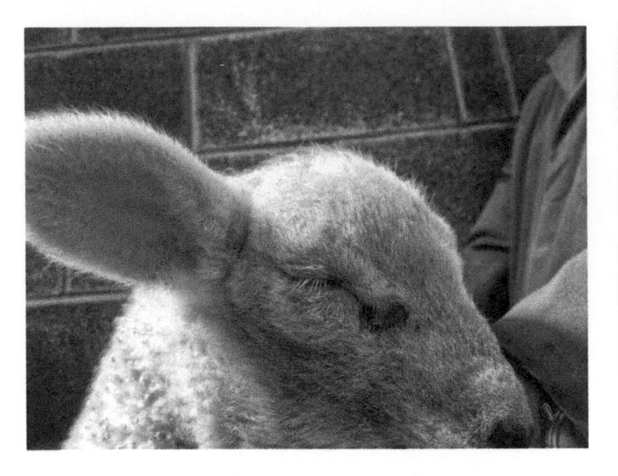

FIGURE 6.61 A lamb with entropion holding its eye closed due to the discomfort.

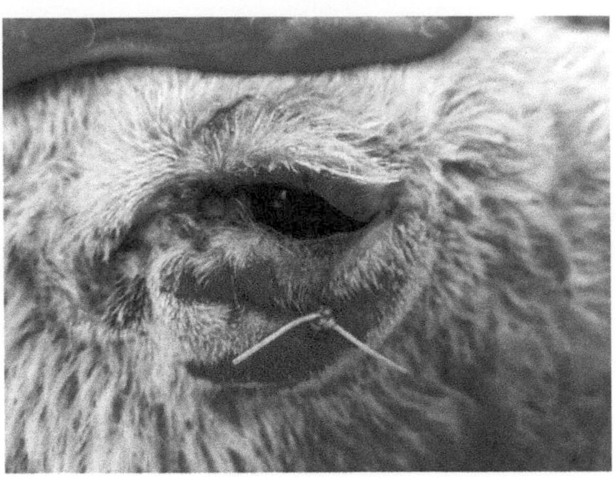

FIGURE 6.63 Corrective sutures can be put into the eyelids of affected lambs by a veterinary surgeon.

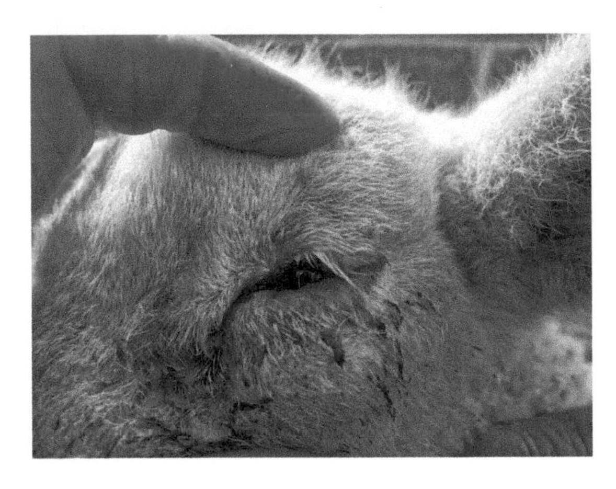

FIGURE 6.62 The lower turned-in eyelid of a lamb with tear staining below the eye.

If there are changes to the surface of the eye, affected lambs should be examined by a vet. Otherwise, correct the position of the eyelid by gently placing a finger on the eyelid and moving it in the direction that would open the eye, that is, upwards for the top eyelid and downwards for the bottom eyelid. Once this has been done, monitor the eyelid(s):

- If they stay in the correct position for several hours, continue to correct their position several times a day, until they remain in the correct position permanently
- If the eyelids do not stay in the correct position for long, seek veterinary attention

Among other methods, sutures (Fig. 6.63) or clips can be used to hold eyelids in the correct position; these must be monitored closely in case they come into contact with the eye; if this looks likely, a vet should be asked to check them. Metal clips that are in contact with the eye should be removed immediately before taking the lamb to see the vet.

Nephrosis

Occasionally, lambs develop 'drunken lamb syndrome' or nephrosis, which often follows an episode of diarrhoea. Affected lambs are usually between 7 days and a month old; they have a staggering walk, are often drowsy and are reluctant to suckle. Without treatment they normally die within 48 hours.

Once the diagnosis has been confirmed by a vet, the most effective treatment is 4 g of sodium bicarbonate, or bicarbonate of soda, in 50 ml of lukewarm water, given by mouth or stomach tube. Your local vet may also recommend that these lambs be given antibiotics.

Septicaemia

Infections from the guts, navel or wound, that spread into the bloodstream can become generalised, affecting multiple organs. In these cases, lambs become very depressed and refuse to suckle. These lambs need immediate veterinary attention, but may not survive. See the section on 'Joint ill' above for details of predisposing factors and prevention.

Meningitis

Infections that get into a lamb's bloodstream can also spread to the brain and cause meningitis. Meningitis results in stupor, anorexia and eventually seizures. Affected lambs often die within a short time. Details of risk factors can be found above in the 'Joint ill' section. These lambs require immediate veterinary attention.

Hairy shakers

Unborn lambs in ewes that are infected by border disease virus during pregnancy, will end up in one of the following categories:

- Unaffected and go on to live normal lives
- Born with the virus and spread it throughout their lives; these lambs may not grow as well as the rest, or they may appear perfectly normal
- Some will be reabsorbed or aborted and the ewe will have no lambs that year
- 'Hairy shakers' – these lambs have a 'hairy' coat, which is longer than normal and less wool-like; they also have a slight tremor, especially when they are active. Some of these lambs will learn to cope with the condition, but will never fully recover
- Other deformities can also occur

Vets can test for border disease virus, but if it is found in a flock, what is done depends on the flock's size and purpose. Options should be discussed with your vet to work out the best plan for your situation.

Cow colostrum-related anaemia

If cow's colostrum is fed to lambs, it can occasionally cause anaemia in those lambs. This can be prevented by pooling colostrum from several cows or testing the colostrum from one cow before it is used. Cow colostrum is extremely beneficial for lambs that do not receive adequate ewe colostrum, but speak to your vet before using it. Affected lambs will stop suckling, become lethargic, weak, eat unusual things, drink water, breath rapidly and will have white or yellow gums.

Lambs with weak or paralysed legs

Weakness or paralysis make it difficult for an animal to stand on and move the affected legs; they may drag these limbs along the ground. The back legs are more likely to be affected than the front legs. Affected animals must be examined by a veterinary surgeon, as the causes are difficult to distinguish from each other. See 'Leg weakness and paralysis' in the 'Behavioural changes' section of Chapter 7 for details of the common causes.

Congenital abnormalities

Variations during embryo development can cause defects in a lamb before it is born; some of these foetuses will not survive the pregnancy and are reabsorbed or aborted. Others will be born alive, but with deformities that are not compatible with a good quality of life – these lambs often need to be born by caesarean section and require immediate euthanasia.

Some deformed lambs can survive and have a good quality of life, provided that it is easy for them to eat, drink and move around without help; they also should be free from discomfort – a vet can help with this decision. If any of these factors should change, the vet must be re-consulted and if the animal is suffering, euthanasia must be considered. Be aware, and make any associated children aware, that these lambs may not live as long as other sheep. Breeding from them is not recommended.

Exposure to certain infections or treatments during pregnancy can cause lamb deformities and if unsure, sheep keepers should seek veterinary advice on specific treatments before using them in pregnant ewes.

7

SICK SHEEP

This chapter will only deal with the most common diseases that are seen in sheep in the UK. The remit of this section is to provide a basic understanding of common diseases in sheep so that sheep keepers are able to recognise when veterinary attention is needed and are also able to take preventative measures for some of these diseases.

HOW TO SPOT SICK SHEEP

Sheep are prey animals so they will often hide signs of disease or pain and because of this it can be difficult to spot sheep that are unwell. Some of the subtle signs to look out for include:

- Drooping ears (the normal ear position is breed-specific, so this indicator is drooping relative to normal)
- Standing or lying away from the rest of the group (Fig. 7.1)
- Not eating – adult sheep spend most of their waking life eating or 'chewing the cud'
- Unresponsiveness or being slow to respond
- Lounging uncomfortably with the eyes half open, rather than asleep
- Healthy sheep often stretch as they stand up after lying down; animals in pain may not do this

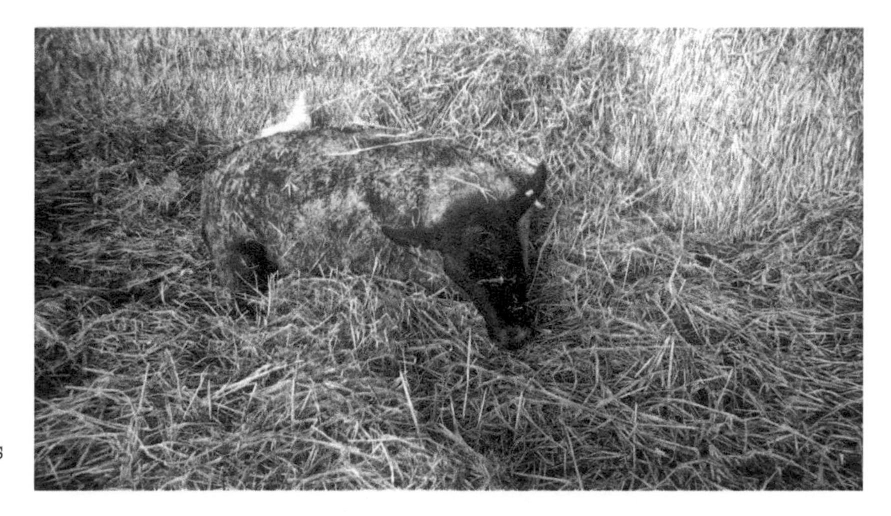

FIGURE 7.1 A sick ewe lying on her own, she is unresponsive and appears depressed.

- Avoiding using the painful part of their body, for example:
  - Limbs – lameness
  - Jaw or teeth – struggle to eat
  - Udder – will not allow lambs to suckle
- Vocalising – sheep will only vocalise when they are in extreme distress, therefore it should not be assumed that a silent sheep is not in pain

WHEN TO CALL THE VET

Once it is established that a sheep is sick, it is important to understand when to call out the vet. If there is any doubt at all, the vet should be called. If a visit is not necessary, vets are normally willing to offer advice over the telephone. The following are examples of when a vet should be called, but these are not exclusive and it is important to exercise judgement with ill sheep, as the owner will know the flock best:

- For listless, unresponsive animals
- For sheep that are not eating
- If an animal, or group of animals is known to have gorged on grain or concentrate feed
- When a lambing is not progressing as expected (see 'Calling out the vet' in Chapter 6)
- For ewes after lambing that are depressed or have a smelly discharge from their vulva
- For lame sheep with no visible lesion or a lesion that is unknown (see 'Lameness' below)
- When a treatment is not working as expected and the animal is:
  - Deteriorating in any way, for example stops eating, can no longer stand, is breathing more rapidly, and so on
  - Not improving in the expected time frame (if the timescale for expected improvement is unknown then the vet should be called early for advice)
- Any animal that is having a seizure or fit (around lambing time give fitting ewes an injection of magnesium under the skin while waiting for the vet to arrive)
- Blowfly strike
- Wounds that are more than skin deep – look at wounds carefully to work out how big and deep they are – they can be hard to assess in sheep due to the wool
- Abnormal behaviours

Please be aware that this list is only intended for guidance and the vet should be called if there are any concerns about the health or welfare of your animals.

TREATMENTS

Strict legislation governs the use of veterinary medicines, especially in animal species that are traditionally used for food in the UK. There is a legal obligation to adhere to these regulations regardless of the intended end-point for the sheep. The main requirements are:

- Only medicines that are licensed in food producing animals should be used – the local vet will have access to the list of these medicines
- Records must be kept of details for all veterinary medicines used in farm animals
- The relevant 'withdrawal period' (measured in hours or days) must be allowed to pass after treatment, before milk can be taken from an animal for human consumption, or

it can be slaughtered for human consumption – the local vet will be able to advise of these time frames

Details of the records to be kept for farm animal treatments are stipulated in the Veterinary Medicines Regulations. Pre-prepared medicine record books or computer templates are available to help with this essential recording.

At the time of writing, there is no legal requirement to record the reason for giving treatment to an animal. But if this is recorded, it can be useful information to review with your vet, as it highlights the dominant diseases in a flock (this is an example of best practice because experience dictates that it is difficult to remember this information without writing it down at the time).

Injection technique

Injections are relatively easy to master, however, it is also easy to do them badly and as such they can be potentially damaging to an animal. Therefore, it is important to ask someone with significant experience to supervise the first few injections given to ensure that the correct technique is used with minimal impact on the animal. Ideal people to supervise the first round of injections that someone gives are veterinary surgeons and qualified veterinary nurses. If there are any doubts or if an owner is not confident with injections, then help should be sought without hesitation. Some people never become comfortable with giving injections and this is perfectly acceptable; if this is the case, find somebody confident with injecting sheep who is willing to assist.

When giving injections it is essential to:

- Check how it should be administered – either into the muscle or under the skin (any injections for intravenous use should be given by a local vet)
- Check that the medicine is thoroughly mixed – if it has separated check with the vet that this is normal for the medicine in question; if so, shake thoroughly to mix it
- Make sure the site for injection is clean
- Use a clean, sharp needle: 18 or 19 gauge and 1 inch in length
- Use a clean syringe; if you want to re-use a syringe ensure that it has only been used for the same medicine as the current injection, looks clean and was first used within the preceding few days

Injections under the skin

- These can be given anywhere that loose skin can be found, including the side of the neck or the side of the chest behind the front leg (Fig. 7.2)
- Pull the skin out slightly and direct the needle into the side of the 'tent' that has been created, avoiding any muscle or bone lying underneath
- Without moving the needle, pull the plunger on the syringe back a little to check that no air or blood comes into the syringe:

    - If air comes into the syringe, the needle tip has come out of the skin at the far side of the 'tent', so the needle must be pulled back slightly and then rechecked by withdrawing the plunger
    - If blood comes into the syringe, take the needle out of the skin, move to a slightly different site and start again. There is no need to change the syringe, needle or injection if this happens

- Inject the medicine, being careful to:
    - Not move the needle while making the injection
    - Not push so hard that the needle comes off the syringe – check that it is securely attached before starting. If the needle does come off then it is necessary to replenish the syringe with the amount of medicine lost and start again
    - Check that the injection is not running down the side of the sheep – if this does happen, fully replenish the syringe and start again

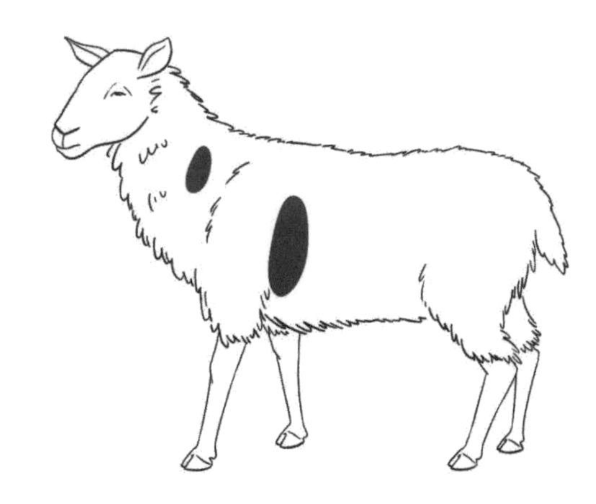

FIGURE 7.2 The areas highlighted in blue are good sites for injections given under the skin.

Picture courtesy of Miss Amanda Aiken.

Injections into the muscle

- These can be given into the:
    - Neck – two thirds of the way from the head towards the shoulder (closer to the shoulder) and two thirds of the way up the neck (furthest from the feet)
    - Rump – feel for a good area of muscle, away from any bones (Fig. 7.3)
- Do not push the needle in too deep, it must stay within the muscle and not touch bone. The depth of muscle will depend on the size and body condition of the sheep being injected. Use 1-inch-long needles, inserting half to three-quarters of the length into the muscle in adults, but only a quarter in lambs
- If the needle hits something hard it is likely to be bone, so withdraw the needle a little
- Without moving the needle, pull the plunger of the syringe back a little to check that no blood comes into the syringe, if it does, withdraw or redirect the needle slightly and re-check

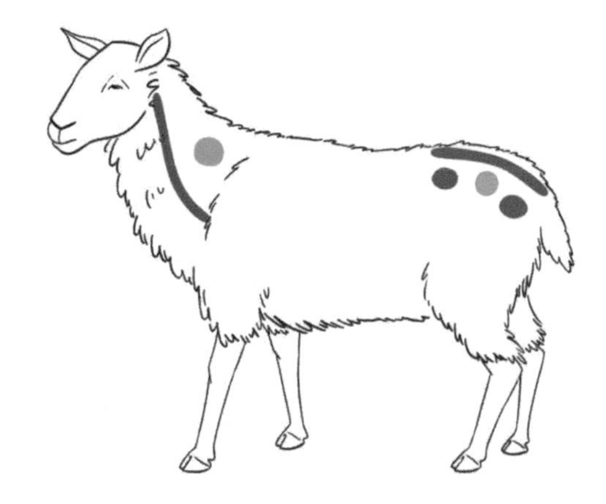

FIGURE 7.3 The areas highlighted in green are good sites for giving injections into the muscle; care must be taken to avoid the red areas, which overlie bone. Some of these bones can be felt through the skin.

Picture courtesy of Miss Amanda Aiken.

- Inject the medicine, being careful *not* to:
    - Move the needle while injecting
    - Push so hard that the needle comes off the syringe – check that it is securely attached before starting. If the needle

does come off, replenish the syringe with the amount of medicine lost and start again

- Rub the injection site firmly with a clean hand to stop the injection from coming back through the needle hole

Using anti-inflammatory drugs

Anti-inflammatories provide good pain relief and they can also reduce tissue damage and swelling, for example in respiratory infections and after difficult lambings. However, care must be taken when using these treatments as excessive or repeated doses can damage the digestive tract and kidneys, especially in young or dehydrated animals. Therefore, always be conservative when working out the dose of anti-inflammatory treatments.

No anti-inflammatory treatments are licensed for use in sheep at the time of writing, therefore they must always be used under the guidance of a veterinary surgeon.

Anti-inflammatories are useful for the following conditions:

- Ewes with
  - Difficult lambings
  - Mastitis
  - Prolapses
  - Twin lamb disease
- Lameness – all painful lesions
- Blowfly strike
- Raised body temperature
- Respiratory diseases
- Injuries

DO NOT OVERDOSE ANTI-INFLAMMATORIES!

Using antibiotics

Antibiotic resistance is becoming a serious problem in veterinary and human medicine, therefore these drugs should be used with care and under the guidance of your local vet.

Antibiotics are necessary to maintain good animal welfare by prompt treatment of disease. Below is a guide to their use that will help to minimise the development of resistance.

- Only use antibiotics when necessary – discuss each case or new outbreak of disease with your vet
- Prevent disease by using vaccines, good hygiene, removing hazardous objects that may cause injury, good colostrum management, good navel treatment, and so on
- Give the right dose for the weight of the animal, avoid under-dosing:
  - It is best to weigh an animal, calculate the correct dose of antibiotic and add 1–2% to ensure that the animal is not under-dosed
  - If weigh scales are not available, look up average breed weights for your sheep or ask a vet who has seen the sheep recently for an estimated weight. Calculate the dose of antibiotic and add 5–10% to account for the estimated weight
- Give a long enough course of the antibiotic. Either:
  - Give a long acting preparation, and if the animal has improved but is not completely better, repeat it after the correct number of days; or

- Give a daily antibiotic every day for a minimum of three days; continue treatment until at least two days after the problem has resolved

- If the problem is not improving within three to five days, call the local vet to reassess the animal
- Use the right antibiotic – consult the local sheep vet for your particular situation

DO NOT UNDERDOSE ANTIBIOTICS!

Fluids

Water is obviously essential to the survival of all mammals. Sheep should have a constant supply of clean, fresh water and if for any reason a sheep cannot move to attain water, some should be placed within immediate access of that animal. Fluids are also useful in diseased animals, to maintain hydration when excessive liquid is lost, for example through diarrhoea, and to maintain good circulation in cases of septicaemia (generalised infection) and shock.

How to give fluids

Sheep that need supplementary fluids, but are not collapsed, can be given these fluids by mouth. This is known as drenching. Collapsed sheep need to be seen by a vet and may require intravenous fluid therapy. A syringe or dosing gun can be used to drench sheep over a couple of weeks old and a stomach tube can be used for young lambs (see 'Stomach tubing a lamb' in Chapter 6). When drenching sheep with fluids by mouth, it is vital that it is done carefully and slowly, allowing the sheep to swallow small amounts of the rehydration solution at a time. The sheep's head should be held securely at a 45-degree angle, with the nose pointing upwards, the syringe in line with the sheep's head and directed towards the back of the tongue. If there is any doubt about this technique, or about whether a sheep requires fluids, do not give the drench but seek veterinary support.

It is important that drenching is done accurately because an erroneous technique may result in fluid going into the lungs, which can cause serious complications.

When to give fluids

Animals need additional fluids when:

- Sheep are too unwell to access water; these animals need veterinary attention, such as ewes with listeriosis, twin lamb disease, severe toxic mastitis or womb infection (see Chapters 6 and 7 for details)
- Lambs are suffering from severe watery diarrhoea:

  - If the lamb cannot stand or is dull and depressed, seek immediate veterinary assistance
  - If the animal can stand, fluids can be given by mouth – use warm water with rehydration salts or powder. Give 50 ml per kg of the lamb's body weight at a time, several times a day, alternating with milk feeds. If there are any concerns have the animal seen by the local vet

- Fluids have been inaccessible for a prolonged period:

  - For newborn lambs this can be a matter of hours without access to milk

- For adult sheep it could be as little as 24 hours in dry conditions
- Fluids should be reintroduced gradually, with small amounts (0.5% of the animal's body weight) given hourly
- If the animal will not drink, seek veterinary help immediately

What should be in rehydration fluids

Fluids given by mouth need to contain salt and sugars to help the sheep's body to retain the additional fluid and provide energy. Pre-prepared rehydration powders or tablets contain these at the correct concentrations and the manufacturer's instructions should be followed when preparing and using them. Homemade rehydration solutions can be used in an emergency; to make one of these add half a teaspoon of salt per litre of warm water for adult sheep; and for lambs under 3 weeks old add half a teaspoon of salt, six teaspoons of sugar and one teaspoon of bicarbonate of soda (baking powder) per litre. Ensure that these are thoroughly dissolved before the solution is given.

LAMENESS

Sheep have soft, tender feet, so great care must be taken when handling them. Anything that causes lameness will reduce feed intake, lamb growth rates, and the fertility and milk production of adults, as well as impairing the welfare of the animal. Therefore, prevention and prompt appropriate treatment of lameness are essential.

How to spot a lame sheep

Lameness is an indication of pain and discomfort, therefore most lame animals will have some level of pain in the affected leg. The speed with which a lame sheep must be attended will depend on the severity of the lameness, that is, the level of pain it is experiencing. Remember that sheep are prey animals by nature and they do not show pain in the obvious ways that might be expected. For instance, when in pain, sheep rarely vocalise, so other symptoms must be sought. Some of these are listed below.

- Walking:

  - A mildly lame sheep might walk oddly or seem uncomfortable when walking
  - A moderately lame sheep will obviously nod its head while walking and it may be possible to spot which leg it is trying to avoid walking on
  - A severely lame sheep will hold the lame leg off the ground and try to avoid putting it down at all; these sheep are often reluctant to walk
  - A sheep that is lame on multiple legs can be difficult to spot; the only signs may be that it is unwilling to walk or appears generally unwell, as described above

- Standing still:

  - A lame sheep will often stand with the lame leg only just touching the ground with the tip of its toe (Fig. 7.4). This is not a normal position for resting sheep, unlike horses
  - If one or both front legs are painful, sheep will often graze resting on their knees rather than standing (Fig. 7.5)
  - With severe lameness, a sheep will stand with the affected leg lifted off the ground

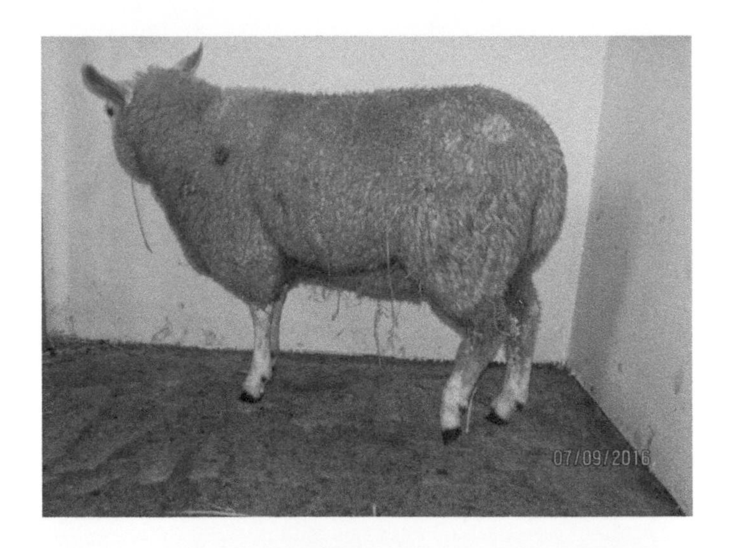

FIGURE 7.4 A lame lamb stood resting its lame leg with only its toe touching the ground.

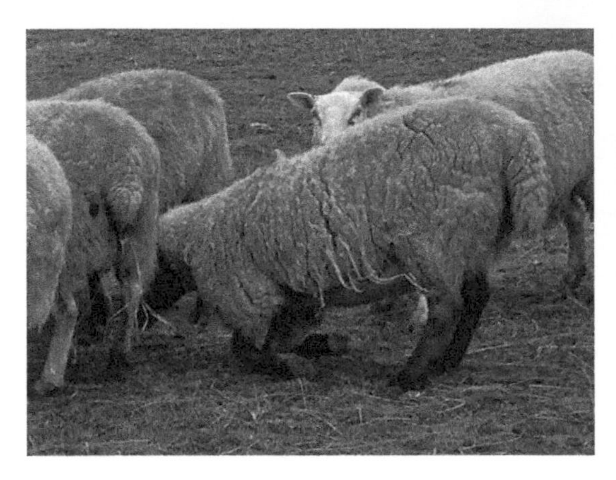

FIGURE 7.5 A ewe with painful front feet kneeling to eat.

- Lying down:
  - Lame sheep will usually spend more time lying down than normal
  - Severely lame sheep can be observed having difficulty lying down and standing up again

Lame sheep can be difficult to identify when they are moving faster than a walk, although they may struggle to keep up with the rest of the group.

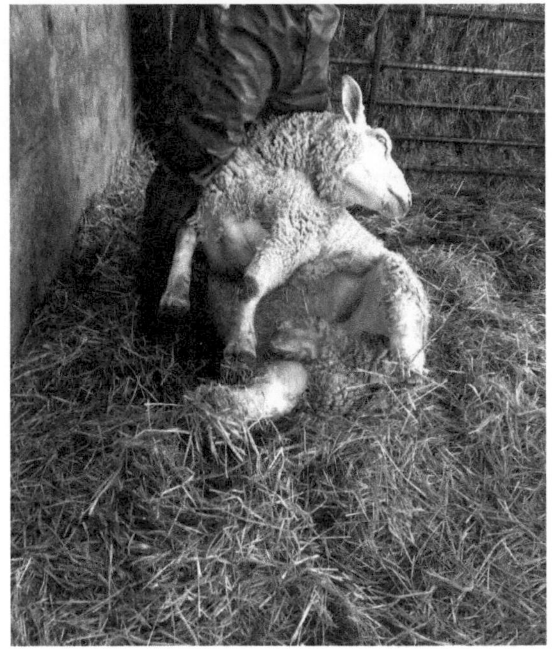

FIGURE 7.6 A ewe turned over to examine the feet.

What to do

For infectious causes of lameness, which are common in sheep, prompt treatment can significantly reduce the spread of infection, therefore for each lame sheep the ideal protocol is:

Catch

- Ideally, the sheep should be caught within three days of becoming lame, unless there are signs of severe lameness in which case immediate attention is needed (Fig.7.6).

- Clean away dirt from the foot with a paper towel. Do not trim any horn unless the lesion cannot otherwise be seen, and where this is necessary remove as little horn as possible. Thoroughly clean the shears afterwards.

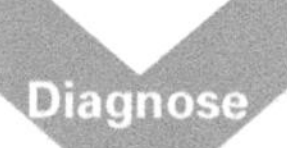

- the cause of lameness with veterinary involvement. A veterinary visit or well-lit photographs of the feet are useful.

Treat

- for the correct condition (according to veterinary advice) and give any anti-inflammatories and pain killers as advised.

Mark

- the affected leg and record the tag number of the sheep.

Cull

- animals that are repeatedly lame to prevent them (and prevent the spread of infections to other sheep).

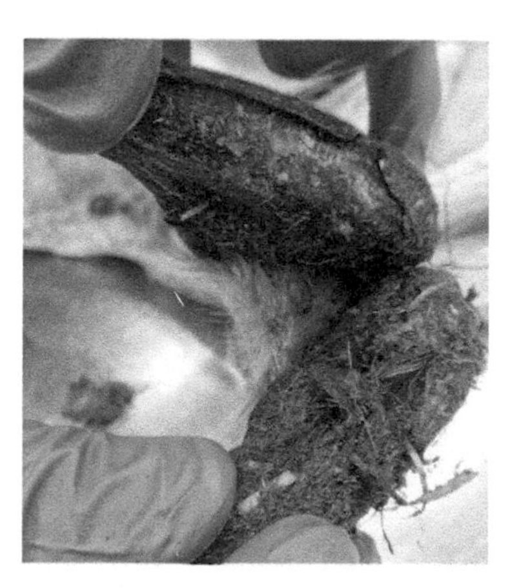

FIGURE 7.7 A normal, uninfected foot, with hair growing between the claws.

For lame animals without foot lesions (Fig. 7.7), the local vet should be called out to locate the problem in the leg.

Common causes of lameness

Due to the experience and training of veterinary surgeons, they will often be able to provide much additional help and advice when visiting a flock. Therefore, the cost of a vet visit, even for something that could be a small consideration, can be money well spent. However, if veterinary advice is desired but it is not necessary for a

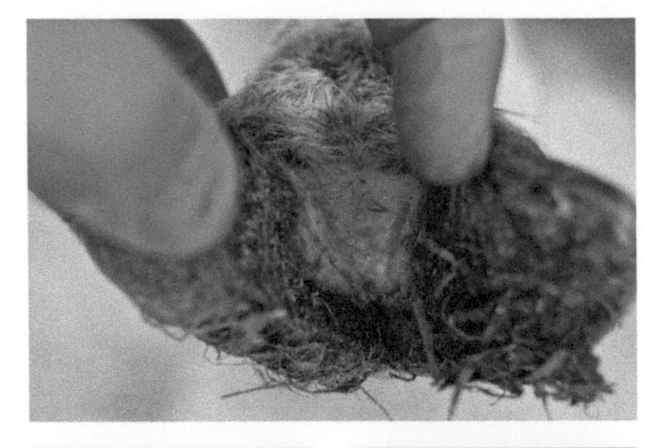

lame sheep to be examined by a vet, it is also possible to show the vet well-lit photographs of lesions, as these can also be very useful to get the appropriate advice.

For animals that appear to have lost the function of one or more of their legs, see the section on 'Leg weakness and paralysis' below in 'Behavioural changes: brain, nerve or muscle problems'.

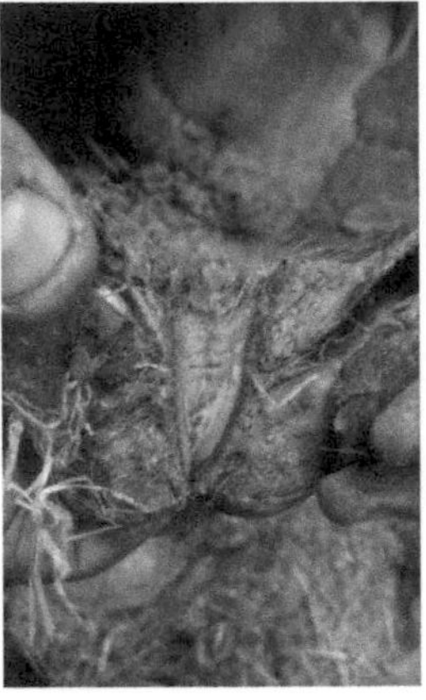

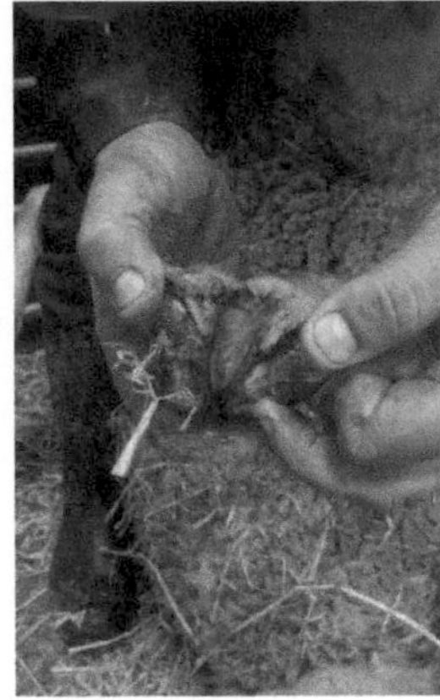

FIGURE 7.8 and 7.9 Scald affects the skin between the claws.

FIGURE 7.10 A foot with scald needs to be sprayed generously with antibiotic.

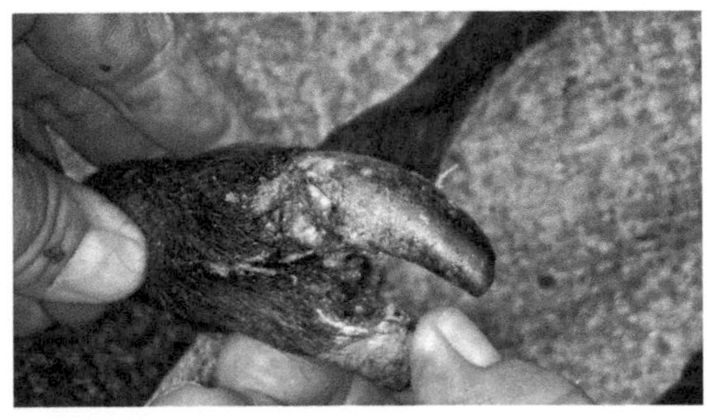

FIGURE 7.13 CODD causes a red, raw lesion at the top of the horn, which spreads downwards.

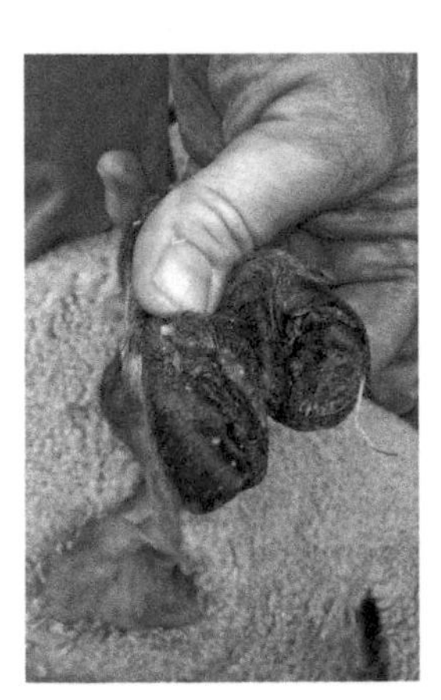

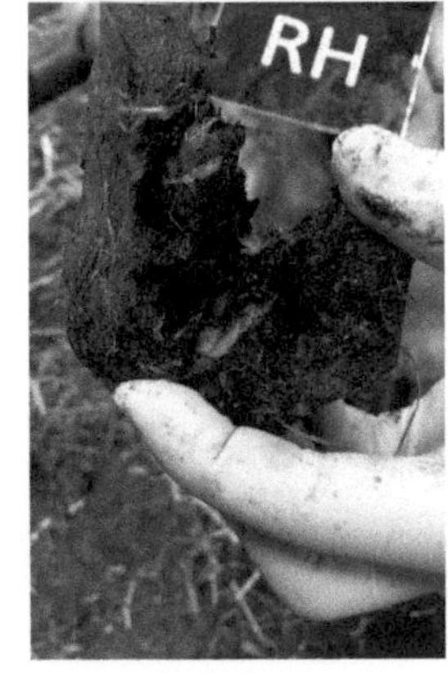

FIGURE 7.11 and 7.12 Footrot is an extension of severe scald, which underruns the horn of the claws and has a distinctive smell.

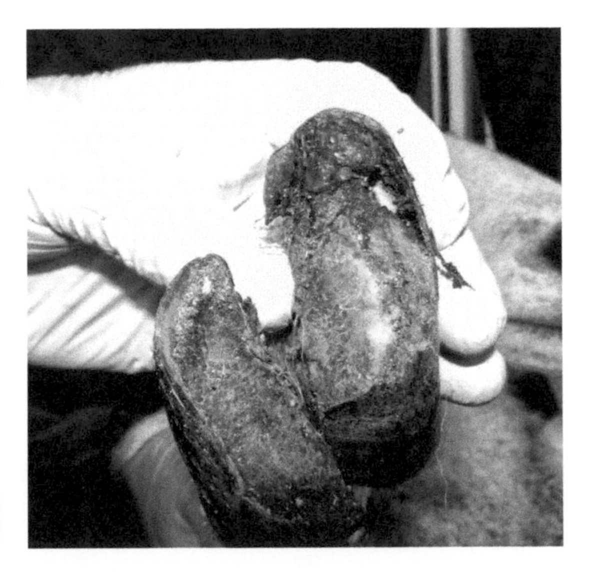

FIGURE 7.14 Toe granulomas are very painful.

Table 7.1 Common causes of lameness.

DESCRIPTION	LIKELY CAUSE – GET YOUR VET TO CHECK	POSSIBLE TREATMENTS (IN CONSULTATION WITH YOUR VET)
Very lame, the skin between the toes is moist, pink or white, and hairless.	Scald (Figs 7.8, 7.9)	Individuals: Spray with antibiotic spray (oxytetracycline or chlortetracycline; (Fig. 7.10). Group outbreaks: footbath the group and move to a 'footrot-clean' field if possible, that is, one that has not had sheep in for over a month. Adult sheep also need a long-acting injection of oxytetracycline.
Dark smelly lesion between claws with under-running of the horn.	Footrot (see Chapter 8 for details of prevention; Figs 7.11, 7.12)	Long-acting oxytetracycline injection. Spray with oxytetracycline/chlortetracycline. Anti-inflammatories (*do not* trim horn). For the first case, any unresponsive cases or an outbreak, get veterinary assistance.
Red, raw 'strawberry-like' lesion breaking out at top of hoof; the hoof horn eventually falls off. Very lame.	Contagious ovine digital dermatitis (CODD; Fig. 7.13)	Long-acting amoxicillin injection, given twice two days apart. For your first case, any unresponsive cases or an outbreak, get veterinary assistance.
Prominent, raw mass protruding from horn or damaged hoof surface, often red and very sore. Prevention: avoid over-trimming feet and keep sheep away from thorns and sharp objects.	Toe granulomas (Fig. 7.14)	Call the vet. Pain relief is necessary.
A thorn stuck into the horn or a stone wedged between the claws. Nail or other longer, sharp object.	Foreign body	Thorn: remove the thorn, give long-acting antibiotics and anti-inflammatories according to the vet's advice. Stone: remove the stone. If it has damaged the skin or horn between the digits, treat as above. Nail or other longer, sharp object: call the vet immediately.
Swelling on the side of the foot just above the horn, severe lameness.	White line abscess (Figs 7.15, 7.16)	Call the vet. (Trapped abscesses form inside the hoof and make their way up to the top of the horn to burst out.)
A cavity running up the inside of the hoof wall; not smelly or inflamed; the horn and sole of the foot look normal; the gap can become packed with mud.	Shelly hoof	Trim off just enough loose horn to stop dirt from gathering in it; do not go near the softer tissues – if in doubt, call the vet.
Lambs with swollen joints that are not keeping up with mum and are hobbling along or lying down a lot; the lamb is often thin. (See Chapter 6 for details.)	Joint ill	Anti-inflammatory and antibiotic therapy according to veterinary advice, ideally antibiotic treatment should last ten to 14 days. Keep the lamb, its mum and sibling(s) in a small pen or paddock for the duration of treatment so that they are easy to catch.

Table 7.1 continued.

DESCRIPTION	LIKELY CAUSE – GET YOUR VET TO CHECK	POSSIBLE TREATMENTS (IN CONSULTATION WITH YOUR VET)
Gradually increasing stiffness with occasional periods of more severe lameness. More common in older animals.	Arthritis	Have the sheep checked by a vet to confirm the diagnosis. Anti-inflammatories can be given periodically when lameness is bad and then more often as the stiffness increases. Have the sheep checked regularly so that the vet can advise when and how to do this.
Severe lameness, with the leg held off the ground; with or without wounds or abrasions. The leg may feel 'loose' when the foot is inspected. Do not inspect any further if a broken leg is suspected.	Broken bones	Call the vet immediately.
Sheep stand with their feet at an unusual angle because of excess horn. It can be flapped over the sole of the hoof or come curling out of the front of the toe.	Overgrown hooves (Fig. 7.17)	Check the whole foot for the infections described above, treat these and delay hoof trimming until the infection is gone (unless the hoof capsule is hanging off and just requires a small snip to remove it). If no infection is present, carefully trim the excess flaps of horn away, no closer than 3 mm from where it joins the hoof. Only attempt this under veterinary instruction and if you have previous supervised experience.

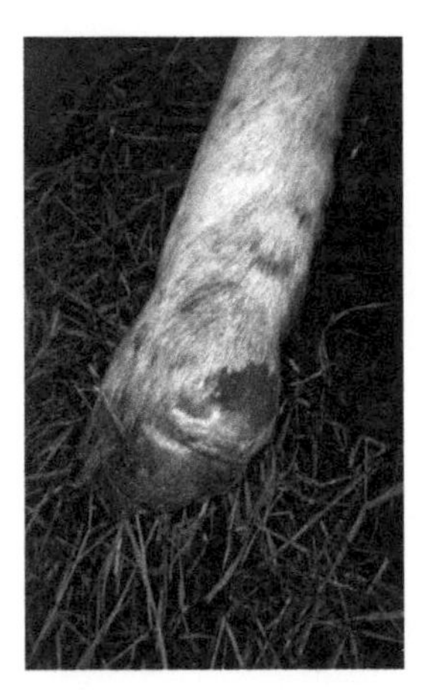

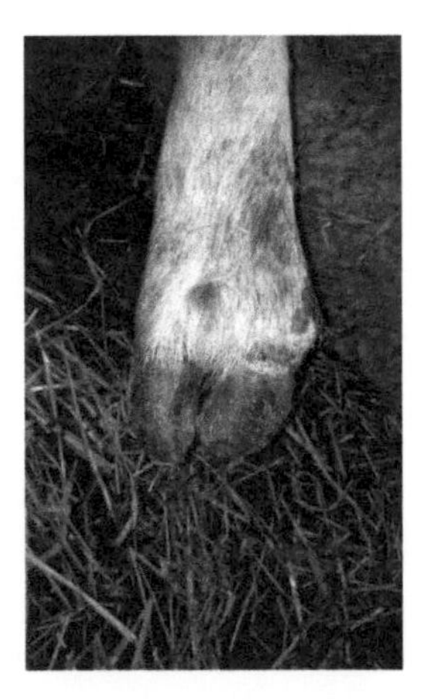

FIGURE 7.15 and 7.16 Abscesses cause swelling above the horn and eventually burst, releasing pus and blood.

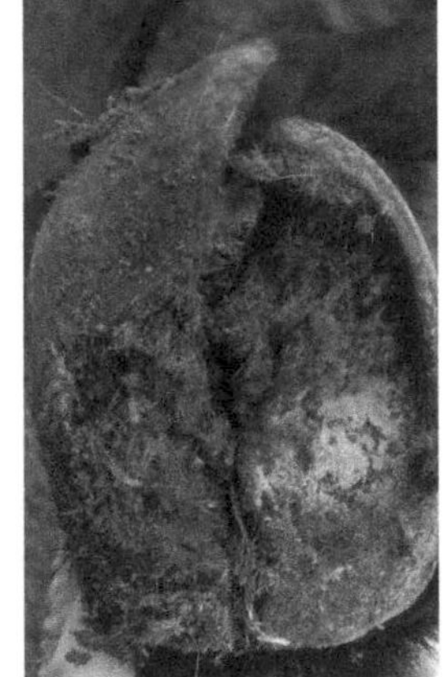

FIGURE 7.17 A flap of overgrown horn. This is unlikely to cause lameness and will wear away naturally.

RESPIRATORY DISEASE

How to spot respiratory diseases

Diseases that affect breathing, or respiration, vary in severity and in the rapidity with which they progress, therefore how soon veterinary attention is required varies. If there is any doubt, seek veterinary assistance at the earliest opportunity.

Signs of respiratory diseases include:

- Depression
- Lack of appetite
- Drooping ears (compared to normal for the breed or individual sheep)
- A reluctance to move, especially to move quickly
- Coughing
- Increases in the rate of breathing, when moving or at rest
- Increase in the effort put into each breath, when moving or at rest
- Breathing with the mouth open
- Noisy breathing

Some of the common respiratory diseases that affect sheep are discussed below.

Pasteurellosis and shipping fever

Pasteurella-type bacteria cause a range of syndromes in sheep, including respiratory disease, septicaemia and sudden death, especially in sheep under 1 year old. Under normal circumstances, these bacteria live in the environment and in the airways of sheep without incident. They only cause disease at times of stress, for example when the weather changes suddenly or there is an abrupt management change, or when respiratory tissues have been damaged by other diseases, for example MV or OPA. Examples of stressors include:

- Transport
- Overcrowding
- Weaning
- Housing
- Stressful handling
- Sudden diet changes
- Handling in wet weather

The symptoms of pasteurellosis appear quickly and include:

- Depression/dullness
- Coughing
- Rapid breathing
- Lack of appetite
- Drooping ears

These symptoms generally respond well to antibiotic and anti inflammatory treatment. The exact treatment and dosing regimen should be guided by advice from a vet. The animal(s) must be seen by a vet if:

- The affected animal is struggling to breathe
- The symptoms increase in severity, for example the breathing becomes more laboured or coughing becomes more frequent
- Signs do not begin to resolve within 12 to 24 hours of treatment
- Several animals are affected

The following suggestions can help to reduce, but not eliminate, pasteurellosis:

- Good ventilation in housing
- Reduced stocking densities in housing
- Minimal stress during handling

- At weaning, move the ewes away, so that the lambs remain on a familiar field for the first week
- Change diets gradually wherever possible
- Use of a Pasteurella vaccine

Mycoplasma

Young adult sheep are most at risk of pneumonia (lung infection) caused by *Mycoplasma ovipneumoniae*. In the majority of cases, this is a mild, soft, dry cough and is often seen in the autumn as the weather changes. Treatment is not necessary in mild cases but seek veterinary advice as other diseases may be involved.

Lungworm

The lungworm *Dictyocaulus filaria* spreads through a flock in a similar way to most gut worms. Immature stages are deposited on pasture in sheep faeces and develop to infective larvae in warm, moist conditions. These worms can cause a cough in late summer or autumn. A vet will be able to test faecal samples for this worm and will advise you about treatment. Most standard wormers will treat lungworm, but the choice of wormer will depend on the time of year, which animals are affected and whether other worms are present in these animals.

Muellerius capillaris and *Protostrongylus rufescens* are also types of lungworm; these require slugs and snails for their development, but rarely cause significant problems in sheep.

Chronic pneumonia/abscesses

Chronic pneumonia and lung abscesses occasionally affect individual sheep; these are debilitating conditions that require intensive treatment. Unresolved bacterial infections of the lungs cause ongoing damage, reducing the amount of functional lung tissue and causing continual ill health. Affected sheep cough frequently, struggle to move fast, become short of breath easily and lose weight. Long courses of treatment are required, under the direction of your local vet. Humane euthanasia should be considered if breathing becomes difficult, or improvements in alertness, breathing and coughing are not apparent in the first seven days of treatment. This should be discussed with the vet. If improvements are noticeable in the first week, continued treatment is justified.

Slowly progressing viral infections

Two slowly progressing viral infections cause permanent changes in the lungs which can eventually cause severe respiratory disease. See 'Slowly progressing viral infections' below in 'Thin sheep' for more details.

Laryngeal chondritis

Some sheep breeds, especially those with short necks such as the Texel and Beltex, are prone to inflammation of the larynx, or voice box. Affected animals breathe noisily and can struggle for breath, standing with their necks and heads pointing straight out in front of them. These animals need prompt veterinary attention, but if they are severely affected the vet should be asked to visit the farm to avoid transporting the animal to the surgery. Some sheep will never fully recover from this condition or have repeated episodes of respiratory distress and should be euthanased to prevent suffering.

DIARRHOEA

Any diarrhoea has the potential to contain organisms that affect human health, therefore when handling faeces or diarrhoea always wear gloves and then wash hands with disinfectant before eating, drinking or smoking.

How to spot diarrhoea

Severe cases of diarrhoea may have the following signs:

- Newborn lambs might have wet back ends, stained yellow, green, black or even red. These lambs need immediate veterinary attention
- A pipe-stream of watery faeces might be seen coming from a sheep with severe diarrhoea

Moderate diarrhoea:

- Newborn lambs' faeces may form a watery paste
- Young lambs with yellow pasty faeces can become blocked if the tail becomes stuck to their backside, stopping faeces from being passed – monitor lambs for this and relieve them by unsticking the tail
- Older lambs or adult sheep may have caked green or brown back ends, where faeces are caught in the wool (Fig. 7.18)

Diagnosing the cause of diarrhoea requires veterinary involvement. Animals with diarrhoea need immediate veterinary attention if:

- They are newborn lambs with severe diarrhoea of any sort

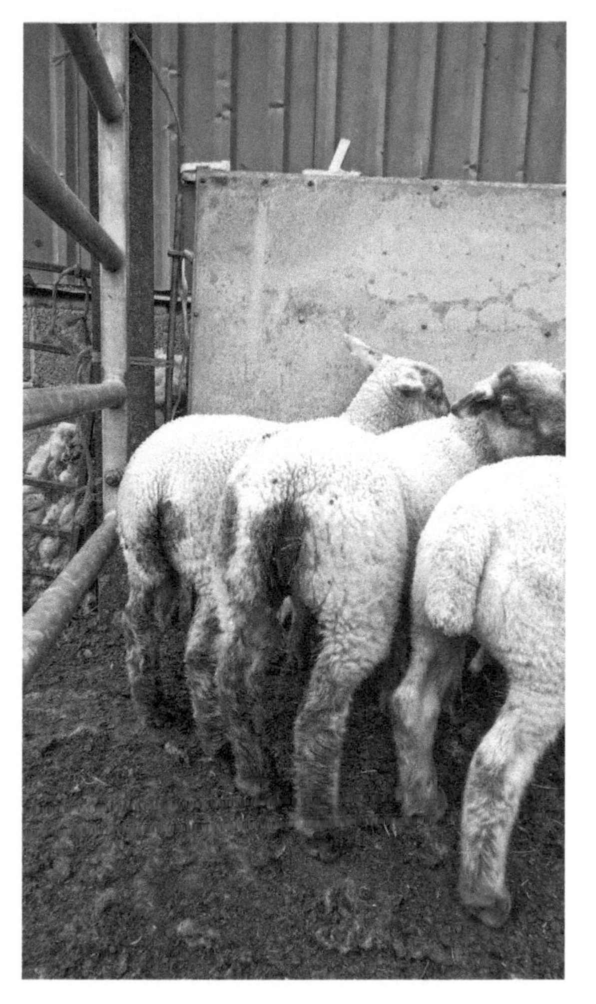

FIGURE 7.18 Lambs with diarrhoea will have stained bottoms.

- There is blood in the faeces
- They are dull or depressed

Nutrition

A sheep's digestive tract can be disrupted by what they eat, just like with people; too much rich food, sudden changes of diet or spoiled feed can all cause problems.

Table 7.2 Causes of diarrhoea in sheep of different ages.

SYMPTOM	POSSIBLE CAUSES
Lambs with scour	
A few days old	*Escherichia coli*, *Cryptosporidium*, Rotavirus, Lamb dysentery
Over 3 weeks old Indoors, on a yard or at grass	Coccidiosis
Over 6 weeks old at grass	Coccidiosis, nutritional (too much lush grass), nematodirosis, parasitic gastroenteritis
Late summer/autumn at grass	Parasitic gastroenteritis, nutritional (change in diet), nematodirosis, coccidiosis
Adult sheep with scour	
Green scour	Nutritional (too much lush grass or change in diet), parasitic gastroenteritis
Scour with blood	Bacterial infection
Scour with grains of cereal or granular	Nutritional, grain overload

Changes in diet

The microflora in the gut of sheep and other ruminants are more sensitive to the type of food they receive and its continuity than the microflora of humans. Therefore, when the major constituents of a sheep's diet are changed suddenly, the microflora can take some time to adjust, particularly if the change includes an increase in the carbohydrate content of the diet, for example concentrate feed or lush spring grass and a decrease in the overall fibre content. A disruption in the availability of feed can also affect the microflora.

Sheep that have had a change of diet may show signs such as:

- Dirty back ends due to diarrhoea
- Loss of appetite
- Change in behaviour

Sheep with a loss of appetite or changes in behaviour (even up to two weeks after the change in diet) must be examined by a vet. Provided the new diet has sufficient fibre content, symptoms should resolve within a few days. However, actions that can be taken to rectify or prevent this include:

- Inclusion of additional fibre in the new diet, such as hay, straw, fibrous haylage/silage or grass from a permanent pasture
- Reintroduction of the original diet and changing it gradually, over the course of a week
- Reduction of the overall concentrate/grain content of the diet

Any animals with unresolved diarrhoea after ten days should also be examined by a vet.

Grain overload

Diarrhoea due to changes in diet reflect the relative differences between the respective diets, however, ruminants (including sheep) can develop diarrhoea, depression and stomach pain (indicated in sheep by watching their bellies) because of an absolute excess of cereal grains or concentrate feed. This excess of high carbohydrate feed can be continual, due to inadvertent overfeeding, alongside inadequate dietary fibre or short-term, due to accidental access to large amounts of these feedstuffs.

Diarrhoea may be seen within 24 to 48 hours; if whole grains are fed some of these may appear in the faeces or the faeces can have a granular texture; the animal may appear depressed. However, in these cases, diarrhoea is of secondary importance; bloat is the most serious potential consequence and can be fatal – see 'Whole abdomen enlargement' below in the 'Lumps and swellings' section.

Animals that have inadvertently received too much concentrate feed should be examined and treated by a vet as soon as possible. They are likely to treat the animal with antibiotics, anti-inflammatories and oral fluids containing probiotics specifically designed for ruminants.

Gut worms – roundworms

In sheep there are several different types of gut worm and there are four main ways that these can cause disease, which are:

- Nematodirosis, which affects lambs in spring or early summer, and occasionally in autumn, when a cold spell is followed by a few days of warm weather. *Nematodirus* can cause a sudden outbreak of severe diarrhoea and rapid dehydration, which can be fatal
- Parasitic gastroenteritis, which affects lambs in mid to late summer and autumn, causing poor growth rates and diarrhoea, but is occasionally fatal
- Adult parasitic gastroenteritis: adults with reduced immunity due to other diseases or undernutrition (lack of food) can suffer from diarrhoea and weight loss due to an excessive load of gut worms, just like lambs
- Haemonchosis, which can affect lambs, and adults that have never been exposed to it before; diarrhoea is not typically seen, instead sheep become lethargic due to anaemia and some may die

Nematodirosis

Nematodirosis is caused by one type of worm, *Nematodirus battus*. It affects lambs over 5 weeks old that are at pasture. The worm eggs are deposited on the grass in lamb faeces; these eggs hatch en masse during a warm spell after cold weather, therefore they normally hatch during the following spring. However, this pattern is changing slightly as the parasites evolve and disease can now be seen in autumn in some parts of the UK.

Hatched larvae are eaten by the lambs and cause inflammation in the guts, resulting in:

- Severe watery green diarrhoea
- Lambs that suddenly look gaunt and dull
- Severe dehydration
- Some lambs dying within as little as a couple of days

This condition can progress rapidly, so veterinary attention should be sought as soon as severe diarrhoea is noticed in lambs, especially those that are 6 to 12 weeks old in spring or older lambs in autumn. Lambs can be affected by several parasites at the same time, therefore a veterinary diagnosis is needed. Your vet may wish to include any or all the following in their investigation:

- Examination of affected lambs
- Testing lamb faeces
- Post-mortem examination of lambs that have died (within the previous 12 hours)

If no other parasites are present in the affected lambs, a white wormer (a benzimidazole) is generally recommended for treatment. All the lambs in the group must be treated, even those that are not affected yet. Severe cases may require fluid treatment; see 'Fluids' above for details.

Fields that are grazed by young lambs every year are high risk for this condition, therefore break the cycle of transmission by rotating the fields that are used for ewes with young lambs. Also, monitoring the weather and online parasite forecasts can help to predict when preventative treatments might be needed; seek veterinary advice at these times.

Lamb parasitic gastroenteritis – summer and autumn

Several species of gut worm can be involved in parasitic gastroenteritis (PGE). The eggs of these worms are deposited on pasture in sheep faeces and hatch in warm, damp weather. The larvae are eaten by lambs and develop into adult worms in the lamb's gut, which in turn produce eggs. Since young lambs do not have any immunity to these gut worms, they produce a lot of eggs and the number of worms can build up quickly if the climate is right. A large number of gut worms are needed to cause the disease, parasitic gastroenteritis, however, if a lamb only receives low levels of infection through the summer and autumn, it will develop immunity to worms without suffering from any related disease. Therefore, disease can be prevented by avoiding a build-up of worms.

Parasitic gastroenteritis causes:

- Reduced weight gain
- Reduced feed intake
- Diarrhoea
- Occasional lamb deaths

Action to take:

- Take fresh lamb faeces samples to your local vet each month; take ten samples per group of lambs, placing each sample into a separate container or bag
- It is important that the correct wormer is used, so speak to your local sheep vet before treating
- See 'Anthelmintics' in Chapter 8 for more information about treatments

Preventing parasitic gastroenteritis includes:

- Worming pregnant or lactating ewes at lambing time – speak to your local sheep vet about when to treat and what to use (do not use a white drench)
- Good nutrition
- Graze lambs on low-risk pastures, such as:
    - New grass leys
    - Fields previously grazed by cattle or adult sheep (not lactating ewes)
    - Fields recently used to make hay, haylage or silage – known as 'aftermath'

Adult parasitic gastroenteritis

Gut worms normally have little effect on adult sheep, but if their natural immunity becomes reduced, worm infections can increase. Things that can cause this drop in immunity include:

- Late pregnancy and early lactation – known as the 'peri-parturient rise'
- Other disease
- Inadequate nutrition
- Rams have a reduced immunity compared to ewes, so may sometimes suffer from PGE

Adults with PGE show similar signs to lambs, such as weight loss and diarrhoea. For adult sheep with diarrhoea, discuss potential causes with the local sheep vet and take faecal samples to the vet to be tested for worm eggs. If a significant worm burden is present, it is useful to discuss potential background issues with the vet.

Haemonchosis

Haemonchus contortus is another gut worm, but one that causes anaemia rather than diarrhoea. This parasite is generally found in warm climates; outbreaks of haemonchosis are seen in the south of the UK during warm summers and occasionally in other parts of the country. It is possible for adult sheep to be affected by this worm as well as lambs, and it can be spread to sheep fields by goats, cattle, deer or alpacas.

Signs of haemonchosis include:

- Lethargy and reluctance to move
- Heavy breathing
- Pale gums or membranes around the eyes
- Diarrhoea is not normally seen

Other diseases can have similar symptoms to haemonchosis, so ask your local sheep vet to examine affected animals and confirm a diagnosis with laboratory tests. This parasite is effective at developing resistance to worm treatments, so consult the sheep vet again if treatments do not seem to be working.

Tapeworms

Sections of white tapeworms are often seen in lambs' faeces (Fig. 7.19), but this is not normally an indication that the lambs need to be wormed. In the UK, the control of roundworms (worms that cause PGE – see above) generally prevents a build-up of tapeworms, therefore they are rarely harmful for sheep. Very rarely, tapeworm numbers can build up to such an extent they form a blockage in the guts of a lamb. Consult your local sheep vet if you have any concerns.

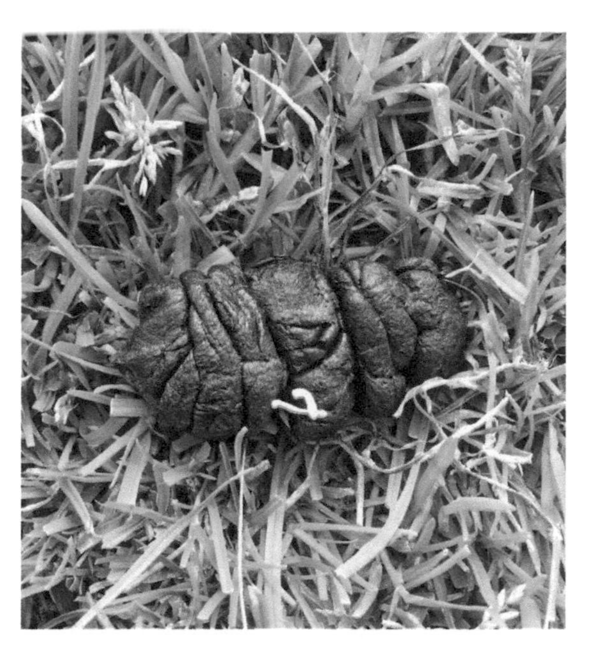

FIGURE 7.19 Tapeworm segments in lambs' faeces are not normally an indication of serious disease.

Coccidiosis

Coccidiosis is caused by single-cell parasites of the *Eimeria* family. Adult sheep shed the parasite at low levels, contaminating the environment; these are picked up by the lambs and multiply rapidly causing damage to the lamb's intestines. Disease is normally seen in the youngest lambs, which are exposed to high levels of infection after older lambs have acted as multipliers for the parasite.

Risk factors for coccidiosis include:

- Lambs born later in the lambing period
- Lambs over 3 weeks old and normally less than 3 months old
- Overcrowded, damp, dirty sheds
- Heavily stocked fields with short grass
- Bad weather that forces lambs to congregate in small areas of a field

Coccidiosis in lambs can cause:

- Watery diarrhoea, sometimes bloodstained or black
- Dehydration
- Depression
- Loss of appetite
- Weight loss

Early veterinary attention is needed for this condition as it can progress rapidly. The local vet will need to investigate an outbreak of diarrhoea in lambs (as for nematodirosis), because lambs can suffer from several parasites at the same time.

There are several treatments available for coccidiosis, which have different dosing regimens, and options for treatment should be discussed with a vet. If coccidiosis is diagnosed, all of the lambs in a group must be treated, even those that are not showing signs yet, and the lambs should be moved to a clean environment or have their shed cleaned out. Severe cases may require fluid treatment; see 'Fluids' above for details.

Prevention of coccidiosis includes:

- Good hygiene
- Avoiding overcrowding
- Providing shelter in bad weather
- Preventative treatments, as a last resort; discuss these with your vet

Newborn lambs

Young lambs with diarrhoea are very susceptible to dehydration because of their small size, therefore early treatment and fluids are essential. There are several causes of diarrhoea in young lambs, including sudden diet change, poor nutrition and infectious diseases (viruses, bacteria and parasites).

In mild diarrhoea, lambs can have pasty faeces that give them a dirty rear end; in newborn lambs, this can be a sign of high milk production by the lamb's mother; in older lambs, it can be a sign of lush grass or parasites. Pasty faeces need to be monitored and for lambs over 2 months old, the faeces should be taken to the vet to test for parasites.

Severe diarrhoea is watery and comes in a stream, making the lamb's rear end wet as well as pasty. The lamb may stop eating and become dull or depressed.

Fluids are the basis of treatment for severe diarrhoea. If the lamb is able to stand, use oral fluids at 50 millilitres per kilogram of the lamb's body weight per feed. The fluid should be given at body temperature with rehydration powder or salts mixed into it (see 'Fluids' above for details). Alternate these fluid 'feeds' with milk. In severe cases, feed the lamb every two hours until the scour stops (once the lamb appears brighter and livelier the frequency of these feeds can be reduced). Fluids can be given by stomach tube; see 'Stomach tubing a lamb' in Chapter 6 for details.

Veterinary involvement is needed for:

- Investigating the cause of diarrhoea
- Providing, and advising on, additional treatments
- Treating lambs that are unable to stand
- Lambs that are not improving within 24 hours despite intensive treatment

Diarrhoea in newborn lambs can be prevented by:

- Good hygiene
- Good colostrum management
- Keeping affected lambs away from other lambs to reduce the spread of infection

Less common causes of diarrhoea in sheep

Tick-borne fever/louping ill

Lambs 3 to 6 weeks old in tick-infested areas may suffer from severe bloodstained diarrhoea, weakness and loss of appetite. Preventing these diseases requires reducing the lambs' exposure to the ticks or using chemical tick prevention while they are grazing tick-pasture.

Listeriosis

Silage that is contaminated with soil and then stored without adequate air exclusion can become infiltrated with *Listeria monocytogenes*; when this is fed to sheep a number of diseases can occur, one of which is severe diarrhoea. If there are any concerns about silage intended for sheep, seek veterinary advice.

Salmonella

Adult sheep with blood in their faeces may have a serious bacterial gut infection, so the vet should be called to investigate this as soon as is practicable.

THIN SHEEP

There is a huge range of diseases that can cause weight loss in sheep, but the first thing to consider in this situation is whether they have access to enough appropriate food. Appropriate food varies depending on the age and stage of reproduction of the sheep in question; see Chapter 4 'Diet and nutrition' for more detail.

Below is a summary of what to do if sheep do not have the expected body condition required, along with a brief overview of the most common causes of ill thrift (thin sheep).

How to spot a thin sheep

It can be difficult to tell whether sheep are thin, fat or at the correct body condition, especially if they have a good fleece. How to assess an adult sheep's body condition is discussed in the 'Body condition score' section of Chapter 2. For young lambs, this may be easier because of the lack of wool. Signs of weight loss include:

- A hollow-looking abdomen
- Being able to see sharp outlines of some of the bones, for example the ribs, hip bones and spine – these should be rounded or not visible when lambs are in good condition

Signs to look for and actions that can be taken by a sheep owner are laid out in Figure 7.20.

If any of these thin sheep die, the vet should be asked to perform a post-mortem examination.

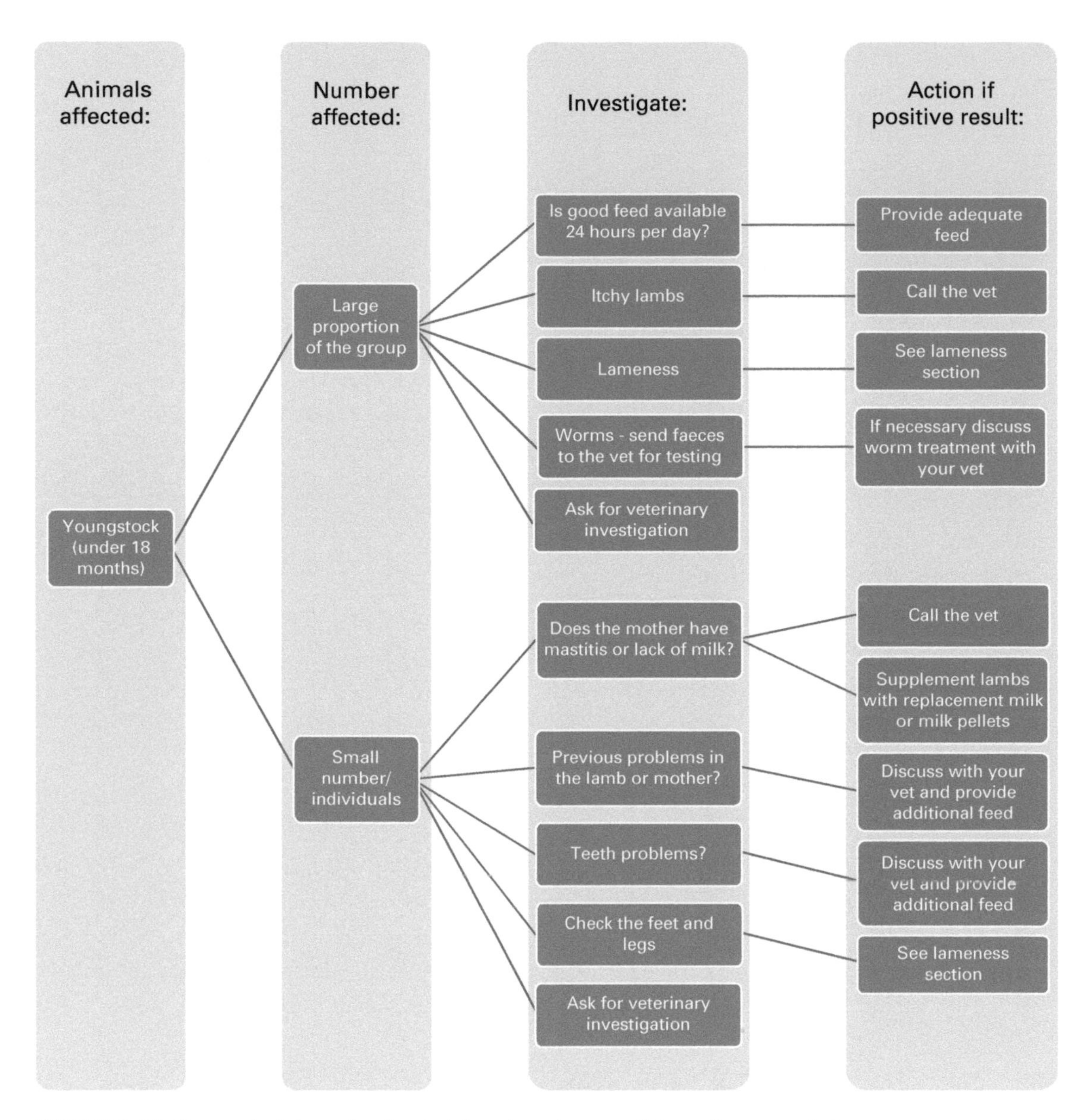

FIGURE 7.20 Signs to look for and action to take when sheep are thinner than expected.

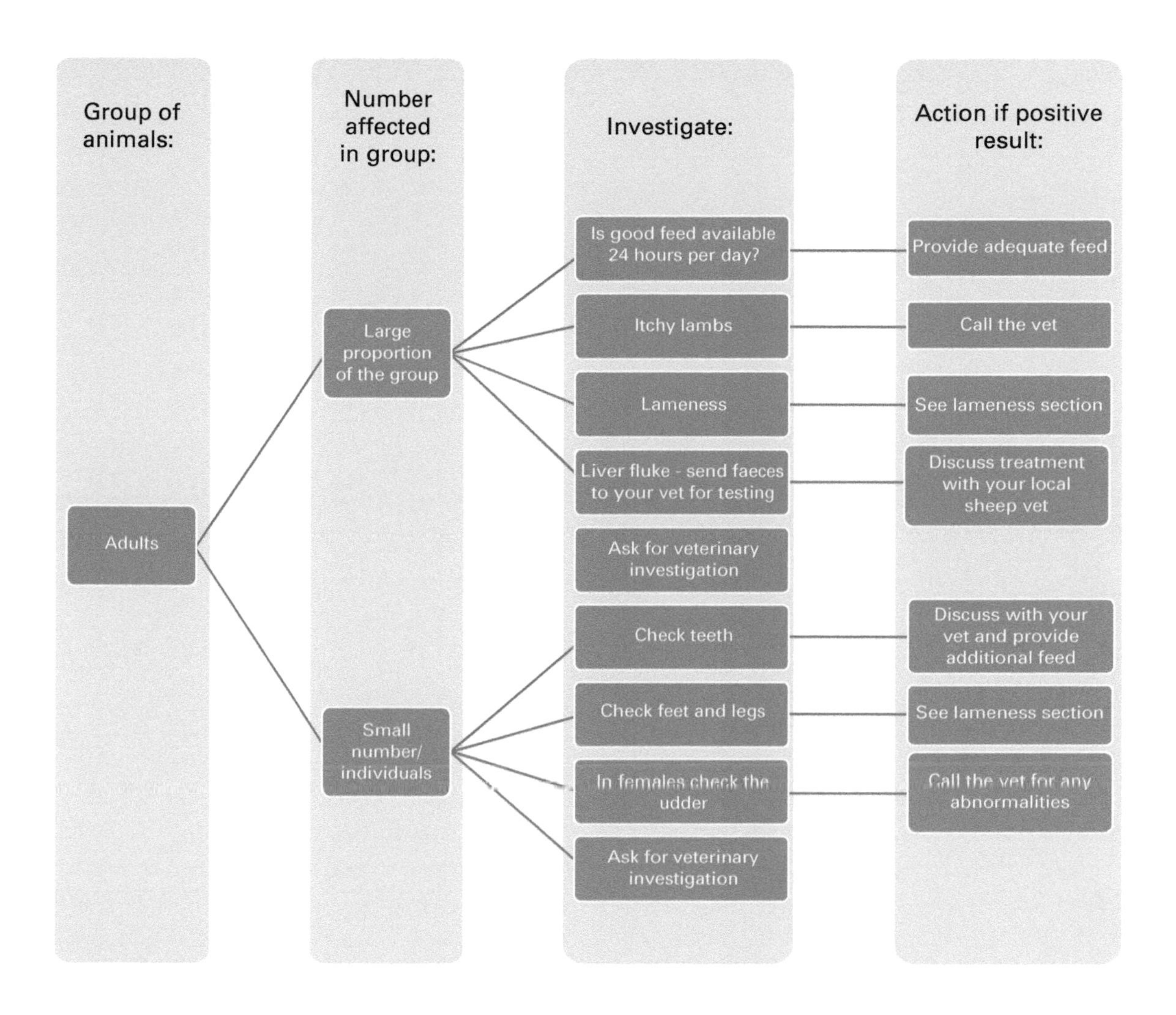

Common diseases of thin adult sheep

Inadequate nutrition

Sheep need a constant supply of food that is high in fibre and contains sufficient energy, protein and micronutrients to sustain them. Lack of nutrition is a common cause of poor body condition in sheep and so the diet of a flock should be constantly monitored and assessed.

Chronic pneumonia

Chronic pneumonia is a common cause of weight loss in sheep. See 'Respiratory disease' above for details.

Dental problems

Problems with teeth affect a large number of sheep, but diagnosis can be tricky because most of the teeth in a sheep are difficult to examine;

the vet will be able to help with this. Some dental diseases are hereditary and are seen in young animals (for example, an overshot or undershot jaw), but others, such as worn down front teeth, are age-related and only seen in older sheep.

Signs of dental problems include:

- Difficulty with getting food into the mouth
- Dropping food while chewing
- Food collecting in the cheeks
- Jerky jaw movements
- Difficulty swallowing
- The mouth staying slightly open, even during chewing
- Swellings along the jaw, top or bottom

Sheep need a constant supply of feed, with high levels of fibre, but animals with dental disease will not be able to eat short grass or unprocessed root vegetables. This can affect their overall feed intake and the fibre content of their diet. Therefore, the diet must be managed when dental problems are identified with careful feeding, until the animal can no longer sustain itself. When a sheep can no longer maintain a reasonable body condition it needs to be humanely euthanased.

Feed management can include:

- Long grass, 6–8 cm high – some affected sheep will cope with this alone
- Supplementary feeding, including any of:
    - Alfalfa
    - Bran
    - Beet pulp
    - Concentrate feed

Occasionally, dental treatment can be attempted by a veterinary surgeon, but only certain conditions are treatable and only if the correct equipment is available and not all practices will be able to attempt this kind of work.

Check the mouths of rams and ewes for hereditary dental problems before they are used for breeding. Ask a vet to demonstrate how this inspection is carried out. Avoid inserting fingers into a sheep's mouth as their teeth are very sharp and sheep have powerful jaws.

Other mouth problems

Other mouth problems can also stop sheep from grazing or processing feed effectively, which may result in feed dropping out of the mouth while a sheep is eating or a reluctance to eat or swallow. Call the vet if a sheep is struggling to eat.

Liver fluke

Liver fluke is a parasite, *Fasciola hepatica*, which damages the liver of sheep and other ruminants; it causes severe disease, especially in sheep as they have small livers and never develop good immunity, so they can be affected multiple times and at any age. Liver fluke eggs are deposited on pasture; if this pasture is wet and contains the dwarf mud snail, *Galba truncatula*, then liver fluke will develop in these snails (Fig. 7.21). The stage of liver fluke that infects sheep comes out of the snail several weeks or months after initial infestation, normally in late summer and autumn, although the timing is variable depending on the weather. The symptoms caused by liver fluke and the time of year that they are seen depend on the level of pasture contamination:

- On heavily infected pastures, disease is often seen in late summer, autumn or early winter; the symptoms include:

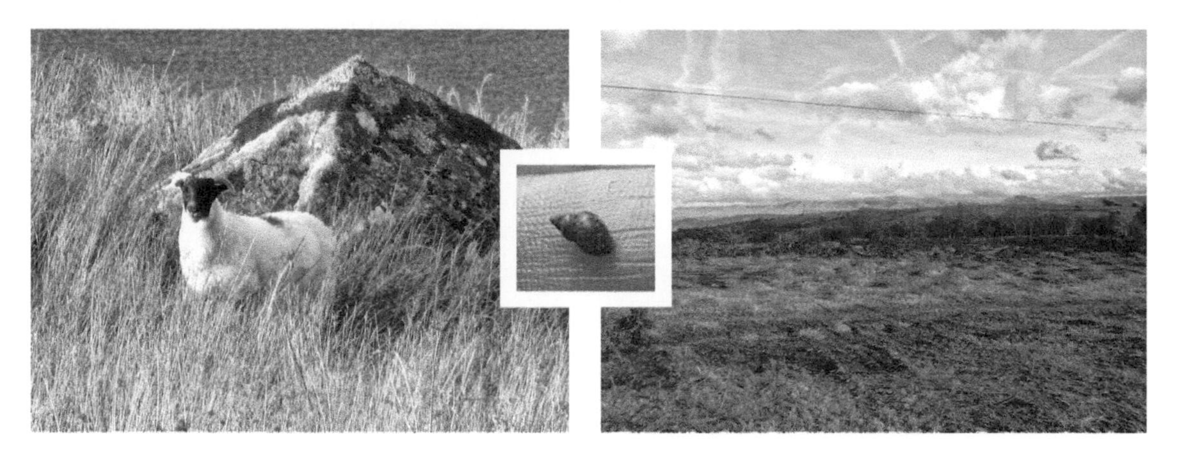

FIGURE 7.21 The liver fluke life cycle, which relies on snails, particularly the 'dwarf mud snail', *Galba truncatula*.

- Sudden deaths
- Rapid, shallow breathing
- Pale gums
- Dull, depressed animals
- Severe pain and unwillingness to move

- For mild to moderately infected pastures, affected sheep in winter or spring:

  - Become thin
  - Have pale gums, are lethargic and breathe heavily
  - Develop a swelling under the jaw in the advanced stages (known as 'bottle jaw' (Fig. 7.22)
  - Might have low pregnancy rates

A veterinary diagnosis is needed because many of these symptoms are also seen in other diseases. Discuss treatment with the vet as well, because choosing the best medicine relies on knowledge of when the sheep became infected (see Chapter 8, the 'Liver fluke' section). When liver fluke is diagnosed, all sheep that have been grazing wet pasture should be treated.

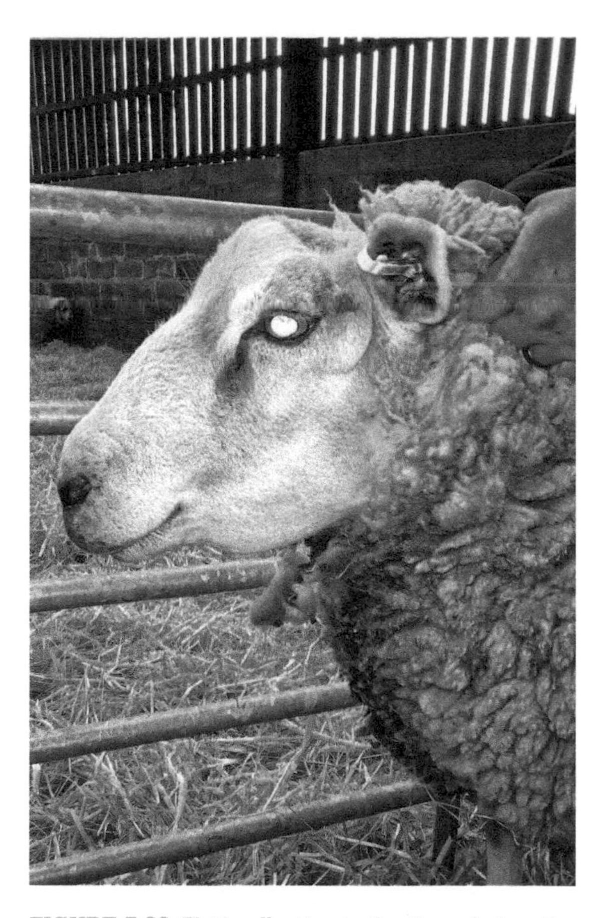

FIGURE 7.22 Fluid collection in the tissue below the lower jaw is known as 'bottle jaw'. This is sometimes, but not always, associated with liver fluke infection.

In some circumstances, it is possible to prevent liver fluke infection, for example:

- If there is a mixture of wet and dry pasture, keep sheep away from the wet pasture at high-risk times, such as autumn
- If wet areas of ground are small, they can be fenced off to prevent access by sheep – searching for the snails can help identify these high-risk areas
- If wet areas of ground are small, they can be drained to remove the snail habitat
- Fence boggy areas around streams and provide drinking water in troughs
- Treat sheep and cattle for liver fluke in the spring to remove the egg-laying adults and reduce pasture contamination for the next fluke season

If any sheep in the flock are sent straight to the abattoir, you may be able to find out whether those sheep have fluke in their livers, which will help to indicate whether liver fluke is present on the fields that they had been grazing. It may also indicate how advanced the infection is since the pattern of liver fluke infection changes from year to year, depending on the weather.

Slowly progressing viral infections

Two viruses cause slowly progressive disease in sheep. These take months or years to develop and are not treatable. These viruses are summarised in Table 7.3.

Johne's disease

Johne's disease is a slowly progressing bacterial infection of the small intestine, caused by *Mycobacterium avium* subspecies *Paratuberculosis* (MAP). Active disease is normally only seen in animals over 2 years old. These animals lose weight despite having a good appetite. There are no other symptoms until the final stages of disease, when it may cause 'bottle jaw'. Diagnosing Johne's disease in individual animals can be problematic and the bacteria can survive in the environment for a long time; both of these factors make it a difficult disease to control. Therefore, if sheep in a flock are affected by Johne's disease, it may be worth considering using the vaccine – see Chapter 8 'Vaccines' for details. Your local vet will be able to provide more information about diagnosis, control and the vaccine.

Scrapie

Scrapie can cause weight loss and behavioural changes in adult sheep. This condition is discussed in more detail in 'Behavioural changes: brain, nerve or muscle problems' below.

Other chronic diseases

Inflammation, infection and long-term tissue damage can affect any part of the body, including the udder of females, testicles of males, the heart, liver, kidneys, bladder, guts, feet and joints. Ongoing tissue damage anywhere in the body will eventually lead to weight loss.

In most cases of weight loss, a vet will be able to find the cause through a clinical investigation, and will then work with the sheep keeper to develop a plan for the affected animal and the flock. Some diseases are difficult to diagnose, for example Johne's disease, and expectations of what can be achieved need to be realistic. Unfortunately, not all attempts to find out what is wrong with a live animal will be successful and not all conditions can be treated. The vet is

Table 7.3 A summary of two viral diseases of sheep, OPA and MV.

<table>
<tr><th></th><th>JAAGSIEKTE VIRUS, CAUSES OVINE PULMONARY ADENOCARCINOMA (OPA)</th><th>MAEDI VISNA (MV) VIRUS</th></tr>
<tr><td>Risk factors</td><td colspan="2">Bought in sheep may carry these viruses and infect others in the flock.
Lambs born to an infected mother are at greater risk of contracting disease.
High stocking densities, e.g. during housing, increase the spread of disease between sheep.</td></tr>
<tr><td>Signs of disease</td><td>Increased effort to breathe, especially during exercise.
Weight loss.
Repeated episodes of pneumonia.
In advanced cases, lowering the head results in clear or frothy fluid running down the nose.</td><td>Increased effort to breath, especially during exercise.
Weight loss.
Repeated episodes of pneumonia.
Dragging of the back legs.
A firm, unproductive udder.
In some countries, lameness and swollen joints are a symptom, but currently not in the UK.</td></tr>
<tr><td>Treatment</td><td colspan="2">There is no effective treatment; therefore, it is best to remove infected sheep from a flock as soon as possible to protect the other sheep.</td></tr>
<tr><td>Prevention</td><td>Try to buy sheep from farms known to be free of OPA (this is difficult).
Good biosecurity – see Chapter 9 'Preventing disease from entering your flock'.</td><td>Test new sheep during quarantine.
Buy sheep from accredited farms.
Good biosecurity – see Chapter 9 'Preventing disease from entering your flock'.</td></tr>
<tr><td>Prevention on infected farms</td><td colspan="2">Reduce the stocking density.
Do not use troughs to feed concentrates and change the area used for feeding daily.
There are many options for dealing with these diseases – discuss them with a sheep vet, as each situation will be different.</td></tr>
</table>

likely to find this just as frustrating as you do. However, there must be a focus on working together to get the best outcome for the animal involved and the flock as a whole. For the individual animal, humane euthanasia may be necessary to prevent suffering. In such cases, a post-mortem examination can help to determine what is going on, providing information that will benefit the rest of the flock.

Growing lambs

A number of the conditions discussed above can also affect lambs and prevent them from thriving, including inadequate nutrition, liver fluke, pneumonia, teeth problems and chronic infections. However, some additional lamb diseases that do not normally affect adult sheep include:

- Gut worms and coccidiosis. See the section above on diarrhoea. These conditions can cause long-term damage to the digestive tract, resulting in reduced food conversion efficiency and slower growth rates even after effective treatment

- Nephrosis or daft lamb disease: Lambs with a history of diarrhoea can develop a condition of the kidneys, which causes them to become thin, dull and dehydrated. They will sometimes stagger as they walk and may continue to have diarrhoea; if untreated these lambs often die within a week
- Limited availability of milk, due to disease in the mother, for example:
  - Mastitis
  - Poor body condition – see 'Thin sheep' above for possible causes
- Disease as a newborn lamb: If a lamb suffers from disease in the first couple of weeks of life, he or she may have long-term damage that prevents them from growing well later in life
- Trace element deficiencies: In some geographical locations, weaned lambs do not receive enough selenium and/or cobalt from grass, resulting in thin lambs despite good grazing and worm control. Other signs of this include:
  - Increased susceptibility to other diseases
  - Cobalt-deficient lambs have an 'open' or unkempt fleece and weepy eyes
- Border disease: If this virus is in a flock it can cause a variety of signs, one being a proportion of lambs that do not grow well – these lambs are likely to spread the virus to other sheep, so should not be kept in the flock. See 'Hairy shakers' in Chapter 6 for more details

BEHAVIOURAL CHANGES: BRAIN, NERVE OR MUSCLE PROBLEMS

Conditions that affect the brain or nerves can result in a wide range of symptoms, including:

- An unusual walking action, for example high-stepping or dragging feet along the ground
- Walking in circles
- Compulsively walking forward until a solid object is reached (Fig. 7.23)
- Inability to bear weight on front or back legs
- Muscle twitching – ears or eyelids may flicker
- Shaky head movements or tremors
- Constant jaw movements
- A head tilt
- Blindness
- Sitting like a dog, staring at the sky – 'star-gazing'
- Pressing the head against a solid object
- Depression
- Seizures or fits
- Unusually aggressive behaviour
- Changes in normal behaviour

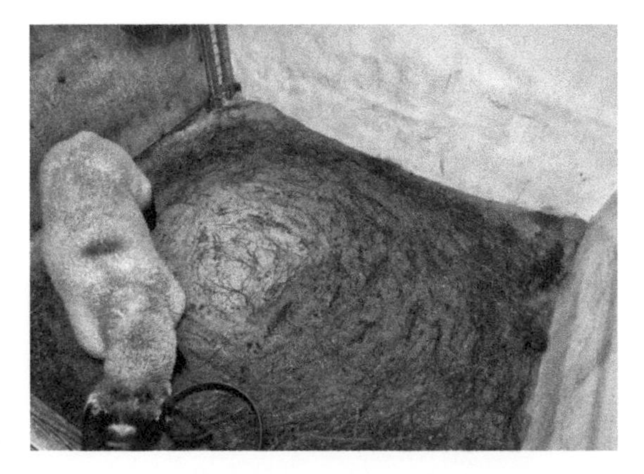

FIGURE 7.23 Circling and compulsive walking can appear similar if an animal is confined in a small space.

For all these symptoms, veterinary involvement is advisable to determine the cause and put together a treatment plan. However, while waiting for the vet to see heavily pregnant ewes with any of these symptoms, treat them for 'twin lamb' disease, hypocalcaemia and in the case of seizures, hypomagnesaemia. Do not attempt to treat aggressive animals.

Common causes of behavioural changes

Listeriosis

Listeriosis is caused by *Listeria monocytogenes*, which is found in the soil and in spoiled silage. Affected areas of silage can often be identified by visible patches of mould. Rarely, sheep can pick this bacterium up while grazing muddy fields, but most will contract it from eating silage. Listeriosis causes several different syndromes in sheep: abortion, silage eye, neurological listeriosis and diarrhoea. Neurological listeriosis has a distinctive appearance. Affected sheep:

- Are withdrawn in the early stages
- Walk in circles or walk forwards compulsively
- Have lopsided faces – one side of the face droops, including the ear
- Drool
- Lack appetite
- Eventually lie down and become unable to stand

Veterinary confirmation of the diagnosis is necessary and the vet will help to plan treatment and prevention of future cases. There is a delay between infection and the development of symptoms, so some sheep will become affected even after the source has been removed.

Brain cysts or lumps

Brain abscesses, tumours and cysts are known as 'space-occupying lesions'; these result in a variety of signs depending on the site of the lesion. Some of the most common signs include depression, circling, blindness in one eye and the inability to navigate small spaces. A dog tapeworm, *Taenia multiceps*, can cause cysts in the brain of sheep (coenurosis cysts or 'gid') and is common in mid Wales. Discussion with the vet and veterinary examinations will determine the most likely cause of symptoms, but the diagnosis can only be confirmed by post-mortem examination of an affected animal.

Possibilities for the prevention of space-occupying lesions include:

- Treating dogs for tapeworms every three months
- Not allowing dogs to eat raw sheep meat
- Prevention and prompt treatment of other infections

Middle ear infections

Occasionally, sheep develop middle ear infections; signs include:

- Head shaking and apparent discomfort
- Tilting of the head to one side
- Circling
- Loss of balance

The local vet should examine affected animals and will be able to advise you about treatment.

Sudden diet changes (cerebrocortical necrosis or polioencephalomalacia)

Sudden diet changes can disrupt the natural balance of microbes that live in the rumen of sheep (and cattle, goats and other similar animals), resulting in a lack of vitamin B_1, also called thiamine. This vitamin is vital for brain function and a shortage of it results in behaviour changes, such as blindness, aimless wandering, 'star-gazing' and death. This can be treated, but not all affected animals survive. Adequate fibre in a new diet can help to prevent this condition.

Meningitis

Meningitis is an infection of the tissues that surround the brain; it is serious and often fatal. Young lambs are most likely to contract meningitis. The infection spreads to the brain from infected tissue elsewhere in the body, for example a wound, the umbilicus, lungs or guts. Signs of meningitis include:

- Depression
- Lethargy
- Seizures

Immediate veterinary attention is necessary, but some affected animals will die even with good treatment. The prevention of meningitis requires prompt treatment and prevention of other infections in newborn lambs, for example good hygiene, colostrum and navel management.

Water restriction

Lack of access to water can result in 'salt poisoning', which will cause diarrhoea, abdominal pain and behaviour changes, such as tremors, circling, incoordination and seizures. This condition can easily become fatal and requires immediate veterinary attention.

Scrapie

Scrapie has received a lot of media attention and research because of its relationship to bovine spongiform encephalopathy (BSE). A blood-testing campaign in the UK, to detect sheep that are genetically susceptible to scrapie and remove them from the national breeding flock, has significantly reduced the disease. Signs of scrapie develop very slowly over months or years, with weight loss, vagueness, head tremors, incoordination and unexplained itchiness.

This is a notifiable disease, therefore if a vet suspects that a sheep is suffering from scrapie they are obliged to report it to the authorities.

Liver disease

Occasionally, severe liver disease will cause changes in behaviour, because of the accumulation of toxins, such as ammonia, in the blood. These toxins disrupt the function of the brain. In sheep, common causes of liver disease include 'twin lamb' disease in pregnant ewes and liver fluke. Prompt veterinary attention is required.

Hairy shakers (lambs)

Some lambs, born to ewes infected with border disease virus during pregnancy, are born with an unusual fleece and a tremor; they are referred to as 'hairy shakers'. These lambs are unlikely to thrive and will often spread border disease to the rest of the flock. Border disease diagnosis and control should be discussed with a vet.

Louping ill

A virus carried by ticks causes louping ill. This virus enters a sheep's system when an infected tick feeds on the sheep. The virus can affect the brain, causing incoordination, paralysis and convulsions. It is a difficult condition to treat and affected animals should be seen by a vet; some animals will need to be humanely euthanased to prevent them from suffering a distressing death. If this virus is a problem locally, tick control and louping ill vaccination should be considered for your flock; discuss these with your local sheep vet.

Leg weakness and paralysis

Weakness or paralysis make it difficult for an animal to stand on or move affected legs; they may drag these limbs along the ground. Back legs are affected more frequently than front legs, and lambs more often than older animals. Affected animals must be examined by a veterinary surgeon.

Common causes in lambs include:

- Spinal abscesses: infection spreads to the spine from other parts of the body. This can happen in two ways: through the bloodstream, or by local spread from a wound close to the spine, e.g. docked tails or injection site abscesses
- Swayback in young lambs is the result of copper-deficient diets in pregnant ewes. Lambs become increasingly incoordinated and weak, especially in the back legs. Treatment and prevention require copper supplementation, but do not provide sheep with supplementary copper unless a vet has confirmed copper deficiency in your ewes, because excessive copper is poisonous to sheep
- White muscle disease in lambs is due to dietary selenium deficiency, especially in the diet of the ewes before the lambs are born. Lambs will experience sudden stiffness and pain in the limbs, or suddenly die. Treatment and prevention require selenium supplementation, but do not provide sheep with supplementary selenium unless a vet has diagnosed a deficiency on your farm, as too much selenium is toxic to sheep

Sheep 6 to 18 months old can suffer from sarcocystosis, caused by *Sarcocystis tenella*, a single-cell parasite deposited onto sheep pasture in dog faeces. This condition can cause loss of function of the back legs and sometimes the front legs. To reduce the risk of this disease, prevent dogs from eating raw sheep meat and remove dog faeces from sheep pasture wherever possible.

Adult sheep rarely have trouble with limb paralysis and weakness. However, some of the conditions implicated when these symptoms are seen include:

- Kangaroo gait, in ewes with lambs at foot, is a temporary loss of function of the front legs; the cause is not fully understood. The ewe needs to be examined by a vet and kept on a soft surface, with good-quality feed and water until she recovers, which can take up to six weeks. The lamb(s) should be weaned onto artificial milk replacer, and/or lamb pellets and forage
- Maedi visna can occasionally cause the slow deterioration of limb function. See 'Slowly progressing viral infections' above for more details

- Scrapie can cause the slow deterioration of limb function. See above for more details

UNPREDICTED DEATHS

How to know whether a sheep is dead

It can sometimes be difficult to be sure that an animal has died, but it is less distressing once the death is certain. Here are some of the things that can be done to confirm a death. When making these checks, gloves and other personal protective clothing should be worn:

- Watch the sides closely to see whether there is any movement to indicate breathing
- Feel immediately in front of the nostrils to check for movement of air
- Find something very light and thin, for example a soft piece of hay or a strand of cotton wool; hold this over one nostril at a time to see whether it is blown away from the nostril by a breath
- Make a loud noise close to the ear
- Touch the eye to see whether there is a reaction
- Pinch the nose or put a piece of straw up the nose and watch the eyes for a reaction

If you are still unsure, call out the local vet to check.

When a dead sheep is found

- Do not allow other animals or children access to the body
- Only handle the body with sufficient personal protective equipment, such as overalls and gloves
- Request a professional post-mortem examination by the vet or local post-mortem provider; or
- Dispose of the carcass by appropriate means according to local regulations

There are lots of reasons that a sheep might die, with or without any previous signs of disease. This can be distressing for those of us who are fond of our animals. However, an unexpected death, whilst unfortunate, can be used to protect the rest of the flock. Good communication with your local sheep vet and a post-mortem examination can help with putting the right preventative measures in place to limit any further losses.

Predation by foxes, badgers, dogs and even eagles can result in the death of sheep. However, signs of predation do not confirm that the predator killed a sheep; these predators will also take advantage of animals that are sick or already dead. A carcass with signs of predation that is subjected to post-mortem examination may give some useful information about the health status of the sheep if the majority of the carcass is still intact. However, if the majority of the carcass is damaged, a post-mortem will not be beneficial.

Whilst a post-mortem examination is a useful exercise to protect the rest of a flock, do not be disheartened if it does not always give a conclusive answer – even a negative post-mortem finding can be of value. For example, finding no signs of liver fluke in a sheep is positive information for the flock as a whole.

Infectious causes

Clostridial diseases

Bacteria belonging to the *Clostridium* family are found in soil everywhere and cause disease throughout the world. The majority of these bacteria usually cause sudden death, therefore prevention is essential.

There are a number of vaccines available against clostridial diseases and when used according to the manufacturer's instructions, these provide good protection (see 'Vaccines' in Chapter 8). Soil disturbances increase the likelihood of these diseases occurring, so sheep must be up to date with their clostridial vaccines if earthworks are planned in fields that they graze.

Liver fluke

Infection by large numbers of liver fluke in a short space of time will cause rapid death in sheep; this is normally seen in late summer, autumn or early winter. See above in 'Thin sheep' for more detail.

Pasteurellosis

Pasteurella-type bacteria cause a range of syndromes in sheep, including respiratory disease (see 'Respiratory disease' above), septicaemia and sudden death, especially in sheep under 1 year old. These bacteria live in the environment and in the airways of sheep under normal circumstances; they only cause disease at times of stress, for example when the weather changes suddenly or there is a sudden change of management.

Haemonchosis

This gut worm does not cause diarrhoea but anaemia, weight loss and sometimes sudden death. Severely affected sheep are pale, depressed, weak and breathe rapidly. See 'Diarrhoea' above for more details.

Feed-related

Grain overload

Sheep that have found large quantities of cereal grains or concentrate feed to eat may become bloated and die within 24 to 72 hours (see the 'Whole abdomen enlargement' section of 'Lumps and swellings' below).

Brassica feeding

Many vegetables from the brassica family make good forage crops for sheep (Fig. 7.24) – these can be grazed straight out of the ground. However, if sheep are suddenly moved onto a diet made up solely of brassicas, disease and death can result. Signs of toxicity include red-coloured urine, breathlessness, weakness and skin swelling or irritation. To reduce the risk, sheep can be introduced to the diet gradually over a week; and should be given an alternative feed source alongside the brassicas, for example a small area of grass to graze or forage such as straw, hay or silage.

Sudden diet changes (cerebrocortical necrosis or polioencephalomalacia)

Sudden diet changes can disrupt the natural balance of microbes that live in the rumen, resulting in a lack of vitamin B_1, also known as thiamine, an essential vitamin for brain function. See 'Behavioural changes' above for more details.

Magnesium deficiency ('staggers')

Heavily pregnant or lactating ewes on fast-growing grass are at risk of magnesium deficiency. Affected animals are normally found dead because they die very quickly. If they are found

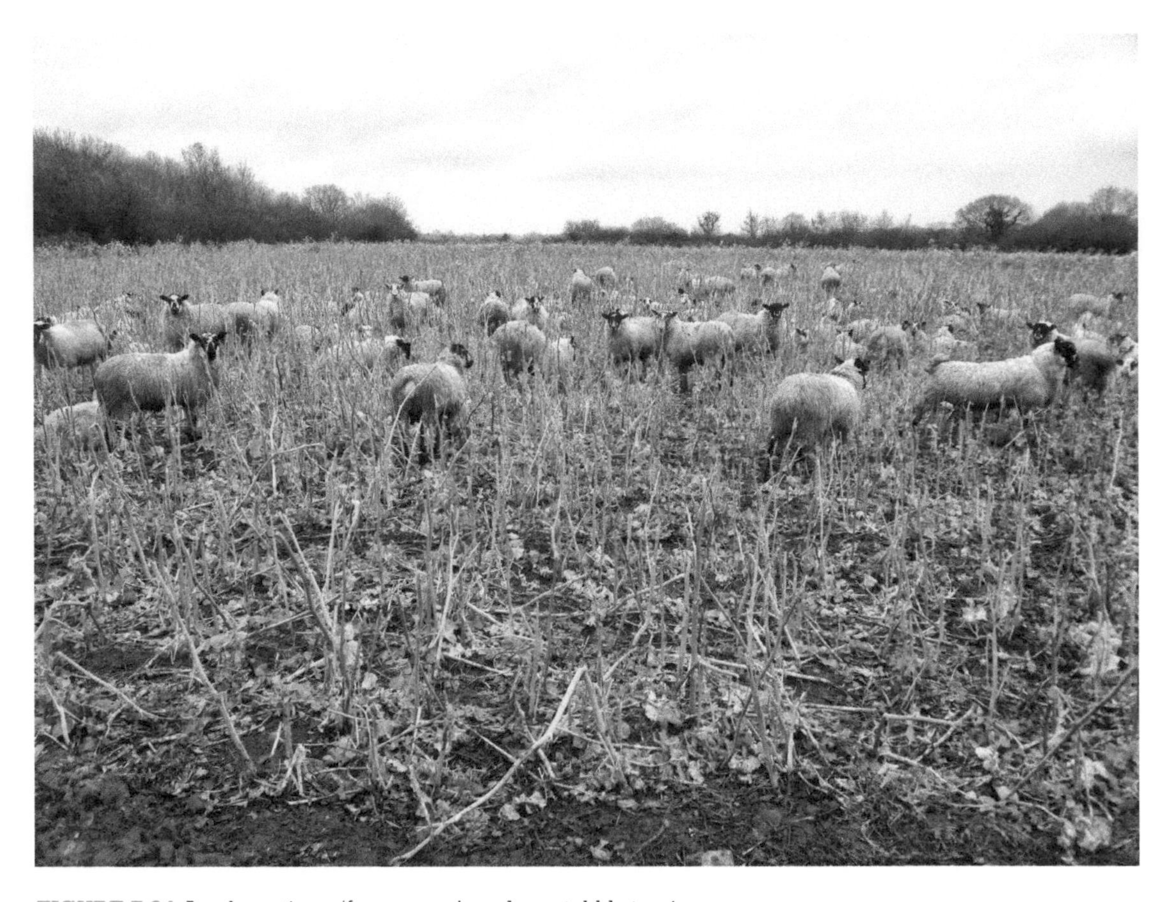

FIGURE 7.24 Lambs eating a 'forage crop', such as stubble turnips.

alive, symptoms can include muscle twitching, seizures and paddling the legs while lying flat. Treatment is needed immediately, so call the vet. If there is injectable magnesium available, this should be administered at the recommended sheep dose under the skin while waiting for the vet. If the vet has diagnosed this disease on your farm in the past, it is worth discussing methods of magnesium supplementation with them.

Hypocalcaemia and twin lamb disease

Insufficient calcium and/or energy in the diet of heavily pregnant ewes can cause diseases that are fatal, unless they are treated promptly. See 'Diseases of ewes around lambing time' in Chapter 6 for more details.

Selenium/vitamin E deficiency ('white muscle disease')

Selenium deficiency tends to occur in defined geographical areas. The animals at greatest risk from this syndrome are rapidly growing lambs, especially if their mothers had a selenium- and/ or vitamin E-deficient diet during pregnancy. Affected lambs suffer from muscle contractions. Symptoms include:

- Sudden stiffness, discomfort and an inability to keep up with the rest of the group, if limb muscles are affected
- Sudden death if the heart muscle is affected

The local sheep vet will be able to diagnose this disease by examining affected animals, and taking samples from live and dead animals. Appropriate treatment and prevention should be discussed with the vet, but sheep should not receive any supplements unless this condition has been confirmed because over-supplementation is toxic.

Redgut

Lambs can suffer from major disruption of the guts, which causes them to die rapidly. This happens in young orphan lambs being fed artificial milk replacer and lambs on energy-rich diets. The vet will be able to confirm the diagnosis via post-mortem investigation. Lambs must be fed milk/high-energy diets, so preventative measures can include provision of high fibre forage, such as hay or straw; feeding orphan lambs milk little and often, rather than large infrequent feeds; and feeding milk cold from 7 days of age (decrease the temperature gradually so that they become accustomed to it).

Poisoning

Plant poisoning

Apart from normal feed substances, many ornamental plants and trees are poisonous to sheep, as shown in Table 7.4.

Table 7.4 Common plants in the UK that are poisonous to sheep.

PLANT	SIGNS OF POISONING	COMMENTS
Rhododendron and laurel	Vomiting, depression, nervous signs, lying down, seizures and death	
Bracken	Blindness, ill thrift, depression, exercise intolerance, reduced appetite, anaemia and tumours	Sheep are less likely to eat large quantities of bracken than cattle
Yew	Sudden death	
Laburnum	Pain, muscle spasms, salivation, incoordination, regurgitation and diarrhoea	
Hemlock	Diarrhoea, regurgitation, salivation, breathing alterations (fast or irregular), incoordination, weakness	
Green potatoes	Diarrhoea, incoordination, seizures and death	
Acorns	Abdominal pain, anorexia, weight loss, swellings and constipation followed by black, tarry faeces	Storms can increase the number of acorns and oak leaves on the ground. Individual sheep may get a taste for them
Buttercups	Drooling, blistering in the mouth, coughing, diarrhoea, incoordination	Sheep do not choose to eat buttercups unless no other food is available

Table 7.4 continued.

Dock leaves	Incoordination, weakness, muscle spasms, nasal discharge, abnormal breathing	Sheep do not choose to eat docks unless no other food is available
Dog's mercury	Dullness, green diarrhoea	Sheep do not choose to eat this unless no other food is available
Nightshades – deadly, black or woody	Dry, scaling skin, thirst, incoordination, death	
Ragwort	Liver disease	Normally only eaten when dried, for example in hay or silage, but is still toxic
Privet	Colic, lying down, loss of use of hindlimbs, death	Access to tree/hedge trimmings can be a source
Other ornamental shrubs: oleander, pieris	Death	Access to garden trimmings can be a source

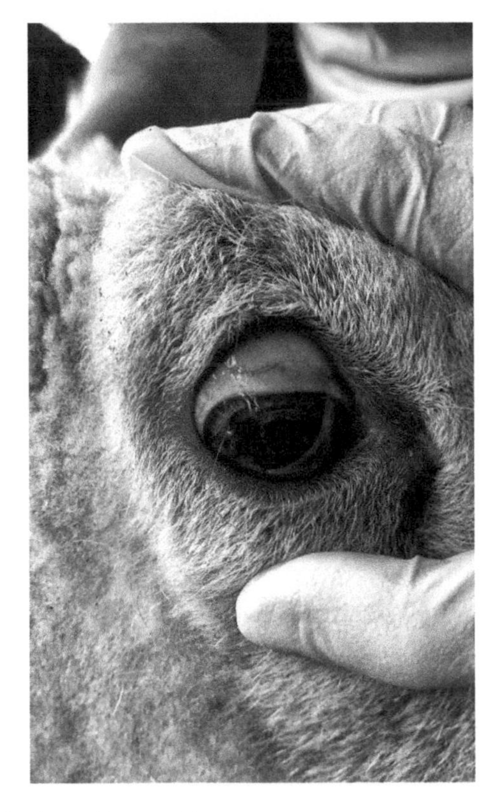

FIGURE 7.25 Sheep with copper poisoning normally become jaundiced, turning yellow around the eyes and inside the lips.

Non-plant poisoning

COPPER

Copper toxicity is normally seen after sheep have received an excess of copper in the diet over several weeks or months; the resulting disease and death are very rapid (Fig. 7.25). Some breeds of sheep are particularly susceptible to copper poisoning, for example Texel and North Ronaldsay. Common sources of extra copper for sheep include cattle feed, pig feed (sheep should not be fed either of these) and unnecessary supplementation. Some affected sheep will have a brief period of depression and anorexia before death, but most are found dead with orange discolouration of the gums and the white part of the eyes. A veterinary post-mortem is needed with subsequent laboratory testing to confirm the diagnosis. Speak to a vet about possible sources of copper if copper toxicity is found in a flock.

LEAD

Sources of lead for sheep:

- Old fashioned lead paint
- Battery packs
- Fields on the site of disused lead mines

Signs of lead poisoning:

- Anorexia
- Colic
- Incoordination and stiffness

Action:

- Call your vet immediately

Prevention:

- Remove all sources of lead from stock housing and fields
- Do not disturb soil around disused lead mines

SELENIUM TOXICITY

Selenium toxicity is unusual in the UK as selenium-rich plants are not common, however over-supplementation is possible and should be avoided by proper testing and, if supplementation is needed, providing only one source of selenium.

SKIN DISEASE

How to spot an itchy sheep

Abnormally itchy sheep, or as vets call them 'pruritic' sheep, need to be distinguished from those that just have a quick scratch. Like humans, sheep get an occasional itch that needs scratching, but where humans have hands to do this, sheep will use their hind hooves, teeth or horns if they can reach, otherwise they use fence posts, gates, trees or other solid items in their environment. Pruritic (abnormally itchy) sheep:

- Keep scratching for longer than normal
- Will scratch repeatedly
- May have a moth-eaten appearance, where areas of wool or hair have been rubbed
- Will eventually acquire bald patches, where the wool or hair has been rubbed away
- May have areas of raw and inflamed skin due to scratching
- Might suddenly move or run away from nothing, as though they feel uncomfortable in a certain area of their body

Skin signs for which the vet should be called

- Any itchy sheep
- Crusty, dry, flaky areas of skin with hair loss, and maybe wart-like growths
- Darkened, damp areas of fleece, which when parted reveal an unpleasant smell, discharge or maggots
- Maggots
- Ticks
- Any unpleasant discharge (fluid) coming from any lesion, i.e. smelly, white, yellow, brown, green, red or black in colour
- Swelling of the head, ears or legs
- Sore, raw-looking lumps or ulcerations around the mouth, eyes, teats or feet
- Wounds around the face, neck, anus, scrotum, penis or udder and deep wounds on the legs
- Wounds that go deeper than the skin
- Anything that causes concern or where the animal is evidently unwell or uncomfortable

Sheep scab

Sheep scab is caused by a mite called *Psoroptes ovis*, which burrows through the skin. These mites cause extreme irritation for sheep, therefore in the UK it is a legal requirement to treat the disease as soon as it is found. Some parts of the UK have more regulation than others, so it is important to be aware of the regulations in the local area. Information on this should be available from the local sheep vet.

Risk factors for sheep scab:

- Contact with infected sheep, for example:
    - While grazing common land
    - New sheep brought into the flock
    - Sheep belonging to neighbours, through fencing
    - Birds dropping infected wool on fields from other farms
- Places that infected sheep have inhabited less than 17 days previously (this is the length of time that the mites can survive in the environment, for example on posts, the ground, gates or trees)

Since it takes time for the number of mites to build up on newly infected sheep, there is a time delay between animals catching sheep scab and becoming itchy; this delay can be from several weeks to a few months.

Signs of sheep scab:

- Extreme scratching/itching, but it can be less extreme if the animal has been infected with sheep scab before
- Patches of wool loss
- Crusty, yellow scabs form on the skin
- Weight loss
- The condition is normally seen when the wool is long in winter or spring

Action to take if there are abnormally itchy sheep in your flock:

- Call the vet for testing and treatment advice
- Once sheep scab infection has been confirmed, all the sheep that have been in contact with the affected animals within the previous few months must be treated
- The available treatments are discussed in Chapter 8, 'Sheep scab'

Other mites

There are a number of other mites that can cause discomfort and infection in sheep. These have a variety of impacts and some of the more common mites are listed below.

Chorioptic mange mites can cause mild itchiness with thickening of the skin and crusting on the lower parts of the legs, the head and the scrotum. These mites are particularly problematic in rams because infection of the scrotum can adversely affect their fertility, so look out for signs of thickened skin and itchiness when buying new sheep. Seek veterinary advice if any abnormally itchy sheep are noticed in the flock.

Demodex mange mites can cause hair loss, nodular lumps and scaling of the skin on the face. Sometimes these areas are also itchy. This rarely causes severe problems in sheep but can mimic other skin diseases, so it is important to ask a vet to confirm the diagnosis.

Forage or harvest mites come from hay, straw or pasture and cause mild itchiness wherever they go on the body. This can lead to hair loss or a moth-eaten appearance of the wool.

Control is very difficult, but if the source can be identified it is best to prevent sheep from having contact with it. These mites can be seen with the naked eye as bright orange dots about the size of a pinhead.

Lice

Lice generally live on the shaft of the wool or hair and tend to move away from light if the wool is parted. They either chew the skin (the most common type in the UK), or suck blood (less common) and cause mild irritation. Lice normally become problematic when an animal's immune system is not functioning very well. Common things that can result in this immunosuppression include:

- Stress – mixing groups, bullying, high stocking density, etc.
- Poor nutrition
- Other diseases

Signs of 'chewing' lice include:

- Moderated itchiness – this can be confused with sheep scab, so the vet should be called as a veterinary diagnosis is always necessary
- Chewing lice are about 2 mm long and can be seen with the naked eye in woolly areas
- Later winter and early spring

Strategies for reducing the number of lice on an animal can include turning them out into heavy rain as the majority of the lice will be destroyed by the soaking. However, for debilitated animals that are unwell for other reasons, this action is not recommended. Alternatively, pour-on treatments are available and can relieve an animal of the burden of heavy lice infestation. Shearing also reduces the number of lice in a flock. Seek veterinary advice about treatment for lice.

Preventing excessive lice burdens in sheep involves maintaining good general flock health through:

- Good nutrition
- Reduced stress
- Control of other diseases
- Shearing in late spring

Other types of lice are rarely seen in the UK but some of these might be visible on the head or legs if they are present. If there are any concerns about the health of a flock, the local vet should be called.

Blowfly strike

Fly larvae, or maggots, can cause severe, even fatal, disease in sheep and this is colloquially known as blowfly strike. It is an extremely painful condition that must be prevented whenever possible, and treated promptly when it does occur. Blowfly strike can occur whenever flies are active, therefore late spring, summer and early autumn are high-risk periods, but exact timings are climate and weather dependent; the warmer the conditions, the longer the period of fly activity. The blowflies, like other types of fly, are attracted to dirty, damp wool or wounds where they lay their eggs (Fig. 7.26). Larvae hatch from these eggs 24 to 48 hours after they are laid and grow into visible maggots within 72 hours (Fig. 7.27). Ideal conditions for blowflies can be created by:

- Diarrhoea staining of the fleece
- Urine staining

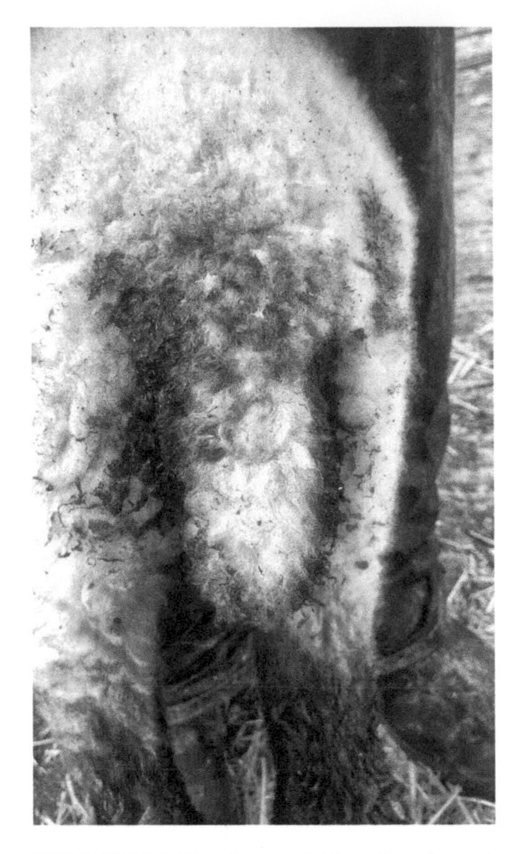

FIGURE 7.26 Blowfly eggs laid on dirty fleece in a lamb with diarrhoea.

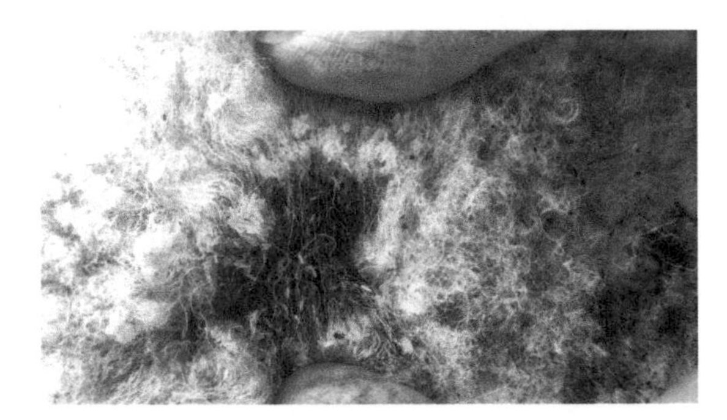

FIGURE 7.27 Hatched blowfly larvae.

- Dipping with dirty sheep dip
- Footrot or CODD lesions in feet (Fig. 7.28)
- Infected feet sitting next to the skin underneath a sheep while they are laid down

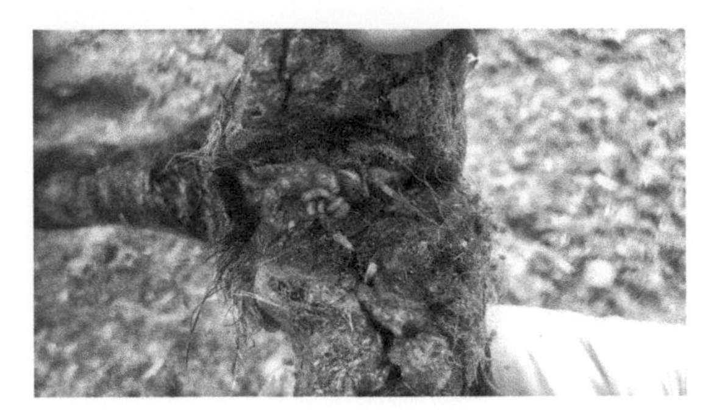

FIGURE 7.28 Maggots in a sheep's foot – call a vet to attend these cases as soon as possible.

The maggots feed on the tissue around them in a wound, destroying muscle or other organs in their path and releasing toxins that make the affected animal extremely unwell. Signs of these migrating maggots include:

- Uncomfortable, irritated sheep that appear to run away from nothing
- A patch of slightly discoloured, damp wool
- An unpleasant smell
- Dullness and depression in later stages of disease
- Tail wagging

Lesions can be very extensive under the wool, with large areas of underrun skin, therefore veterinary involvement is necessary to assess and treat the animal. The following steps may be included in your vet's treatment plan, and it is possible to perform steps 1 to 4 and 6 while waiting for the vet to arrive:

1. Remove the wool over the wound by clipping or shaving it, until there is a 10-cm gap of normal skin around the lesion – this can help to avoid underestimating the size of the wound.
2. Remove all of the maggots.

3. Flush the wound with disinfectant diluted in warm water, using a syringe (do not scrub the wound, just flush it).
4. Pat the area dry.
5. Give antibiotics, anti-inflammatories and apply wound dressing according to the vet's advice.
6. Provide good food (e.g. hay and a small amount of concentrate feed, or good grass) and fresh water within easy reach of the animal.
7. Monitor the sheep carefully for several days.

Many sheep with large blowfly strike lesions will not survive, therefore, in some cases, the vet may decide that humane euthanasia is in the best interest of the animal in order to prevent unnecessary suffering. Discuss this option with the vet, as they will be able to assist in the decision as to whether the sheep is likely to survive. Where a decision is made to treat the animal but it continues to deteriorate, it may be necessary to reassess this decision within one or two days. The reassessment should also be discussed with the vet.

Prevention of blowfly strike can include:

- Shearing at the appropriate time
- Preventing wounds
- Protecting wounds from flies with:
    - Fly repellents
    - The application of blowfly strike preventative treatments around wounds (not in them)
    - Housing the sheep
- Controlling diarrhoea
- Prevention and prompt treatment of lameness
- Blowfly strike preventative treatments (see Chapter 8 'Blowfly strike')

Other flies

Flies that do not cause blowfly strike can still be a nuisance, irritating sheep around the eyes or horns, and making superficial wounds worse. Dipping sheep or applying a small amount of a pour-on to the back of the head can help to control nuisance flies (do not allow the pour-on to go anywhere near the sheep's eyes).

Keds

Keds look like flies but have no wings. They are 5–7 mm long and reddish-brown in colour. These insects live on sheep permanently and suck blood; they cause irritation in small numbers and anaemia (blood loss) in large numbers. Most control measures for sheep scab or blowfly strike will prevent keds as well.

Nasal bots/*Oestrus ovis*

This is a fly that is normally found in warm, temperate climates, therefore the southern parts of the UK are most likely to be affected. These large grey flies have black spots and deposit larvae in sheep's nostrils, where they migrate into the sheep's sinuses to develop. The adult flies cause sheep to huddle with their heads close together, press their noses to the ground, run away from the flies, shake their heads and stamp their feet.

Many affected sheep will not show many signs, but a few may have a discharge from one or both nostrils and sneeze or rub their noses on the ground and occasionally more serious signs can follow.

Treatment is rarely needed. Seek veterinary attention for any sheep with a discharge from the nose or sneezing as other diseases can also cause these signs.

Ticks

Ticks in the UK have hard shells and three life stages: larval, nymph and adult. Each life stage will take one blood meal once a year from a mammal or bird before it transforms into the next life stage. The ticks attach to the chosen blood source for a few days before falling off again. Ticks are active in warm (over 7°C), damp conditions, therefore the spring and autumn are times of peak tick activity. However, in some parts of the UK these conditions are present for most of the year and so ticks can be active at any time.

For small mammals, such as young lambs, large numbers of ticks can cause anaemia (lack of blood), but the main problem with ticks is the diseases that they spread from one mammal to the next. These include:

- Tick pyaemia – causing severe joint ill or spinal abscesses in lambs
- Tick-borne fever – causing severe diarrhoea in young lambs and tick pyaemia
- Louping ill – causing brain or nerve-related diseases and abortion in pregnant ewes that have not been exposed to louping ill before
- Babesiosis – transmitted to sheep by ticks but disease is rarely seen in sheep in the UK
- Q fever – causing abortion in pregnant ewes (and women)
- Lyme's disease – a risk to human health (see 'Sheep diseases that can affect humans' below)

Orf

Orf is a painful disease commonly found in young lambs and lactating ewes, caused by a parapox-virus. Orf can cause painful disease in humans as well so it is vital to always wear gloves when handling affected animals, the scabs from sheep or the orf vaccine.

The orf virus causes protruding, raw, pink, hairless areas of skin that are painful, often ulcerated, and sometimes look like multiple inflamed warts clustered together. The location of these lesions affects the impact that they have on the animal:

- Lambs with lesions around the mouth (Fig. 7.29) often stop suckling and eating because of the pain, which:

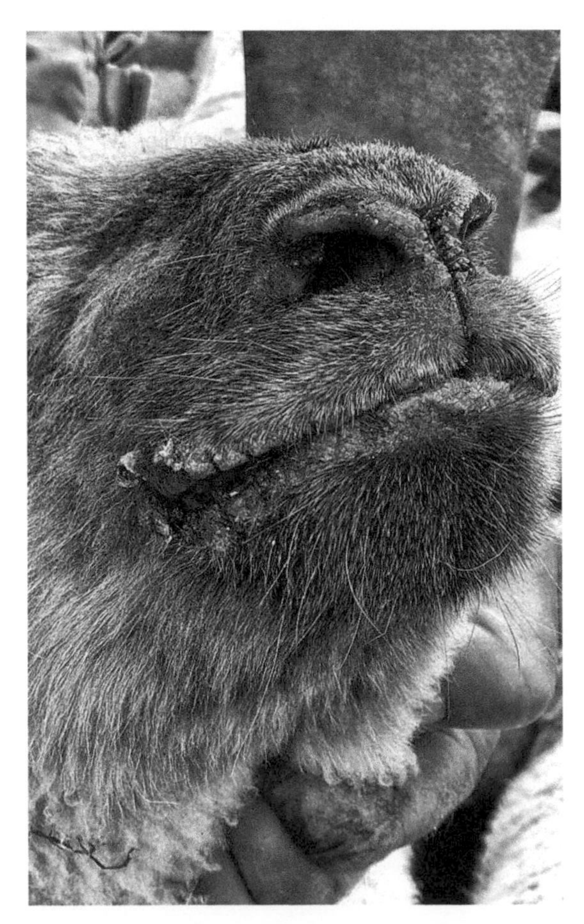

FIGURE 7.29 A lamb with orf affecting the mouth.

  - Reduces their growth rates
  - Increases their susceptibility to other diseases
  - Puts them at risk of dying of starvation

- Ewes can have lesions on their teats and so do not allow their lambs to suckle, so the first sign may be hungry lambs. It also makes ewes more likely to suffer from mastitis
- Lesions can develop on other parts of the body, for example legs (Fig. 7.30), ears or the head – lambs and rams are at most risk of developing these forms of orf and they can take a long time to resolve

Seek veterinary advice early if orf is suspected in a flock. Initial treatment may include:

- Anti-inflammatories
- Antibiotic spray on the affected areas
- Ensuring that lambs are getting plenty of milk, whether the lamb or its mother is affected
- Checking ewes for mastitis regularly and seeking veterinary assistance if this is suspected

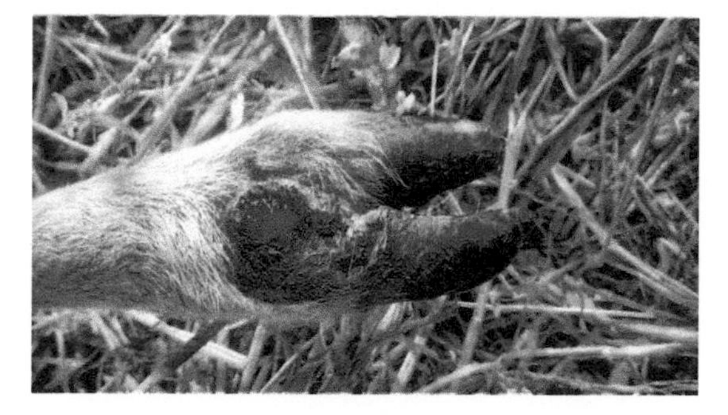

FIGURE 7.30 Orf can affect other parts of the body, including the legs.

Ask a vet to examine cases where:

- It is the first outbreak of orf, so that the diagnosis can be checked and appropriate treatment discussed
- Lambs do not begin to eat within 24 hours
- The lesions continue to grow after a week despite treatment
- Pus (a cream or yellow, thick discharge) is coming from the lesion(s)

The vaccine can be used during an outbreak to help prevent new cases, but must not be used on farms that do not see cases of orf, as it is a live vaccine and will introduce the disease to that farm. See Chapter 8 in 'Vaccines' for more details of the vaccine.

Orf can affect humans, so always wear gloves when handling affected animals or the vaccine.

Lumpy wool

Lumpy wool is a colloquial term for a bacterial skin disease that produces a sticky yellow discharge, which clumps the wool together. The bacteria that causes it is called *Dermatophilus congolensis*; this gets into the skin during prolonged wet weather or from dirty dipping solution.

Signs of lumpy wool include:

- Crusty skin
- Woolly areas: clumping of the wool, held together by yellow or grey scabs
- Face and ears: scaly, lumpy skin with a 'moth-eaten' pattern of hair loss

Treatment is not always necessary, especially in mild cases on the face and ears – however, if these become itchy or the lesions grow in size, ask a vet to examine the affected animals. If the skin of woolly areas is affected, call your local vet, especially if the sheep are at all itchy (see 'How to spot an itchy sheep' above).

Shelter for sheep during inclement weather can reduce the risk of these lesions developing. Forms of shelter can include mature hedges, trees or field shelters.

Other bacterial skin diseases

Bacterial infections of the skin can range from harmless pustules on haired or hairless areas, often seen in lambs and the equivalent to teenage spots, through to multiple hairless nodules in the skin of the cheeks and muzzle that may start to discharge pus. In extreme cases, serious deep invasions of the skin with abscesses that discharge pus or scabs with foul-smelling, green discharge underneath can be seen. Anything more serious than 'teenage spots' will need to be assessed by a vet and the more serious of these may require prolonged treatment.

Photosensitisation

Photosensitisation normally affects the white-haired or hairless areas of sheep and is caused by toxins in the skin being altered by sunlight and producing inflammation; these toxins are either released during severe liver disease or come from certain plants that sheep may eat, for example:

- St. John's wort
- Bog asphodel
- Ragwort
- Buckwheat
- An excess of lush green plants

Symptoms of photosensitisation include:

- Swelling of the face and ears, legs and sometimes the back of thin-fleeced sheep
- These areas become crusty with loss of hair or wool
- The skin eventually peels off

Ask a vet to assess affected animals; if photosensitisation is suspected, move these animals out of direct sunlight for up to three weeks.

Preventing this condition involves:

- Removing toxic plants from grazed pasture
- Ensuring sheep have a source of fibrous forage if they are grazing, particularly lush green grass in spring

Ringworm

Ringworm is a fungal skin disease that can affect many species of animal, including humans, therefore gloves should be worn when handling infected animals and hands and arms should be washed in disinfectant afterwards.

Sheep may suffer from ringworm because they have:

- Come into contact with infected sheep
- Come into contact with equipment or people who have been in contact with infected sheep
- Reduced immunity due to poor nutrition or other diseases

Ringworm usually occurs on haired areas and symptoms here include:

- Dry, flaky skin, often in a roughly circular shape
- Crusting and wart-like lesions

In woolly areas of the sheep it can be hard to see ringworm lesions, but when the wool is parted the skin is moist and inflamed. Ringworm is not normally very itchy, but due to the similarity in appearance of many skin diseases it is best to have affected animals checked by the local vet to confirm the diagnosis. The fungi are sensitive to sunlight, so many cases will resolve spontaneously when turned outdoors. The vet will be able to give advice about other treatment options.

Animals with ringworm should be kept together, away from the rest of the flock until all the lesions have fully resolved to prevent it from spreading. This condition is one of the many reasons to disinfect clothes and equipment and wash hands before and after contact with animals from other farms.

Wool slip

Sheep that have had a serious disease or been under stress can lose their fleece over the ensuing weeks. No treatment is required, but in cold weather affected sheep may need to be housed. If there is no clear reason why an animal is losing its wool, the local vet should be asked to examine the sheep; it is important to be cautious and ensure that they are not suffering from sheep scab rather than wool slip.

Wounds

The extent and location of a wound will determine what kind of treatment is necessary. Wounds around the face, neck, anus, scrotum, penis or udder and deep wounds on the legs will need to be examined by a vet (Fig. 7.31). Wounds that only involve the skin can usually be managed without veterinary involvement, but if there is any doubt, ask a vet to look at your unfortunate sheep.

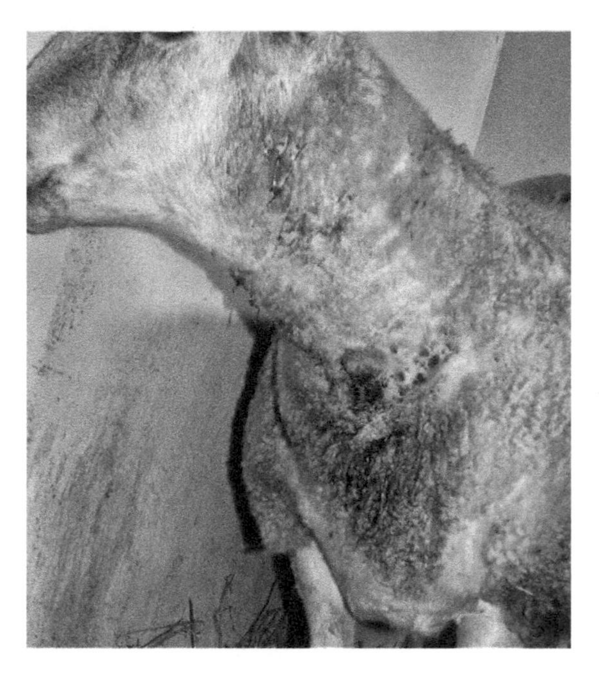

FIGURE 7.31 Dog bite wounds can be more serious than their surface appearance suggests and should be assessed by a veterinary surgeon.

To treat wounds at home:

- Clip away the surrounding wool
- Clean the wound with disinfectant diluted in warm water (povidone-iodine or chlorhexidine), removing any foreign material like grass, soil, hair or wool
- Check how deep the wound is to make sure that veterinary attention is not needed. Do this using a gloved hand that has been thoroughly cleaned in disinfectant
- Spray with antibiotic spray
- Inject the animal with anti-inflammatory and long-acting antibiotic – if the wound appears to be infected, ask the vet to examine it and prescribe the necessary treatment
- During fly season, house the animal or apply fly pour-on to the area around the wound (not on it)

Infected wounds can vary in how they look, so if you have any doubts at all, consult a vet. Any discharges, unpleasant smells or swellings can be indicative of an infection, however, the absence of these things does not mean a wound is not infected.

Bird attacks

Crows and magpies will occasionally take advantage of stationary animals, attacking wounds that are already present and making them worse, or creating new wounds particularly at the eyes and other sensitive parts of the body. Call a vet to assess and treat bird attack wounds as they are often deeper than they appear. After treatment, house affected animals away from these pests or cover the wound with a breathable material by sticking it to the surrounding wool. Check wounds daily.

LUMPS AND SWELLINGS

There are several causes of lumps and swellings in sheep. The most common are not normally life-threatening, especially with appropriate treatment. Some common examples include:

- Cysts
- Bruises
- Blood blisters
- Seromas – fluid-filled masses associated with trauma or bruising
- Abscesses

It is best to have swellings and lumps examined by a vet, especially if they are affecting the animal and you notice any of the following:

- The sheep is not eating or drinking normally
- They are struggling to pass faeces or urine
- There is a discharge from the lump
- There is damage to the skin over the lump
- The lump is painful to touch

A vet should see lumps that are in a sensitive area within a day or two, for example those near the mouth, nose, eyes, anus, udder, vulva or penis. Otherwise, the lump can be monitored for a couple of weeks. If it starts to affect the sheep as described above, or it does not begin to reduce in size within this time, the sheep should be examined by a vet.

Common surface lumps

Abscesses

Abscesses are common in sheep, often developing at the site of a recent injury or injection. Injection-site abscesses are unfortunately common and if abscesses are noticed at recent injection sites then the number of times a needle is used before being thrown away should be reassessed. It is also prudent to keep an eye on how clean the needles are each time they are used (Fig. 7.32). Lumps due to abscesses are often warm to the touch and painful; with time,

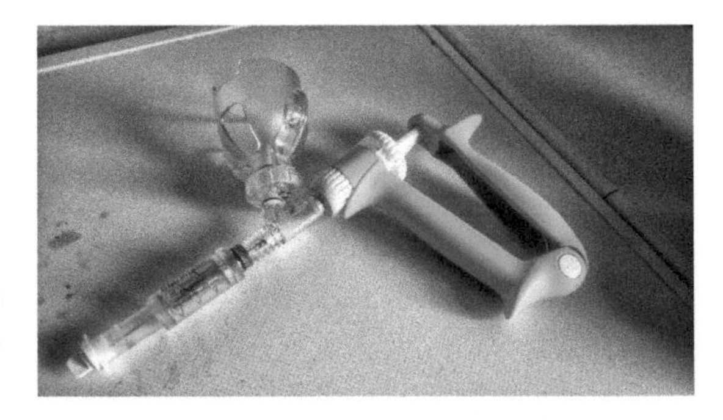

FIGURE 7.32 Needle sanitisation systems can reduce needle contamination when undertaking multiple injections.

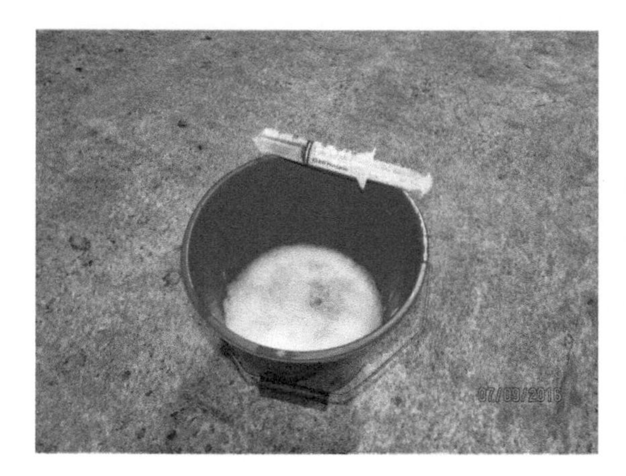

FIGURE 7.33 A large syringe can be used to flush a ruptured abscess with dilute disinfectant or salt water daily.

an area of skin over an abscess may lose its hair or wool, then become soft and discoloured; when this happens, the abscess is normally about to rupture. Ruptured abscesses benefit from daily flushing with salt water, using one teaspoon of salt in a pint of warm water (Fig. 7.33).

Caseous lymphadenitis (CLA)

Caseous lymphadenitis (CLA) is an infectious disease of sheep (and goats) that causes solid abscesses to form in lymph nodes, those either just under the skin or deep inside the body. Those deep inside the body cause more serious problems but are less common in the UK. Bacteria, *Corynebacterium pseudotuberculosis*, cause these abscesses (Fig. 7.34). Veterinary diagnosis requires laboratory testing. If CLA is found in a flock, then a sheep vet will be able to provide advice about control, but for sheep intended to be pets, rather than those intended for showing or breeding, the effect of this disease may be minimal and control might only involve the treatment of affected animals.

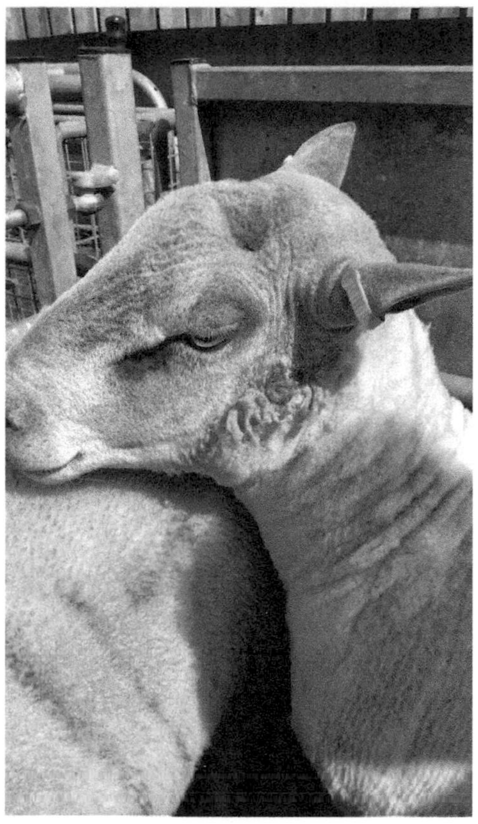

FIGURE 7.34 A ruptured abscess from a lymph node just behind the head of a ram is likely to be caused by CLA and will spread the causative agent into its surroundings.

Cancer

Cancerous tumours are rare in sheep, but become more common in older age. When they do occur, tumours must be monitored closely to ensure that they do not cause unnecessary suffering for the affected animal. Ask the vet to assess any long-term lumps and get them re-checked if anything changes, for example:

- The sheep is struggling to breathe, eat, drink, urinate or defecate
- The sheep appears unwell

- The skin over the lump is damaged
- The lump becomes large and heavy

Some cancerous tumours can be surgically removed, but your local vet will need to decide whether this is feasible depending on the location of the mass, its size and the overall health and age of the animal. When untreatable cancerous lumps affect an animal's quality of life, humane euthanasia will prevent unnecessary suffering. The vet will be able to assist in reaching this decision.

Whole abdomen enlargement

Some diseases can result in the enlargement of the whole abdomen, which is the area behind the ribs but in front of the back legs. Enlargement at the top of this area, along with rapid breathing may indicate a serious condition called 'bloat', which requires immediate emergency veterinary attention.

Bloat

Bloat is due to a build-up of gas or froth in the largest stomach, the rumen; this can compress other organs around it, and is life-threatening. Immediate veterinary attention is needed.

Risk factors for bloat include:

- Animals breaking into a grain or hard feed store
- Accidental overfeeding
- Sick animals leaving concentrate feed for just one or two animals to eat
- Grazing recently harvested cereal fields
- Grazing lush new grass fields with high clover content
- Low-fibre diets
- Occasionally, non-diet-related dysfunction of the digestive tract

Signs of bloat include:

- Depression and listlessness
- Loss of appetite
- Enlargement of the stomach/abdomen, especially at the top on the left hand side
- Rapid breathing, open-mouth breathing in serious cases
- Mild cases may only have diarrhoea with obvious undigested grains 24 to 48 hours later

Animals that have eaten excessive amounts of concentrate feed or cereal grains, or with the signs above, must be examined by a veterinary surgeon immediately. This is an emergency situation, especially when the abdomen is enlarged.

Prevention includes careful control of the diet, by:

- Preventing access to excessive amounts of concentrate or cereal-based feed
- Providing adequate dietary fibre

Excess fluid

Pendulous distention of the lower part of the abdomen may be due to an accumulation of fluid. Veterinary attention should be sought for affected animals, but unless the sheep is otherwise unwell, this is not an emergency.

Pregnancy

Unplanned pregnancies can occur 'out of season' if a ram has had access to ewes.

EYES

How to spot eye problems

Eye diseases need prompt detection and treatment as the eye is a delicate organ, which is easily damaged. However, eye problems can be difficult to pick up from a distance, so closer inspection is sometimes necessary. This can be done in conjunction with other care activities, such as worming.

Seek veterinary advice for all eye diseases, to confirm the diagnosis and for advice on treatment and control. Here are some of the telltale signs of eye problems:

- Weeping eyes – a wet or crusty area below the affected eye(s)
- One or both eyes held in a closed or partly closed position
- Swelling of the eyelids and sometimes the surrounding area
- Reddening of tissues around the eyes, especially inside the eyelids

For any condition of the eyes, seek veterinary attention as soon as practicable.

Infectious keratoconjunctivitis (IKC)

IKC is a common problem that will spread through a group of sheep within a few weeks and will sometimes continue to circulate despite effective treatment of affected animals. The infection spreads between animals when they are in close contact, for example during housing, trough feeding or gathering. Flies can also spread the infection from sheep to sheep.

Signs of keratoconjuncitivitis (Fig. 7.35):

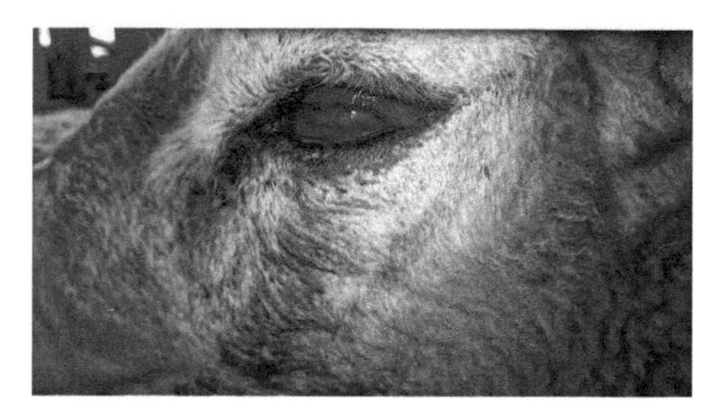

FIGURE 7.35 An infected eye, with a cloudy eye, pink conjunctiva and tear staining.

- Weeping eyes
- Partially or fully closed eyes
- Swollen eyelids
- The conjunctiva (pink mucosa inside the eyelids) looks reddened
- Eventually the eye becomes cloudy
- It can affect either one or both eyes

If these signs are encountered:

- Isolate affected sheep away from the rest of the flock until they have recovered completely
- Have a vet visit and inspect the flock to confirm the diagnosis and advise about treatment and control

To prevent the spread of infection:

- Reduce close contact between sheep
- Apply effective fly control

When buying new sheep, check all their eyes during the quarantine period. If any eye problems are seen, seek veterinary advice and delay moving these sheep into contact with the existing flock for as long as possible.

Silage eye

Listeria monocytogenes is a bacteria that can multiply in poorly-made silage; when this silage is fed to sheep, a number of disease syndromes can result. One of these is infection of the eyes. Signs of silage eye are initially similar to IKC:

- Weeping eyes
- Partially or fully closed eyes
- After a few days, the surface of the eyes become blue-white in colour

Eye injuries

Injury of the eyes or skin surrounding them must be taken seriously as these can quickly result in permanent blindness – seek immediate veterinary attention for eye injuries. Sheep do adapt very well to being partially or completely blind, but even if the eye cannot be saved, pain relief and antibiotic treatment are often needed to prevent excessive discomfort for the sheep.

Entropion – turned-in eyelids in lambs

Lambs with weeping, partially closed eyes could have a hereditary condition known as entropion. See 'Entropion' in Chapter 6 for details.

MISCELLANEOUS DISEASES

Getting stuck on their backs

This is an emergency situation.

Occasionally, adult sheep with a full fleece will get stuck on their backs; this is an emergency and the sheep should be rolled onto its front as quickly as possible. Sheep that have been on their backs for a while may appear disorientated and struggle to stand and may need to be supported for a couple of minutes, but if this has not resolved within 15 minutes, call the vet to examine the animal. There is sometimes an underlying reason for a sheep becoming stuck on its back, which will need to be assessed and treated by the vet.

Bladder stones

This is an emergency: veterinary attention must be sought immediately.

Male sheep fed high levels of concentrates or cereals, little fibre, on pasture that is high in clover or that have limited access to water, can develop bladder stones. Bladder stones are hard deposits of mineral in the bladder. During urination, these pass through the penis and can become lodged at narrow points, obstructing the flow of urine so that the bladder can no longer be emptied. This is often a fatal condition and affected male lambs or rams are in pain and quickly become unwell, separating themselves from the rest of the flock, showing signs of depression and anorexia. They strain to urinate repeatedly, but urine might only drip from the tip of the penis and this is often tinged pink.

Treatment must only be attempted in early cases that do not have evidence of kidney damage. Available treatments can be difficult and expensive, and there is potential for the blockage to recur once the urine begins to flow again. Affected animals must be assessed by a vet. This condition can be prevented by managing the diet of male sheep in consultation with the local sheep vet and/or a sheep nutritionist; always provide plenty of water and high fibre forage.

Rectal prolapses

Lambs can sometimes push a piece of bowel inside out from the anus (Fig. 7.36). This is uncomfortable for the lamb and can cause serious problems if it is not quickly corrected. Rectal prolapses look like pink or red sausages protruding under the tail of the lamb. Veterinary attention is required immediately and potential causes should be discussed. Causes can include:

- Diarrhoea
- Continual coughing
- Urinary conditions
- Tails docked too short

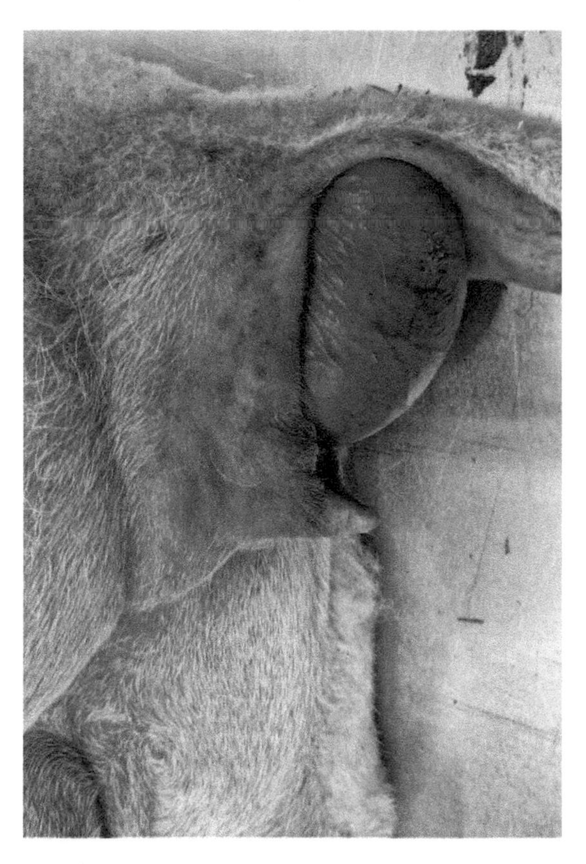

FIGURE 7.36 Rectal prolapses need prompt veterinary attention.

SHEEP DISEASES THAT CAN AFFECT HUMANS

Sheep, along with other animals, can carry microbes capable of causing disease in humans. Therefore it is very important to:

- Wash hands after handling sheep
- Wear gloves when lambing sheep or dealing with aborted material
- Never give the 'kiss of life' to any animal, especially not a newborn lamb
- Wear appropriate protective clothing (for example, wellington boots and washable overalls)

People with reduced immune function are at particular risk of acquiring diseases from animals and extra care should be taken to protect young children, elderly relatives, cancer sufferers and other vulnerable people. Diarrhoea and aborted material can be highly infectious and should be stored out of reach of people, dogs and other animals. Wear personal protective equipment (gloves, washable overalls) when handling this material.

Pet lambs

Newborn lambs are a source of temptation for many people, but weak lambs can carry infectious diseases that are harmful to humans. Avoid having these lambs in the house or being cuddled by small children. Pet lambs for children should be chosen from healthy lambs whose mother cannot support them.

Some of the specific diseases that sheep can pass to humans are discussed below.

Salmonella and *Escherichia coli*

Salmonella and *E. coli* can cause diarrhoea, abortion and septicaemia in sheep, or can be present without any signs at all. These bacteria are a major reason for the need to be vigilant with personal hygiene when handling sheep.

Infectious abortion (Enzootic abortion of ewes (EAE), toxoplasmosis, *Campylobacter, Salmonella*, Q fever)

Make sure that women who are pregnant, or who may be pregnant, do not come into contact with sheep within a month either side of lambing. Neither should they have any contact with clothing or equipment that has been near sheep at this time. Many of the diseases that cause abortion in sheep will cause abortion and serious disease in pregnant women.

Orf

People can catch orf from affected sheep and the orf vaccine. This virus causes very sore swellings of the skin. Gloves, long sleeves and trousers should always be worn when handling animals with orf or handling the vaccine. Ensure that your face is not touched while wearing the gloves!

Ringworm

Ringworm can cause a slightly flaky, reddened, circular area of skin in people, which may be itchy. In most cases it resolves within a few weeks. However, if it continues to grow or the person affected has a compromised immune system, medical attention should be sought.

Tick-borne diseases

There are several diseases that people can contract from ticks; in the UK, Lyme disease is the most common. When in tick areas, avoid contact with ticks by wearing closed shoes and long trousers tucked into socks. If a tick is found, this should be removed by twisting or levering it out the skin, ideally with a specially-designed tick remover (available from veterinary practices or outdoor activity stores), to avoid leaving the head behind. Once a tick has been removed from yourself or a member of your family, it should be kept in a sealed container for a couple of weeks. If you or anyone else feel unwell during this time, seek medical advice and take the tick along to the appointment.

8 PREVENTATIVE TREATMENTS

The purpose of disease prevention is to stop unnecessary loss and suffering in flocks. Preventative measures have general themes that may be applied to all diseases. These include:

- Good nutrition: this is the foundation of good health and welfare; feed quality is as important as sufficient supply
- Controlling the environment
    - Clean water provision
    - Good ventilation in housing
    - Minimising contact with faeces and urine
    - Preventing access to sharp objects
- Minimising stress
    - Avoid overcrowding
    - Avoid stressful handling
    - Provide shelter from inclement weather
- Preventing infection entering the farm from outside
    - Careful sourcing of new livestock
    - Good fencing and gates

WHAT FORMS CAN PREVENTATIVE TREATMENTS TAKE?

This chapter will discuss general products that are currently available, but not specific brands as these change regularly. Your local sheep vet will be able to advise you about specific products that are available. It is important to remember that the non-medical strategies for disease prevention mentioned above are essential and should not be substituted by medicines. These treatments rely upon animals being well fed and not overwhelmed by infection from unsanitary surroundings; they are not effective unless combined with good flock management.

All treatments have the potential to cause side effects as well as benefit an animal. The majority of side effects from medicines are far less harmful than the disease they are intended to treat or prevent: this is especially true of vaccines. Medicines should always be given at the recommended dose; do not adjust the dosage without consulting a veterinary surgeon.

Below is a list of preventative measures:

- *Vaccines:*
  These prime an animal's immune system, so that when the vaccinated animal encounters the disease its immune system already has some of the necessary weapons to fight it. This does not prevent an infection from getting into an animal's system, but should reduce the effect of that infection on the animal and reduce its spread to other animals
- *Antimicrobials:*
  Antibiotics and anthelmintics (or 'wormers') are examples of antimicrobials; these treatments control or kill infections that are already present in an animal. They reduce the damage and suffering that these infections cause and reduce their spread. Resistance[1] to antimicrobials is a growing problem, therefore they must only be used when absolutely necessary and must be used correctly
- *Lameness prevention:*
  A variety of treatments and management practices are combined to reduce the spread of infectious causes of lameness
- *Newborn lamb management:*
  Managing the environment for newborn lambs is very important for the prevention of neonatal diseases, as it is for any newborn animal

1 Resistance means that the chemical – antibiotic or anthelmintic – no longer works as effectively for treating a disease.

MAKING SURE THAT TREATMENTS ARE AS EFFECTIVE AS POSSIBLE

To ensure that treatments have maximum impact, it is important to follow the guidelines below and to ensure that treatments are combined with good health management practices. Treatments must be:

- Given at the correct dose for the weight of the animal
    - Have an appropriate set of weigh scales available
- Given in the correct way, as identified by the treatment instructions
    - By mouth
    - Injected under the skin
    - Injected into the muscle
    - Poured onto the skin
- Given at the appropriate time
- Stored as directed by the manufacturer
- Used whilst still in date/within the correct time from being opened

For smallholders that own just a few sheep, buying preventative treatments can be problematic due to large pack sizes. Often treatments are not expensive even if a pack of excess size needs to be purchased, however, it is possible for smallholders to coordinate treatment programmes and thereby make some cost savings. Working together with the local veterinary practice, it is possible for several smallholders to agree a set date for a specific treatment. The surgery will then open the treatment on that date, allowing each smallholder to collect what is needed for their own flock and split the cost between all parties. If undertaking this option, however, it is important to remember that most vaccines need to be used within a few hours of the bottle being opened, so timing is crucial.

NUTRITION

The quality and quantity of the food provided for sheep is key to having a healthy flock. If animals are well fed, they are better equipped to fight off infections. Sheep need a constant supply of high-fibre feed, in the form of grass, forage or other grazed fodder. Depending on the quality of this feed and the timing of the production cycle, additional energy, protein and minerals may be needed. See Chapter 4 'Diet and nutrition' for more detail.

VACCINES

There are a variety of diseases that sheep can be vaccinated against; which vaccinations are used depends on local risk and the purpose of the flock being treated. When deciding on the vaccination plan to be used, the most important consideration is animal welfare and prevention of unnecessary suffering. For example, pet sheep that are not intended for breeding do not need to be vaccinated against abortion, but breeding ewes in an area with outdoor cats and kittens should be vaccinated against *Toxoplasma* abortion.

Vaccines must be used according to the specific manufacturer's instructions (Fig. 8.1) as the incorrect use of vaccines is a waste of money. It is important that vaccine doses are given at the correct time intervals to ensure efficacy. If a dose is missed, the initial course should be restarted and followed up by timely boosters. It is also important to make sure that all 'at risk' animals are included in the vaccination programme and that the entire flock is suitably vaccinated. For example, many people forget to vaccinate their rams but with the exception of abortion vaccines, rams need the same vaccines as ewes.

Unless the manufacturer's instructions state otherwise, leave a gap of at least two weeks between administering different vaccines. This enables the sheep to produce an effective

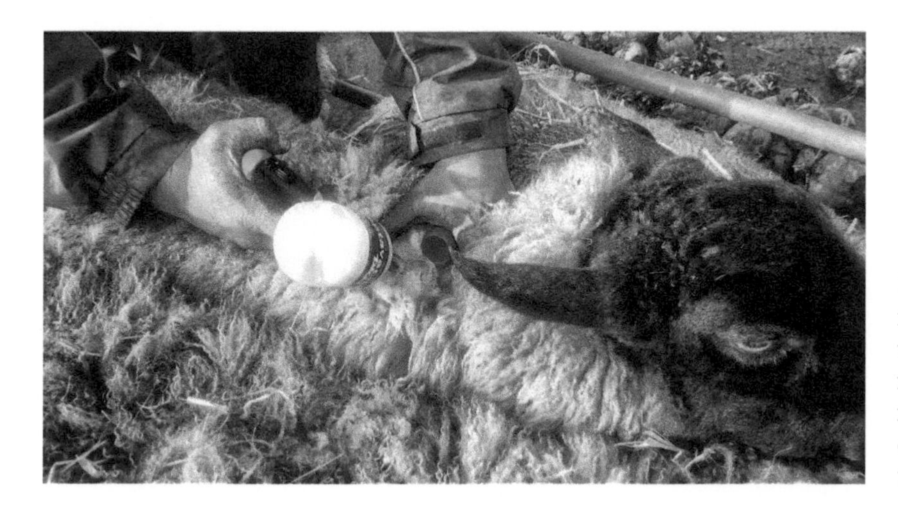

FIGURE 8.1 It is important to give vaccines by the route recommended by the manufacturers, for example by injection under the skin.

immune response to each individual vaccine without them interfering with each other.

Vaccine manufacturers go to significant lengths to keep vaccines at the correct temperature until they reach the client; for the vaccines to be effective, it is important that they remain at that temperature until they are administered. These vaccinations are intended for animal use only, so if human injection or use occurs, it is vital to seek medical advice immediately.

Clostridial diseases

Clostridial bacteria are found in soil and natural surroundings across the world, so it is not possible to eliminate contact with them. Outbreaks of clostridial diseases are generally seen after soil is disturbed in stock fields.

Sheep affected by a clostridial disease usually die quickly, which is why clostridial vaccines are important for all livestock and these vaccines are effective when used properly. There are a variety of products available that will protect vaccinated animals against three, four, seven, eight or ten different clostridial diseases at once, plus or minus two *Pasteurella*-type bacteria (see 'Pasteurellosis' below). All of these products include tetanus vaccination. Some vaccines are designed for lambs that are only intended for meat production, the rest are intended for young and adult sheep alike, so it is important to purchase the correct vaccine for your needs.

All initial courses of clostridial vaccines are composed of two injections, which are followed by annual boosters. Once a brand of clostridial vaccine has been selected, it is important to continue to use this vaccine and not to switch between manufacturers as there is currently no proof that booster vaccinations work across product brands. If you are going to switch vaccine, all sheep must be given a new initial course of the new vaccine (two injections) before starting annual boosters.

If lambs receive adequate colostrum, the first milk that protects newborn lambs from disease, within the first few hours of life from a correctly vaccinated mother, they are protected against these diseases until between 3 and 5 weeks of age. It is best to make use of this protective mechanism, as there is no other way of protecting lambs from clostridial diseases in the first few days of life. Once over 3 weeks old, lambs can begin their own vaccination course.

Pasteurellosis

As well as causing pneumonia, *Pasteurella*-type bacteria can result in sudden death due to septicaemia, so prevention is the best course of action. *Pasteurella* vaccines either come alone or in combination with the vaccinations for clostridial diseases.

Vaccine protection against pasteurellosis does not last as long as some of the other vaccines, so it is best to give them a short time before they are likely to be needed, for example before:

- Housing
- Weaning
- Changeable weather, for example autumn
- Any other period of stress

Vaccination is thought to reduce the disease, but not eradicate it.

Footrot

Footrot is a debilitating disease for sheep, which leads to severe lameness that can cause them to lose weight and become less productive. The footrot vaccine that is currently available includes all ten common UK strains of *Dichelobacter nodosus*, the cause of footrot. Where footrot is the main cause of lameness, vaccination can result in a significant reduction and is a recommended action in the recently developed 'Five-point plan' for footrot control developed by Dr Ruth Clements, a vet from 'FAI Farms'.

This vaccine causes a mild, short-lived fever shortly after vaccination and some animals develop a lump where the injection has been given. Therefore, the vaccine must be used carefully.

- Inject it under the skin of the neck, 2 to 3 inches behind the ear
- Do not use it within six weeks of:
  - Breeding
  - Lambing
  - Before shearing (so that shearing combs do not catch the lumps)

This vaccine can be given during an outbreak of the disease to help control it, however, prevention is still best practice and so should be planned into the management and prevention strategy for the year.

As with some of the other vaccinations discussed, the footrot vaccination programme commences with two initial injections, followed by boosters ahead of times of increased risk, for example when moving sheep into housing or during prolonged wet weather. Footrot boosters can be given from four to 12 months apart depending on the level of footrot in the flock.

Please note, sheep that have been vaccinated against footrot with the current vaccine 'Footvax' (MSD Animal Health™), should never receive an injection of current formulations of 1% moxidectin for parasite control, that is, Cydectin 1% (Zoetis™) or Zermex 1% (Downland™), as some will have an allergic reaction.

Orf

Orf causes painful raw growths around the mouths of lambs and udders of ewes, preventing lambs from suckling and thriving. The current orf vaccine is a 'live vaccine'; this means that it contains the live virus that can cause disease, which raises two concerns:

- Preventing human infection, as orf is very infectious to people as well as sheep. When using the vaccine:
  - Always *wear gloves*
  - Safely dispose of all contaminated materials as soon as possible after use
- Introducing orf into an orf-free flock: do *not* use the vaccine unless orf is already present in the flock

The live orf vaccine causes disease in vaccinated sheep in an area of the body where the consequences are minimal. The vaccine is scratched into the skin and orf should develop within 14 days; the scabs normally drop off within seven weeks. These scabs are infected with the orf virus, so vaccinated ewes should not be moved to the lambing shed or field until at least seven weeks after vaccination.

Read the manufacturer's instructions very carefully to check how to prepare the applicator, administer the vaccine, which animals to vaccinate and when. Both ewes and lambs may be vaccinated:

- Ewes vaccinated before lambing are less likely to develop orf lesions on their udder and pass the disease on to lambs
    - Vaccinate ewes no less than seven weeks before lambing is due to start
    - Do not move vaccinated ewes to the lambing area until seven weeks after vaccination
- Lambs
    - Can be vaccinated for orf at any age
    - Should be vaccinated in batches as the vaccine should be used within a few hours of opening

When applying the orf vaccine, the treatment should be scratched into the axilla, a sheep's equivalent to a human armpit, between the front leg and chest where there is no wool.

Abortion vaccines 1: Enzootic abortion of ewes

Enzootic abortion in ewes is an infectious cause of abortion that spreads between ewes at lambing time; ewes abort within a few weeks of their due date in the subsequent pregnancy. Vaccines for enzootic abortion in ewes (EAE) contain either:

- Live attenuated *Chlamydophila abortus*, which must be given at least four weeks before mating so as not to cause problems in pregnant ewes; or
- Inactivated bacteria. This can be used in pregnant and non-pregnant ewes (vaccinate up to four weeks before or from four weeks after breeding)

Whilst vaccination is effective, because it is possible for EAE to cause abortion a long time after ewes are exposed to the infection (usually at the following lambing), some ewes may be infected before they are vaccinated. Vaccination does reduce the number of these ewes that will abort, but it cannot prevent all these abortions.

Timing of vaccination:

- Over 5 months of age
- Less than four months before mating
- More than four weeks before mating if using the live or inactivated vaccine, and for inactivated vaccines, from four weeks after mating
- Revaccinate every three to four years
- Do not vaccinate ewes on antibiotic treatment with the live vaccine as the antibiotic will prevent the vaccine from working

When first vaccinating a flock:

- Vaccinate all the ewes in the first year
- Vaccinate all new ewes on joining the flock. This should be done annually

Be safe with the live vaccine as it can cause disease in humans:

- Wear gloves when handling the vaccine
- Pregnant women and people with immunosuppression should not handle the vaccine

Abortion vaccines 2: *Toxoplasma gondii*

Toxoplasma is a parasite that can spread to ewes from rodents or young cats and cause embryonic death early in pregnancy or abortion in the few weeks before lambing. The current *Toxoplasma* abortion vaccine is also live and cannot be used either during or within three weeks of pregnancy. When used properly, the vaccine is effective, preventing abortion and early loss of embryos.

Vaccinate ewes:

- Over 5 months of age
- Less than four months before mating
- More than three weeks before mating
- Revaccinate every two years

When first vaccinating a flock:

- Vaccinate all the ewes in the first year
- Vaccinate all new ewes on joining your flock. This should be done annually

Be safe, because this is a live vaccine and can cause disease in humans:

- Wear gloves when handling the vaccine
- Pregnant women and people with immunosuppression should not handle the vaccine
- Handle the vaccine with care – it can cause disease in humans if injected under the skin or squirted into the mouth or eyes

Ovine Johne's disease

Ovine Johne's disease is an incurable cause of weight loss and death in adult sheep, caused by *Mycobacterium avium* subspecies *Paratuberculosis*. Vaccination against *Mycobacterium avium* subspecies *Paratuberculosis* is only used in flocks that have a problem with Johne's disease and has been shown to be one of the most cost-effective ways to control this disease. Vaccination does not rid a farm of disease, but it does reduce the number of sheep affected and reduces the spread of the disease.

The current vaccine is inactivated, so cannot cause disease. To maximise protection, give the vaccine to lambs as soon as possible once they are over 4 weeks old.

The injection should be given under the skin (subcutaneous), not into deeper tissues; reactive lumps often form where the vaccine has been injected, and these can reach up to 5 cm in diameter after a couple of months. Roughly a quarter of animals will still have a lump several years later – in most sheep this is not a problem, unless they are intended for showing. Rarely, a lump might rupture; if this happens, bathe the area with dilute salt water (one teaspoon of salt per pint of water) and seek veterinary advice.

Caseous lymphadenitis

Caseous lymphadenitis (CLA) causes abscesses in the lymph nodes of sheep and goats; for more details of the disease, see 'Lumps and bumps' in Chapter 7. Vaccines for CLA are available in various countries including New Zealand and Australia, but not the UK, therefore a special import licence is required to bring them into and use them within the UK. The vaccines contain several strains of the causative agent *Corynebacterium pseudotuberculosis*, but these are strains encountered in the countries in which the vaccine is available, not necessarily the strains seen in the UK. Discuss vaccine options with your vet.

ANTIMICROBIALS

Antimicrobials are used to treat established infections, rather than stimulate the animal's immune system to attack the disease. It is important to avoid overuse of antimicrobials in order to limit the development of resistance.

This will enable these drugs to continue to prevent disease and death in the future. Therefore, antimicrobials should be used only under the guidance of a veterinary surgeon who has professional knowledge of sheep and knows your farm or smallholding.

Antibiotics

The use of antibiotics to prevent disease rather than treat it should be reserved for outbreaks of disease, when it is too late to control infection by management alone. In the long term, disease prevention is better achieved through good nutrition, hygiene and vaccination.

For example, during the lambing season, it is good practice to ensure that young lambs are born into a clean, dry environment with plenty of clean bedding or into a clean field. If an assisted lambing occurs, then good hygiene, including washing and disinfecting hands, lambing ropes, snares and other equipment, and wearing clean gloves, will contribute to ensuring that the process is as hygienic as possible, which is of benefit to the ewe and the lamb.

Diseases for which preventative antibiotics are used during disease outbreaks include:

- Watery mouth in lambs*
- Joint ill in lamb*
- Navel ill in lambs*
- Abortion due to bacterial infection of ewes
- Infectious kerato-conjunctivitis

*The best prevention for these diseases is good quality colostrum and navel management in the first few hours of life – see 'Newborn lamb management' below.

See guidelines for using antibiotics in Chapter 7.

ANTHELMINTICS

Roundworms – gut worms

Anthelmintics should be just one of the tools used to control gut worm infections, alongside rotation grazing, low stocking densities and high-protein diets. Eradication of gut worms from a sheep farm is not feasible with current technology; previous overuse of wormers, in an attempt to rid lambs of these parasites, has resulted in the worms developing resistance to pharmaceutical treatments, therefore, farmers have now had to learn to live with the parasites, while reducing the effect that they have on livestock.

Additional methods to prevent gut worms

Alternative forms of prevention can include:

- Good nutrition:
  - High-protein feeds aid the immune system
  - Some foods, such as chicory, have shown activity in reducing gut worm infections
- Graze lambs on low-risk pastures, such as:
  - New grass leys
  - Fields previously grazed by cattle or adult sheep (not lactating ewes)
  - Fields recently used to make hay, haylage or silage – known as 'aftermath'

Good practice to reduce resistance when using wormers

The development of resistance discussed above has prompted the sheep industry to set up an advisory group, 'Sustainable Control of Parasites in Sheep' (SCOPS), which brings together the latest research in parasite control, producing best practice guidelines on the use of anthelmintics. See the website, www.scops.org.uk for details. Here is a brief summary of the guidelines:

- Worm sheep only when necessary – see 'When to use worm treatments' below
- When worming, weigh animals and give accurate doses; or weigh and dose the whole group according to the weight of the heaviest in the group (if there is a lot of variation in the size of animals in a group, split them into smaller groups according to weight and dose for the heaviest in each group)
- Calibrate the dosing gun to make sure that it is giving the correct dose. It is possible to make a calibrating cylinder by taking the plunger out of the syringe and blocking the end with a finger
- Correct dosing – drenching
    - Restrain the animal securely, so that it receives the whole dose and does not damage the back of its throat on the dosing gun
    - Gently move the drenching gun or syringe through the gap between the front teeth and cheek teeth and over the back of the tongue
    - Make sure all the dose goes into the back of the mouth
    - Hold the head tilted slightly upwards until the dose has been swallowed
- Correct dosing – injection
    - Restrain the animal securely
    - Make sure you can see the site that you are injecting
    - Inject according to the manufacturer's instructions: under the skin or into the muscle (see 'Injection technique' in Chapter 7 for instructions on giving injections)
- Regularly change the wormer group that you use – the group, not just the name of wormer (see Table 8.1)
- Use good quarantine protocols, to avoid bringing resistant worms onto your farm – see Chapter 9 'Quarantine period' for more details
- Do not treat sheep for worms immediately before moving them onto 'clean' pasture

Table 8.1 Current wormer groups.

GROUP	COLOUR OF WORMER	GROUP NAME	ABBREVIATION	EXAMPLES
1	White	Benzimidazoles	BZ	Albendazole Mebendazole Ricobendazole Oxfendazole
2	Yellow	Levamisole	LV	Levamisole
3	Clear	Macrocyclic dactones	ML	Ivermectin Doramectin Moxidectin
4	Orange	Amino acetyl derivatives	AD	Monepantel
5	Purple	Spiroindoles	SI	Derquantel

(new grass leys or pasture not grazed by sheep for several years). Dose them a few days beforehand or a few days after they are moved. Otherwise, only worms that are resistant to the treatment will survive and infect this pasture
- Test the wormers to make sure that they are working – speak to your vet about this

'White drenches' are usually only used for treating nematodirosis (see 'Nematodirosis' below), because there are high levels of resistance to this group in other worms.

When to use worm treatments

Making the decisions about when to worm sheep and which wormer to use should be done in conjunction with your local sheep vet. Below are some guiding principles that the vet will take into account when making these decisions with a farmer or smallholder.

EWES

Adult ewes have good immunity to roundworms for most of the year, except for a few weeks around lambing time. Most ewes over 2 years old should not need to be wormed except at this time. Even then, well-fed ewes carrying single lambs and some carrying twins that are in particularly good body condition (see 'Body condition scoring' in Chapter 2), should not need to be treated; faeces testing can be used as a guide as to whether a wormer is required. The main purpose of worming ewes at lambing time is to reduce roundworm pasture contamination by ewes, which in turn will lessen the risk for lambs.

Ewes 1 to 2 years old will need to be treated for worms more often than adult ewes; the frequency of this should be tested using faeces and in liaison with a veterinary surgeon. It is important to worm these ewes before breeding to ensure that they are in the best possible health.

RAMS

Rams have a reduced immunity in comparison to ewes and therefore need to be wormed more often. Regular submission of faecal samples to the local vet will enable a worming schedule to be identified. In general, rams are likely to need worming twice a year; in summer and before breeding time.

LAMBS

Ideally, worming treatments should only be used to treat lambs that are being affected by worms. Symptoms of roundworms include:

- Reduced growth rates despite good food
- Scour/diarrhoea
- Worm eggs in faeces

In the UK, the risk period for roundworms is normally from June through to October or November; this period is prolonged by warm autumn weather. To maintain an overview of infection, farmers and smallholders are advised to take fresh lamb faeces to their local vet each month throughout this period.

A reduction in growth rates is normally the first sign of parasitic gastroenteritis (roundworm infection), therefore regular weighing of lambs (fortnightly is a useful frequency) can help target worming to affected animals, early in the disease. Treatment should be provided to:

- Individual lambs that have not grown as well as the rest of the group
- The whole group when the majority of lambs

have not grown as well as expected, if the grass quantity and quality have remained the same

When a whole group of lambs is growing more slowly than expected, other reasons must be considered, for example quality and quantity of nutrition and trace element deficiencies, especially selenium and cobalt (see 'Thin sheep' in Chapter 7).

Grass quality is important in this scenario, because the nutritional value of grass reduces when:

- Long (over 8 cm in height)
- Autumn approaches

How to collect faeces samples

- Move the animals to be tested into a small area, to make it easier to find fresh faeces
- Collect samples only from the animals of interest, that is, if you want to know whether to treat lambs, only collect lamb faeces
- Collect ten samples per group, or one per animal if testing individuals
- Samples must be fresh, that is, warm and cause the bag or container to steam up
- Place each sample into a separate container or bag (Figs 8.2, 8.3)
- Samples can be stored in a fridge if there is a delay between collection and delivery to the practice

Nematodirosis

Nematodirus battus is also a roundworm. It is described in Chapter 7, in the 'Diarrhoea' section.

Fields that are grazed by young lambs every year are high risk for this condition as eggs deposited one year will hatch the following year. It is possible to break the cycle of transmission by rotating the fields that are used for ewes with young lambs. If this is not possible, monitor the weather and online parasite forecasts to help predict when preventative treatments might be needed and seek veterinary advice at these times. If no other parasites are present in the

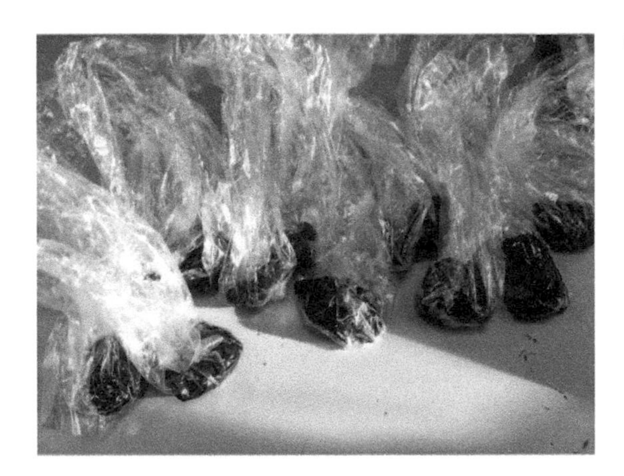

FIGURE 8.2 Collect individual fresh faeces samples into separate containers or bags. Fresh samples should cause the bag to steam up.

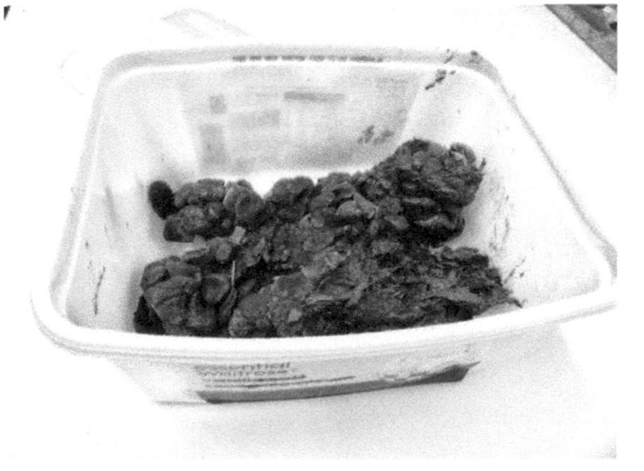

FIGURE 8.3 Do not put all the samples into one container and do not mix ewe and lamb samples together.

affected lambs, a white wormer (a benzimidazole) is generally recommended.

Coccidiosis

Coccidiosis is a cause of serious diarrhoea and ill thrift in lambs, but it can be prevented by good hygiene and regularly moving lambs to clean pasture. If coccidiosis is a problem in spite of these measures, there are a selection of treatments that can be used for prevention or treatment. Many of the treatment options need to be repeated due to the nature of the disease. Discuss suspected disease and prevention/treatment options with the local sheep vet.

It is important to take particular care when using the preventative treatments for this disease as lambs can get coccidiosis after these treatments are stopped, if they have not had enough exposure to infection during treatment to develop a natural immunity.

Liver fluke

Liver fluke treatment is only needed when this parasite is present on a farm.

Investigate whether liver fluke is present on your farm

- If used, ask the local slaughterhouse to look for signs of liver fluke in your sheep. If doing so, it is good practice to warn the slaughterhouse prior to slaughter that this information is wanted
- Ask the local vet to bloodtest lambs in their first summer and autumn
- Take faeces samples to the local vet for testing in late autumn, winter and spring
- Ask your local vet to perform post-mortem examinations on sheep that die in the autumn and winter

When is treatment needed?

For more details of this parasite and methods of preventing infection, see the 'Thin sheep' section of Chapter 7. Unfortunately, liver fluke treatment is not straightforward since the correct medicine choice depends on the length of time that sheep have been infected, as the treatment varies depending upon whether it is immature or adult fluke that are present. This differentiation is largely dictated by the time of year, but also varies according to the weather (Tables 8.2, 8.3).

Vets working with sheep in your area will know what level of liver fluke to expect, but unless the farm has fields that are confirmed as free of *Galba truncatula* snails (see 'Liver fluke' in Chapter 7), specific monitoring is needed. Annual variation in liver fluke patterns, influenced by the weather, make it essential to continually monitor and plan liver fluke control with the local vet, alongside online UK parasite forcasts. The active ingredients of currently available treatments are listed in Table 8.4 for your information.

The development of resistance to triclabendazole in some populations of liver fluke is a concern, as this is the only product that can be used to control the early stages of liver fluke. To avoid resistance in liver fluke populations it is important to:

- Weigh sheep, calibrate dosing equipment and dose stock accurately as described above for wormers
- Do not rely on one product; use the full range of available medicines, at the appropriate times of year, in consultation with your vet

Table 8.2 What to expect with different levels of liver fluke infection.

LEVEL OF LIVER FLUKE ON FARM	SIGNS	COMMENTS
None	No clinical signs. None in livers at slaughter; faeces samples repeatedly negative.	Monitor the situation with the help of your vet, especially in wet years. Give good quarantine treatments for liver fluke (see Chapter 9).
Low	Little or no disease. Occasional positive abattoir and test results.	Few treatments should be needed, mostly in wet years. Seek veterinary advice and regularly monitor with testing.
Moderate	Some fluke-related disease is seen most years. Often positive abattoir or veterinary test results.	Routine treatments are likely to be needed. Discuss a testing and treatment protocol with your local sheep vet.
High	Severe disease/deaths associated with liver fluke seen most years.	Regular treatments are necessary. Formulate a prevention, monitoring and treatment plan with a sheep vet.

Table 8.3 Typical yearly pattern of infection, with some potential weather variations.

TIME OF YEAR	STAGE OF LIVER FLUKE INFECTION IN SHEEP	WEATHER DEPENDENCY
Late summer and autumn	Early immature	In warm, wet years this can start in mid summer. In dry years, infection can be delayed into winter.
Early winter	Early and late immature	
Mid winter	Late immature and adults	In mild winters, early immature stages may still be present.
Late winter/spring	Mature adults	In very mild winters, earlier stages may still be present.

Table 8.4 Active ingredients of liver fluke treatments.

TREATMENT	STAGES OF LIVER FLUKE TREATED	COMMENTS
Triclabendazole	All stages including early immatures	Resistance levels are increasing due to overuse
Closantel	From 6–8 weeks after infection	
Nitroxynil	From 7–8 weeks after infection	
Oxyclozanide	Adult flukes only (and rumen fluke)	
Albendazole	Adult flukes only	

- Use carefully planned quarantine treatments when bringing new stock onto the ground (see 'Quarantine period' in Chapter 9)

Sheep scab

Sheep scab is caused by the *Psoroptes ovis* mite and affects the skin. It is extremely irritating and debilitating for infected animals, so there is a legal requirement in the UK to treat sheep scab as soon as it is discovered. Some parts of the UK have more stringent regulations than others, so it is vital to be aware of the regulations in your area; information on local regulations will be available from the local sheep vet. Veterinary involvement is also required to confirm the diagnosis, so where itchy sheep or sheep losing wool are identified in a flock, they should always be checked by a vet. In the interest of animal welfare, sheep keepers also have an obligation to prevent this disease wherever possible. Strategies for prevention are discussed below.

Keeping sheep scab out of a flock

The mites that cause sheep scab spread through direct sheep-to-sheep contact or via surroundings recently inhabited by infected sheep. They can be prevented from entering a flock by:

- Good fencing that prevents animals escaping into or out of fields
- Double fencing farm boundaries, especially if they neighbour stock fields
- Isolation and quarantine treatment of new stock – see 'Quarantine period' in Chapter 9
- Isolation, and sometimes treatment, of animals that have been in contact with other stock, for example at shows

Once disconnected from a sheep, *Psoroptes ovis* mites can survive in the surroundings for up to 17 days, for example, on the ground, fence posts, in buildings and vehicles, and so on. Therefore, uninfected sheep should not be

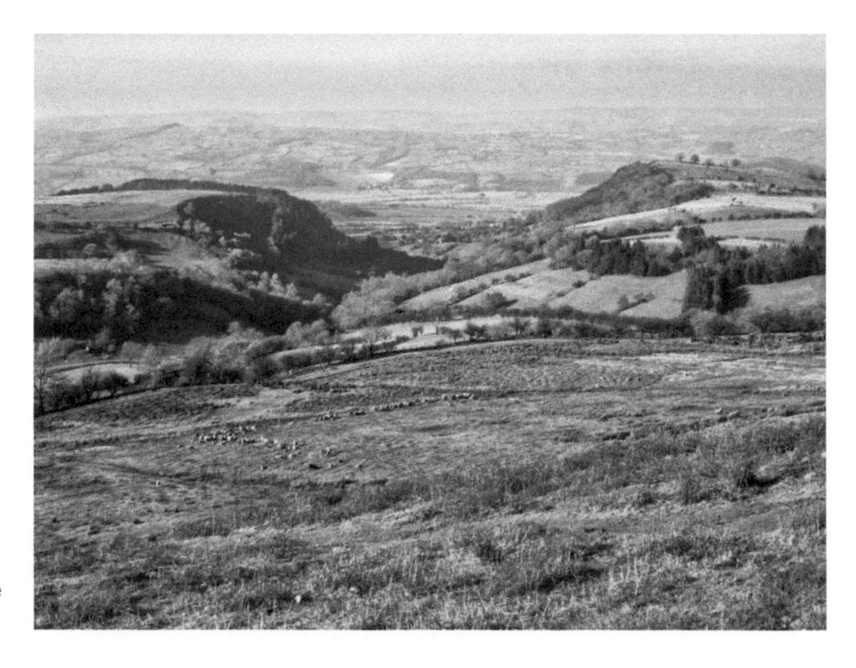

FIGURE 8.4 Sheep on a hill with grazing rights belonging to multiple farms, making disease control more difficult.

Table 8.5 Injectable treatments for sheep scab.

ACTIVE INGREDIENT	TREATMENT	PREVENTION	INJECTION SITE	TIME UNTIL CAN MIX WITH OTHER SHEEP
Ivermectin	Two doses seven days apart Move sheep to a new field/ shed	Not effective	Under the skin	Seven days after the second injection
Doramectin	One dose Move sheep to a new field/ shed Higher dose rate	Not effective	Into muscle	14 days
Moxidectin 1%*	Two doses 10 days apart	One dose (lasts 28 days)	Under the skin	12 days
Moxidectin 2%	One injection	One injection (lasts 60 days)	Under the skin, immediately behind the ear	12 days

*Do not use in sheep that have been injected with Footvax (footrot vaccine)

moved to surroundings that were inhabited by infected sheep within the previous 17 days. In addition, animals treated by injection must be kept isolated from other sheep until a set period after treatment. See Table 8.5 for details.

Where grazing is shared, such as usage of common land for grazing (Fig. 8.4), prevention of sheep scab can be difficult. If there are good relations between those who share the grazing, coordinated treatments can help to control the spread of this disease. However, if sheep scab is seen regularly in animals on shared grazing, routine treatments are likely to be needed; discuss treatment options and the timing of treatments with your local sheep vet. Those sheep that have not been on common grazing, and not had any contact with stock from common grazing, should not need regular treatment.

Medicines to treat or prevent sheep scab

Medicines and the licences that cover their use in farm animals change with time, so always speak to your local vet about available options. Products that will be discussed here include:

- Injectable anthelmintics, the 'clear' wormers in injectable form
- Organophosphate dips
- Organophosphate showers

It is important to emphasise that sheep scab control and treatment must include *all sheep* in a group, because if one infected animal is not treated this will act as a source of infection for the whole flock. The new outbreak can take several months to become evident, but is not a fresh breach of biosecurity. Also, if treatments are used poorly or overused, the mites can develop resistance to those treatments; if it is suspected that a treatment has not worked, your local vet should be contacted immediately.

Injectable treatments

For injectable products, the same treatment principles apply to scab as for gut worms (see 'Good practice to reduce resistance when using wormers' above). The main disadvantage of using injectable treatments for sheep scab is the increased potential for the development of worm resistance. Sheep scab prevention/treatment is normally needed in winter when worm numbers are low and would otherwise not be treated; this can speed up the development of resistance (Table 8.5).

Dips

Organophosphate dips are an effective method of preventing and treating sheep scab as the effects last for several weeks. However, these products pose significant risk to human health and the environment and so are subject to significant legal restrictions. Find out about these regulations from your local authority or relevant government organisation before considering their use.

In order to be effective, organophosphate dips must be used carefully, following the manufacturer's instructions. Dirt and faeces deactivate dip solution, therefore top up or drain and replace the dip at the frequency recommended by the manufacturer and replace it all when further dipping is to be carried out on a subsequent day. If sheep are especially dirty, clean the dip bath more often and if they are wet before dipping, top up the solution more frequently.

Organophosphate showers have become popular in recent years; however, at the time of writing in the UK, dip products are not licensed for use in showers. Showers are not recommended for the control of sheep scab because the mites live in the skin, therefore if the shower does not penetrate the wool as far as the skin, it will not reach the mites. Showering infected sheep will subdue an outbreak of sheep scab but may not remove all the mites. Organosphosphate showers are useful where sheep scab is not present, for the control of lice and blowfly strike.

Blowfly strike

Blowfly strike causes serious problems in sheep and can be fatal, so prevention and early treatment are vital. Disease is seen during warm months when flies are active.

Protecting sheep from blowfly strike

Complete prevention can be difficult, but there are some strategies to reduce the number of sheep affected:

- Shear adult sheep in late spring or early summer, before fly numbers multiply too much (Fig. 8.5)
- Dagging or crutching: shearing the back of the rump and the tail to prevent faeces from getting caught in wool, in autumn or spring (Fig. 8.6)
- Tail docking lambs in susceptible sheep breeds and/or high risk areas
- Trim wool around the prepuce of rams
- Prevent other diseases that can attract flies
    - Footrot
    - Diarrhoea (gut worms, coccidiosis, etc.)
    - Urinary diseases
    - Open wounds
    - Skin diseases

- Remove places that flies will breed, for example:

  - Store carcasses in a sealed container until they are collected
  - Keep rubbish bins sealed, even those containing rotting vegetation
  - Compost faeces and bedding carefully

- Various fly-trapping systems can be used; these may be bought or homemade
- Timely application of blowfly treatments; options include:

  - Plunge dipping in organophosphate, at least three weeks after shearing. However, dirty dip solution will make sheep more attractive to flies, so ensure the dip is clean
  - Shower dipping: contractors will shower dip sheep in many parts of the UK. Again, sheep need two to four weeks of fleece growth and to be clean – allow one minute of shower time for every week since shearing. However, at the time of writing dip solutions available in the UK are not licensed for use in showers
  - Pour-on: these are effective if applied correctly and according to the manufacturer's instructions. Some products are useful for prevention and some for treatment and prevention (Table 8.6)

When treating fattening lambs, remember to take into consideration the meat withdrawal time for the chosen product.

If adult sheep need to be treated before shearing, observe the manufacturer's recommendations for the length of time between

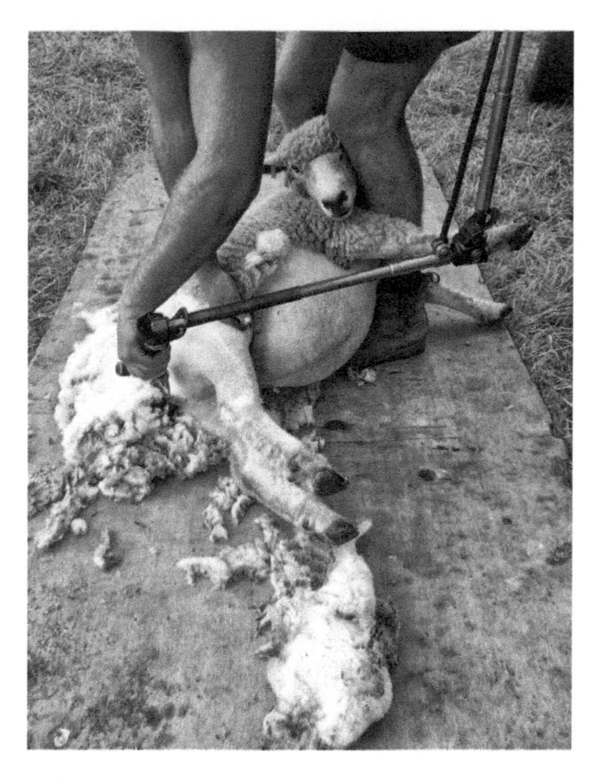

FIGURE 8.5 Timely shearing of sheep helps to prevent blowfly strike.

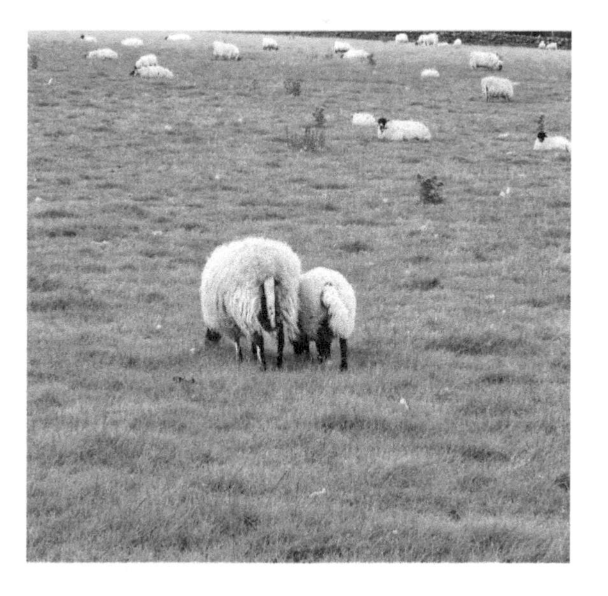

FIGURE 8.6 A ewe's tail has been sheared to prevent faeces from getting caught in it.

Table 8.6 The active ingredients of current medicines for the treatment and prevention of blowfly strike.

ACTIVE INGREDIENT	TREATMENT METHOD	LENGTH OF PROTECTION	BLOWFLY STRIKE
Diazinon	Plunge treatment	3–8 weeks	Prevention and treatment
High-cis cypermethrin	Pour-on	Ranges from 6 to 10 weeks	Prevention and treatment High concentrations needed for blowfly control
Alphacypermethrin	Pour-on	8–10 weeks	Prevention and treatment
Cyromazine	Pour-on	10 weeks	Prevention only
Dicyclanil	Pour-on	16 weeks	Prevention only
Deltamethrin	Pour-on	None	Treatment

treatment and shearing. For some products, this is for the health and safety of the shearers, for others it is to avoid toxic wool residues interfering with the sale and use of the wool.

Ticks

Ticks are not present on all farms; they are most common in moorland and woodland (Fig. 8.7), but it is important to monitor your sheep for the presence of ticks. The purpose of tick control is to prevent the diseases that they carry and transmit; if neither ticks nor the diseases that they can carry are present on a farm, tick prevention is not required.

It can be helpful to keep sheep away from tick-infested areas during times of greatest tick activity, such as in spring and autumn. However, ticks can be active throughout the summer in the UK, especially in mild, wet western areas.

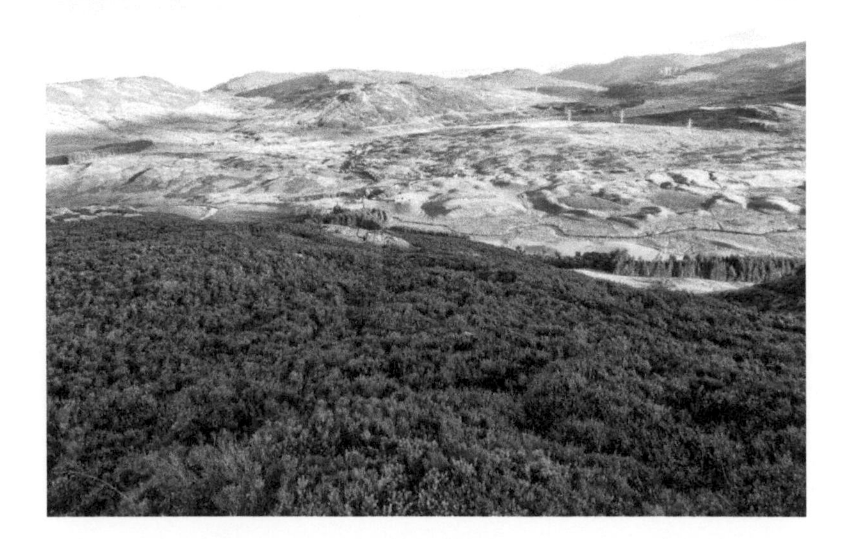

FIGURE 8.7 Moorland forms an ideal habitat for ticks.

Table 8.7 The active ingredient of current medicines for the prevention of tick infestation.

ACTIVE INGREDIENT	TREATMENT METHOD	LENGTH OF PROTECTION
Diazinon	Plunge treatment	6 weeks
High-cis cypermethrin	Pour-on	10 weeks Lambs under 10 kg, 3 weeks
Alphacypermethrin	Pour-on	8–12 weeks

For young animals or new stock that have been moved into a tick area, preventative treatment should be applied at the start of the risk period and maintained throughout this time (Table 8.7).

LAMENESS DUE TO INFECTIOUS DISEASE

Lameness prevention is very important because of the significant detrimental effect that lameness has on animal welfare, body condition, productivity and lamb growth rates. At the time of writing, footrot is the most prevalent cause of lameness in sheep in the UK and prevention of this painful condition is being given much attention by the sheep industry. The main principles for preventing footrot can be seen in Figure 8.8 and are discussed below; some of these also apply to other infectious causes of lameness such as contagious ovine digital dermatitis (CODD).

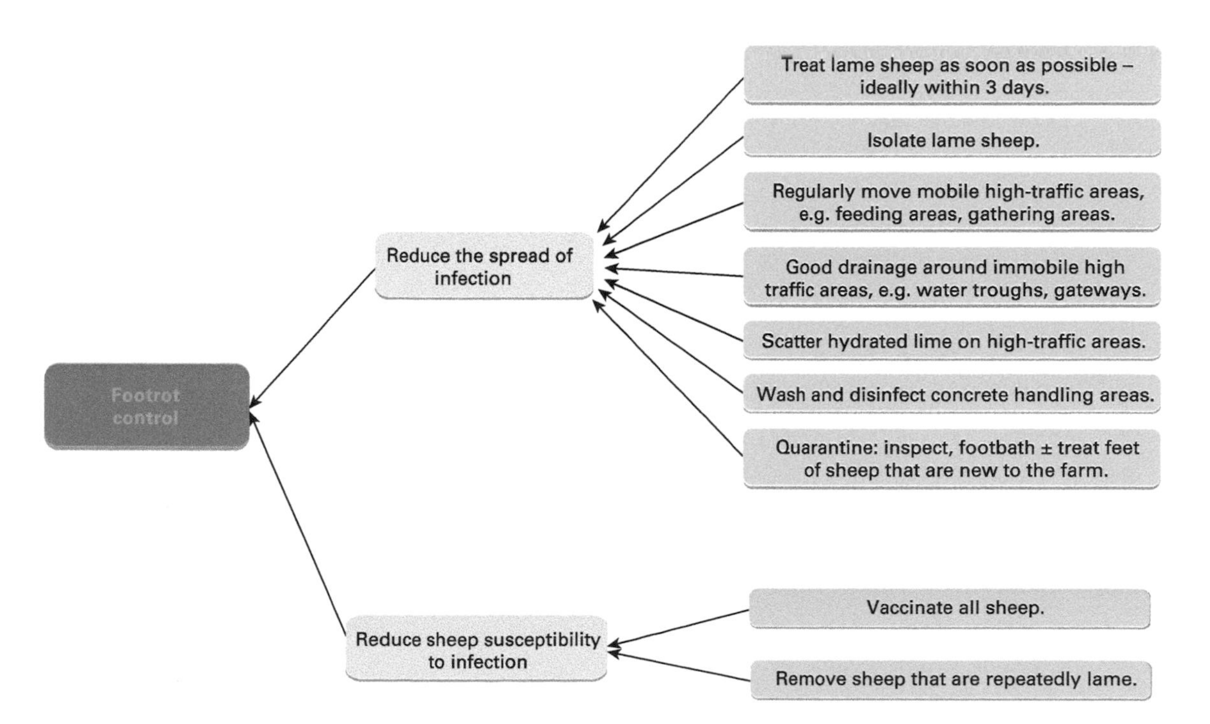

FIGURE 8.8 Strategies for preventing footrot infection.

Reducing the spread of footrot and CODD within a flock

Every footstep taken by a sheep that is affected by footrot or contagious ovine digital dermatitis (CODD) leaves behind some of the causative agents of these diseases, ready for another sheep to step into and become infected. Spread of disease in this way is especially effective in warm, wet conditions.

Infection builds up in areas that sheep go to regularly, for example around water troughs, feed troughs, mineral buckets, gateways and gathering areas, especially if these become wet and muddy; these sites are high risk for unaffected sheep to pick up infection. The build-up of infection can be reduced by:

- Treating affected sheep as quickly as possible, ideally within three days of noticing that they are lame; improves recovery rates and reduces the amount of infection that is shed into the surroundings
- Isolating lame sheep into a separate field or pen. This means that infection is trodden onto ground that will not be used by healthy sheep
- Moving feed areas/buckets/licks/mobile gathering units regularly
- In high-traffic areas, such as gateways, permanent handling systems and around water troughs, laying surface materials that:
  - Allow water to drain away, for example gravel; or
  - Enable easy cleaning, such as concrete
- Washing and disinfecting permanent concrete handling systems between uses and between different groups of sheep; ideally, allow them to dry before use
- Scattering hydrated lime on the ground in gateways and handling areas before use
- Having an effective quarantine plan for new sheep: inspect the feet of all new sheep, treat those with lesions and use footbaths, before these animals are mixed with the home flock (see Chapter 9, section on 'Diseases to consider')

How to make sheep less susceptible to footrot

Even if footrot levels are high, it is possible to increase the resilience of a flock, so that individuals within it are less likely to succumb to the disease. There are two main strategies for achieving this:

Vaccination

In flocks where footrot levels are high, vaccination can be used twice a year. Once the disease has become less prevalent, this can be reduced to yearly boosters. See details above in 'Vaccines'.

Selective breeding

Hoof conformation in sheep varies from animal to animal. Each individual may have naturally strong hooves, weak or misshapen hooves and are either susceptible or resistant to lameness. Breeding a flock with healthy hooves and low levels of lameness requires the removal of sheep that are repeatedly lame and their offspring. Removing repeatedly or continually lame sheep from a flock also removes a constant source of infection from the farm (Fig. 8.9), as most of these lame sheep will continually spread infection wherever they walk.

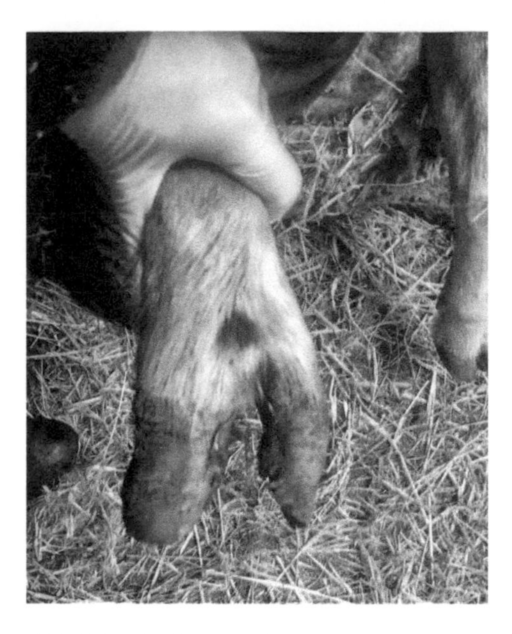

FIGURE 8.9 Sheep with thickened digits are likely to be continually or repeatedly lame and a potential source of infection for the rest of the flock.

Making best use of foot bathing

Footbaths for sheep are a popular way of controlling scald, footrot and CODD. However, to be effective, footbaths must be used well; at worst, if they are used badly, they can increase the spread of infection. To do foot bathing effectively:

- Ensure that the product is used correctly:
  - At the correct concentration
  - The animals stand in the solution for an adequate length of time
  - With or without straw in the footbath – this has a positive effect for zinc sulphate footbaths, but is detrimental for formalin footbaths
  - Consider whether or not the solution can be reused or must be discarded at the end of the day
- Sheep should have clean feet before going into the footbath. A water footbath can be used before the medicated footbath, but if pasture is clean and dry this may not be necessary
- Allow the footbath solution to dry onto the feet by standing sheep on a dry hard surface for 30 to 60 minutes afterwards
- Separate out lame animals and put these through the footbath last

Footbaths can be used:

- At the start and end of a quarantine period
- Every time sheep are gathered
- During an outbreak of footrot, scald or CODD

Footbath solutions

Formalin is frequently used for footbaths. It should be used at a concentration of 2–3% (no higher because it can burn the skin); sheep can walk through this solution – there is no need for prolonged contact time. Formalin is denatured by contact with mud or faeces so it stops working when the solution gets dirty – do not put straw or anything else into the footbath as this will also destroy the formalin. This chemical breaks down quickly, so formalin footbaths cannot be reused on subsequent days, but they are easier to dispose of than some of the other products. Regular use of formalin footbaths can cause sheep's feet to harden and become brittle, so they should be used conservatively. Direct human contact with this chemical should be avoided, as it is carcinogenic; wear appropriate protective clothing when handling it.

Zinc sulphate can be used in footbaths at a concentration of 10% and is a more robust chemical than formalin, so straw can be added to the bath. It is a less noxious chemical, which means it is less painful for lame sheep to walk through. However, the sheep need to stand in the solution for at least 15 minutes and ideally longer. In addition, they must not drink the solution because it is toxic, so sheep cannot be left unattended in the bath. Due to its chemical stability, zinc sulphate can be more difficult to dispose of safely.

Copper sulphate at a 10% concentration is also used in footbaths; as with zinc sulphate, it needs prolonged contact time and is more difficult to dispose of than formalin, and is generally more expensive to buy. Copper sulphate cannot be used in metal footbaths, as it corrodes the metal.

Various *antibiotics* have been used in footbaths for the treatment of CODD, but none are currently licensed in the UK for use in this way, therefore veterinary advice must be sought about these and regular use is not recommended.

Is foot trimming necessary?

Routine trimming

Trimming sheep's feet has become a contentious issue in recent years. Traditional shepherding included trimming the feet of all sheep every year, but there is now evidence that this is not necessary for most sheep that are kept outdoors for most of the year. Also, sheep's feet are easily damaged by trimming because of their small size and the softness of the horn; trimming is liable to cause lameness rather than prevent it.

Sheep that are kept indoors for long periods, however, will occasionally need a small amount of hoof wall trimming away in order to prevent dirt from getting trapped and to prevent the horn from splitting.

It may be necessary to trim the feet of a sheep if they are getting long, misshapen or the horn is splitting. In this scenario, help and advice should be sought from your local sheep vet.

Trimming infected hooves

For lame sheep, if the cause of lameness is not obvious, a little loose horn can be removed to increase visualisation; some trimming may also be needed to remove thorns or to open abscesses (this procedure should be carried out by a vet; owners should not attempt it). If footrot is the cause of lameness, the desire to trim feet must be resisted, because:

- Trimming the hooves of sheep with footrot delays healing and recovery
- The hoof shears can spread infection from one sheep to another, even if they are disinfected in between sheep

Advice for sheep with CODD is similar, except that sometimes the hoof horn ends up hanging on by a very small attachment. This should be snipped off to prevent it from impinging on the inflamed tissue left behind.

Other

Sheep's hooves are thin and soft, especially on the surface closest to the ground, so they can easily be bruised or punctured by thorns or sharp stones. To further protect the flock, famers and smallholders should try to minimise exposure to these hazards.

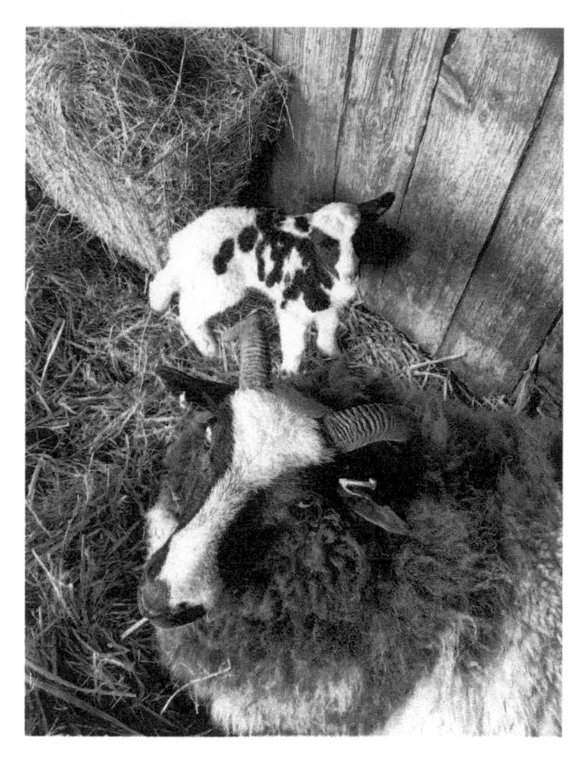

FIGURE 8.10 Lambs born indoors need a clean, dry bed.

Photograph courtesy of Stephanie Bingham.

NEWBORN LAMB MANAGEMENT

To be fit and healthy, newborn lambs need:

- To receive enough good quality colostrum shortly after birth
- A dry, hygienic environment (Fig. 8.10)
- Effective navel treatment/disinfection
- Temperature control – this will depend on the breed of sheep involved: hardy hill breeds (Fig. 8.11) have different requirements to softer lowland breeds

How important are the surroundings?

Lambs born into a clean and dry environment are less likely to suffer from disease than those surrounded by faeces or wet, soiled bedding. A clean, dry shed with plenty of bedding (Figs 8.12, 8.13), such as straw, or a clean, sheltered field (Fig. 8.14) are ideal surroundings for ewes to give birth.

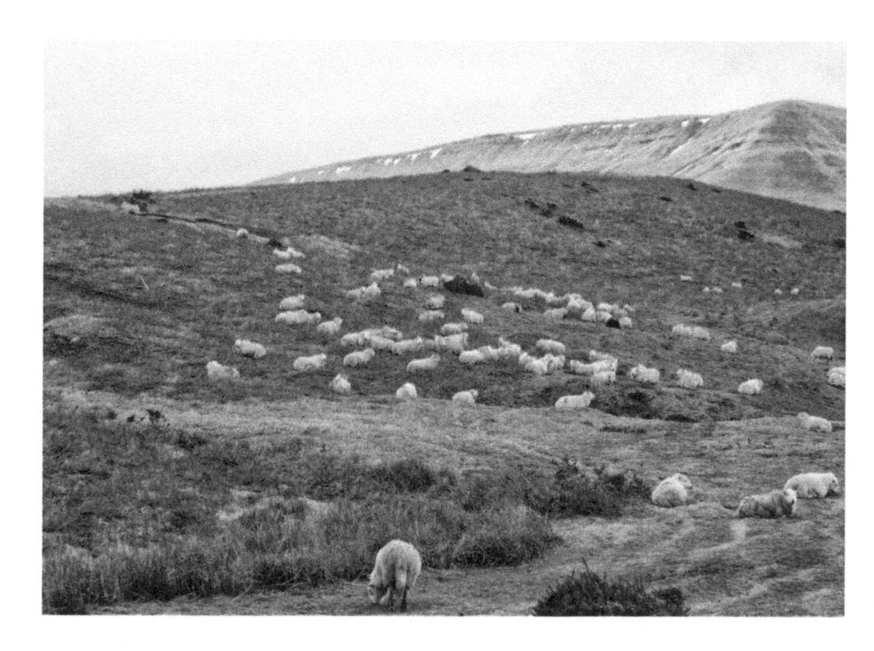

FIGURE 8.11 Welsh mountain lambs from these ewes will be born with a reasonably thick fleece and so will be less susceptible to the cold.

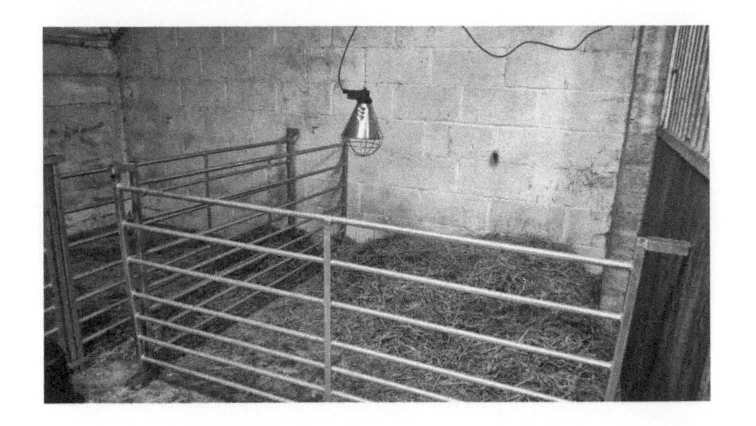

FIGURE 8.12 Clean concrete floors with plenty of clean, dry straw provide hygienic surroundings for newborn lambs. A heat lamp can help keep the lambs warm.

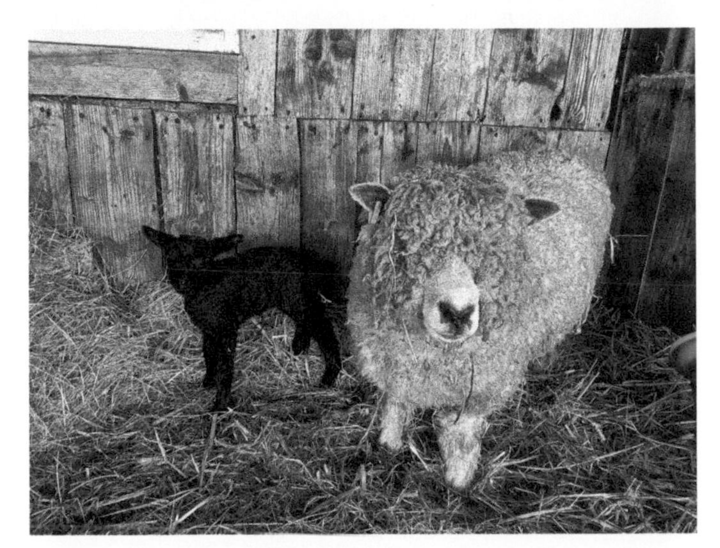

FIGURE 8.13 Plenty of clean bedding helps to keep the environment warm, dry and clean.

Photograph courtesy of Stephanie Bingham.

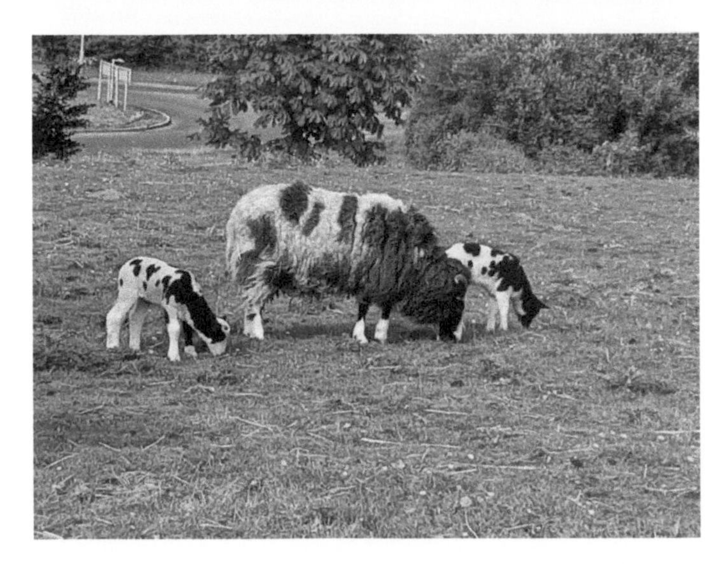

FIGURE 8.14 A sheltered, clean field is an ideal environment for newborn lambs.

Photograph courtesy of Stephanie Bingham.

If lambing pens are used, ideally all the bedding should be removed and renewed between occupants; where possible, allow 24 hours for the area to dry before it is re-bedded.

Various powders are available, claiming to act as disinfectants for lambing pens. Check the label of these products for a recognised active ingredient that is effective in the presence of organic matter (straw, faeces, etc.). Hydrated lime is used in lambing pens on many farms, but a generous layer of straw must cover it as lambs' feet can be burned by contact with hydrated lime.

Does navel treatment matter?

The main access points through which infection gets into newborn lambs are the mouth and umbilicus (navel). The navel of each lamb should be treated with a disinfectant that will help to dry it; a 10% iodine solution is routinely recommended. It is possible to mix the iodine solution with surgical spirit to speed up the drying process (Fig. 8.15).

The solution can be applied by dipping the navel into it or spraying it onto the navel; the same principles apply for both methods:

- Apply the solution as soon as possible after birth
- The navel must be thoroughly covered – all the way around its connection with the body wall and all the way to the tip. It is easy to miss bits when spraying, so it is important to take care and ensure that the procedure is done thoroughly (Fig. 8.16)

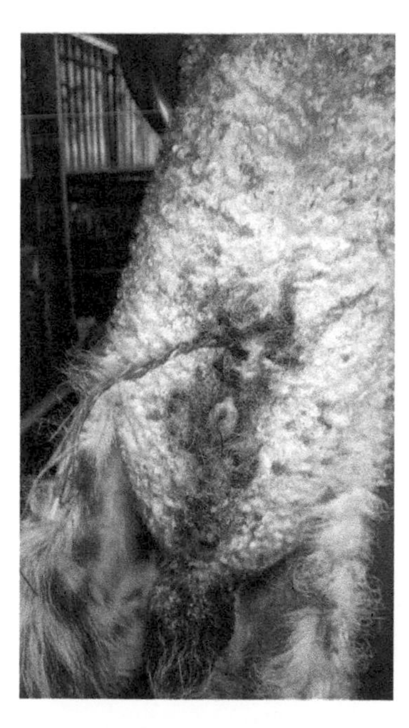

FIGURE 8.15 A dry navel. The navel treatment should help to dry the navel quickly to prevent infection becoming established.

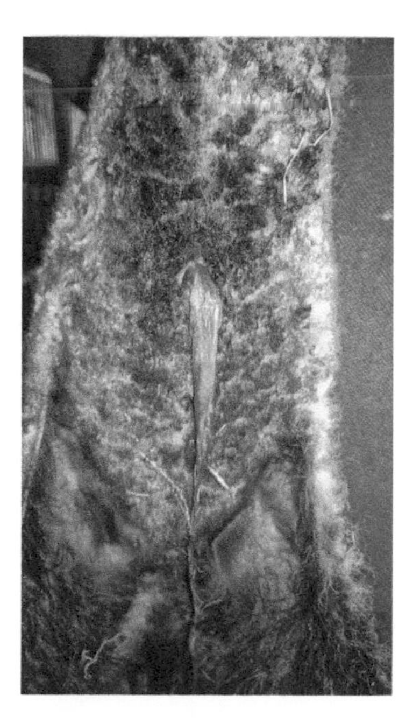

FIGURE 8.16 Make sure that the whole of the navel and its connection with the body are covered in iodine. This lamb also has a rounded stomach, indicating that it is full of colostrum or milk.

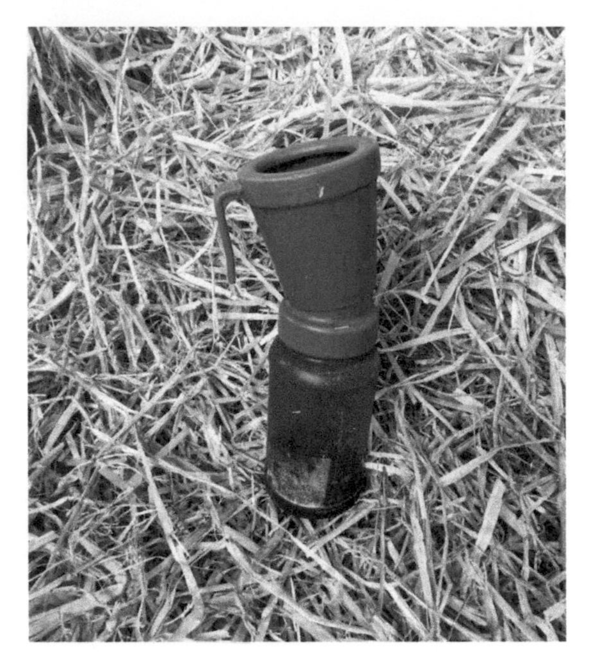

FIGURE 8.17 Dairy cow teat dipping cups can be used to dip lambs' navels, provided the cup does not allow dip solution back into the storage well underneath and the cup is washed daily.

- The solution must be kept clean – when dipping navels into disinfectant, the dipping cup must only hold enough solution for one lamb at a time and any excess must be thrown away (not put back into the storage container; Fig. 8.17).
- The application equipment must be kept clean – ensure that spray tips are clean and dipping cups are washed in warm soapy water at least once a day.

The impact of colostrum

Immunity is the body's ability to fight disease. Young animals develop their own immunity when they are exposed to organisms in the environment, but when they are first born they need some help from their mother's immunity. In sheep, the transfer of immunity from mother to her lamb(s) happens in the first few hours of life when the lamb suckles colostrum (the first milk, which should be thick and yellow). This should happen within the first two hours of life. The quality of the colostrum and protection that it can provide depends upon the health of the ewe and effective vaccination – see the section above on clostridial vaccination.

The best source of colostrum is the lamb's own mother, as she will have immunity to local diseases. But if the ewe does not have enough colostrum for all her lambs, or if her colostrum is thin and pale, the lambs may need supplementary colostrum from another source. If a lamb will not suckle its mother, although she has plenty of milk, the colostrum can be milked off her and given by stomach tube (see 'Stomach tubing a lamb' in Chapter 6).

How much colostrum do lambs need?

- At least 50 ml of colostrum per kilogram of body weight within two hours or birth: an average lowland lamb would weigh 4–5 kg at birth, so needs 200–250 ml; average healthy hill lambs weigh 2–4 kg, so need 100–200 ml.
- A total of 200 ml of colostrum per kg body weight within 24 hours of birth, split into feeds every three to four hours: a 4 kg lamb would need 800 ml, in six feeds of 150 ml each.

The quality and amount of colostrum that lambs receive is not only important because of the protection that it gives against disease, it also provides the energy for them to thrive and keep warm in all except the most severe weather conditions encountered in the UK.

Alternative sources of colostrum

Alternative colostrum sources are listed below in order of suitability, with the most suitable first:

- Colostrum from another freshly lambed ewe in the same flock – usually a ewe that has lambed on the same day with plenty of colostrum and only one lamb
- Frozen ewe colostrum. See 'How to store frozen colostrum' below for details
- Good-quality powdered colostrum with high fat content (over 20%) and high immunoglobulin levels (over 3 g per lamb). This information is available for some products on independent websites; your local sheep vet can advise on this
- Cow colostrum:

    - Taken from a farm that is free of bovine tuberculosis and Johne's disease
    - The colostrum from some cows can contain antibodies that are dangerous for newborn lambs; the colostrum can be tested for these antibodies or they can be diluted by pooling colostrum from several cows
    - Lambs need one third extra volume of cow's colostrum compared with ewe colostrum
    - Ideally, colostrum for lambs should come from cows that have been vaccinated against clostridial diseases

Some diseases are spread to lambs through colostrum, therefore using colostrum from another sheep flock is not advised, unless the flock has been tested for and is free of both maedi visna (MV) and Johne's disease. Also, if MV or Johne's disease are present in your flock, speak to your vet about colostrum management, as it is likely to be different to the advice given above.

How to store frozen colostrum

- Choose a ewe with a single lamb and plenty of colostrum
- Once her lamb has suckled for the first time and obviously has a full, rounded stomach, milk off the rest of the colostrum
- Place the colostrum into containers or bottles of 150 ml each, or ice-cube freezer bags
- Label the containers with the date, 'ewe colostrum' and the ewe's name or number
- Place in the freezer as soon as the colostrum is cool

The immune function of the colostrum is damaged by overheating or exposure to microwaves. To defrost and warm the colostrum:

- Retrieve the labeled colostrum from the freezer, using the oldest first
- Put the container into a bowl of warm water
- Once it has defrosted, change the water, make it a little warmer than body temperature and keep changing the water until the colostrum is at body temperature
- Ice-cube bags work well because they defrost quickly, but if cubes are broken off to use, these will need to be placed in a smaller container inside the bowl of warm water in order to avoid diluting the colostrum

Frozen colostrum can still be useful months or years after being harvested.

Do not microwave colostrum to defrost or warm it.

What kinds of weather can newborn lambs cope with?

Newborn lambs need to dry quickly; a ewe will lick her lamb(s) to help them dry (Fig. 8.18), however, if she is unwell it may be necessary to dry the lambs with clean straw or an old towel. It is worth being aware of the surroundings that lambs are born into; check for the following:

- Draughts
- If so, can lambs escape the draught?
- Wet floors or fields

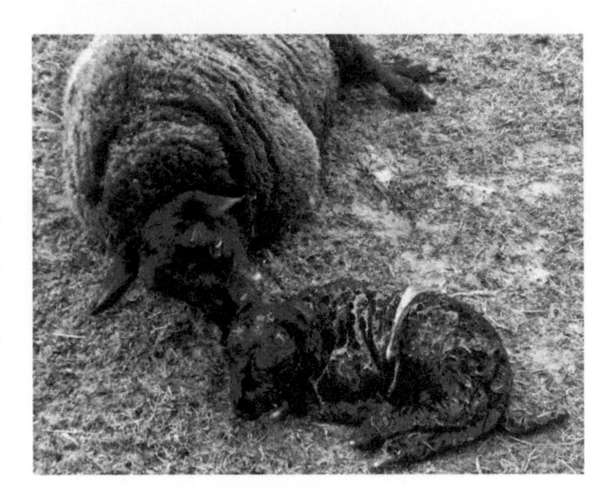

FIGURE 8.18 A ewe licking her newborn lamb.

If little shelter is available, additional windbreaks can be put into fields or sheds, using securely fastened straw bales, pallets or boards; these must not be able to fall or tilt over onto animals sheltering beside them.

Newborn lambs will not survive freezing conditions, whereas well-fed older lambs can cope with these low temperatures, provided that they are well fed and the conditions are not continually wet as well as cold. Shelter or windbreaks are still needed for older lambs.

Ewes must be able to access food at all times and in all weathers in order to survive and provide milk for their lambs. When snow is on the ground, provide outdoor ewes with forage or house them with food.

9 PREVENTING DISEASE FROM ENTERING YOUR FLOCK

BIOSECURITY

The purpose of biosecurity is to prevent new diseases from entering an existing flock or even preventing new strains of an existing disease that may be worse than strains that are already present.

This chapter presents best practice for biosecurity so that you can make an informed decision about the risks that you are willing to take. Some of the suggestions are easier to implement than others and not all are routinely practiced on all sheep farms.

Potential sources of new infections

Diseases can come onto a farm through a variety of routes, including:

- With new livestock that are carrying the disease
- On the wheels of vehicles that have recently been to other farms
- In dirty trailers or lorries
- On people – ruminant diseases are normally carried on the outside of peoples' clothes, for example in faeces attached to footwear or overalls
- In feed and forage
- Dogs, foxes, rabbits
- Birds
- In running surface water
- Through infected insects
- Airborne from neighbouring farms

Minimising potential sources of infection

Although diseases can enter a farm in a number of ways, as noted above, it is possible to minimise exposure of the flock to these contagions. A number of measures are outlined in Table 9.1.

Table 9.1 Measures to reduce the risks associated with sources of infection (except for new livestock).

SOURCE OF INFECTION	RISK REDUCTION MEASURE
Vehicles	Vehicles that do not belong on your property should be parked at its edge or on areas not accessed by livestock. Park 'home' vehicles at the edge of a property or in non-livestock areas when visiting other farms. Wash and disinfect vehicles and stock carriers before re-entering your farm, especially the wheels and stock carrying areas. Have disinfectant-filled* drive-over foam pads at farm entrances. These are especially important in national disease outbreaks, such as foot-and-mouth disease.
People	Provide overalls and footwear, or boot covers, for all visitors. Have disinfectant* footbaths and boot brushes at farm entrances; replace the footbath contents daily or before each group of visitors. Put up signs on footpaths asking dog walkers to remove all dog faeces. Fence footpaths so that they run along the edge of fields rather than through them.
Feed and forage	Acquire feed from a known and reputable source (Fig. 9.1). Store in a dry, cool place. Do not allow rodents or birds to have access to feed. Store silage and haylage without exposure to air.
Birds	Turn feed troughs upside down after feeding to keep bird faeces out (Fig. 9.2). Reduce access to sheep buildings and forage stores with bird netting.
Water courses	Fence natural water sources and provide pipe-filled water troughs (this may be excessive or uneconomical depending on the level of risk and the terrain).
Airborne	Double fence external farm boundary fences; the ideal gap between the two fences is 2 metres.

* Seek veterinary advice about appropriate disinfectants.

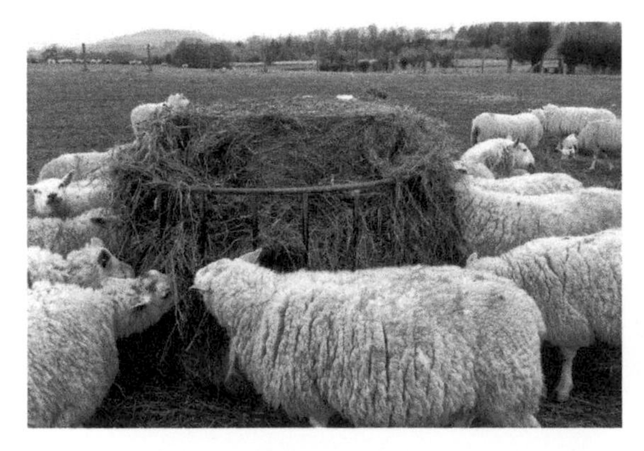

FIGURE 9.1 Source and store forage carefully before feeding it to ewes, to prevent spoilage and listeriosis.

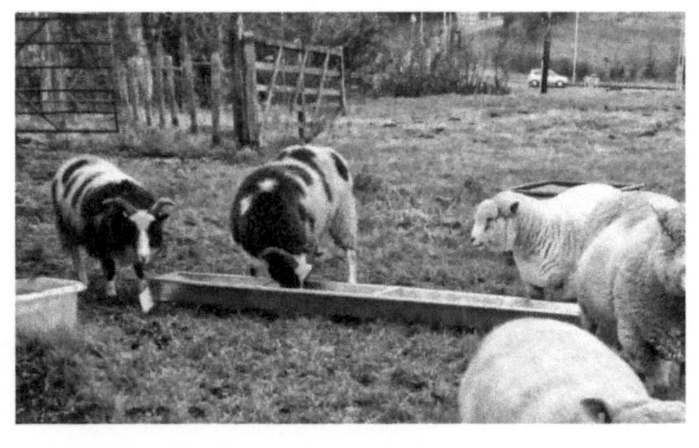

FIGURE 9.2 Turn the feed trough upside down once the sheep have finished eating to prevent bird faeces collecting in the bottom.

NEW LIVESTOCK

Buying new animals is an exciting time, however, in the excitement try not to forget that these animals could bring new diseases onto your farm. The rest of this chapter will discuss ways of limiting the risks associated with livestock movements.

When expanding a flock, use home-bred ewes whenever possible as this avoids the need to buy ewes from elsewhere. However, it is important to take care that these young ewes are not mated to males they are related to, which normally necessitates having a new ram every couple of years.

Livestock to consider

When trying to exclude new diseases, animals that should be taken into account include:

- All new livestock
- Livestock belonging to someone else that will be grazing your land or using your sheds
- Livestock that have been away from home or on ground previously grazed by sheep or cattle
- Livestock that have been grazing shared common land
- Hired or shared rams

Buying new stock

When buying new stock, think about where to buy them from and find out as much information about the farm of origin as possible. Wherever possible, try to buy them directly from that farm. Buying animals straight off a farm has a number of benefits, including gaining an overview of the selling farm and the rest of the flock, including the parents and/or progeny of your prospective purchase(s). It also means that new purchases do not have to go to market, where they can pick up additional diseases. Resist the temptation to buy 'cull sheep' or those being sold as rejects from other farms. These sheep often have multiple problems, which will create work, could introduce disease and may develop to compromise the animal's welfare.

Here are some signs to look out for when buying sheep. Do not buy any animals that:

- Have diarrhoea
- Are thin
- Appear itchy
- Are losing wool
- Are lame
- Have weeping eyes
- Have poor teeth
- Have unexplained lumps (Fig. 9.3)
- Have poor conformation (see 'Hereditary diseases' below)

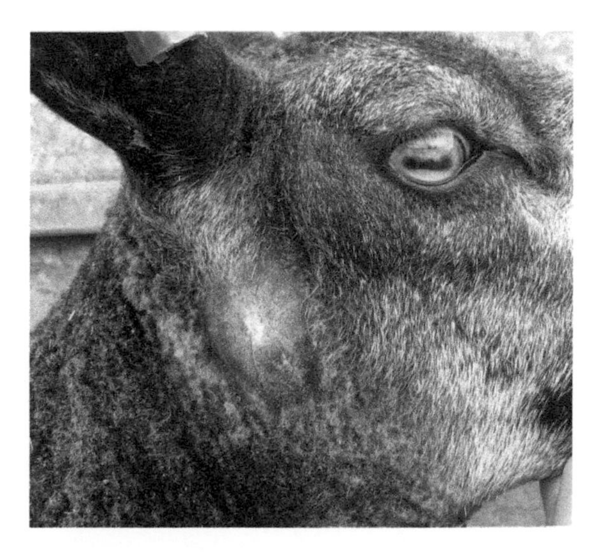

FIGURE 9.3 Do not buy animals with lumps like this, which may be due to contagious lymphadenitis.

Buying breeding rams

When looking at a breeding ram to buy, it is essential to undertake the same checks on it as would be done with your own rams before breeding. This will include checks on:

- Eyesight
- Gait, for lameness or stiffness
- Limb conformation – see 'Hereditary diseases' below
- Body condition
- Testicle size and consistency
- Penis

See Chapter 5 'Breeding sheep' for more detail.

Quarantine period

When newly purchased livestock arrive on a farm, they should be kept away from all other livestock for a period of time (see Table 9.2) and should not initially be turned out onto pasture (Fig. 9.4). The purpose of this quarantine period is to monitor the animals for signs of disease that are not obvious on the first day, to allow treatments and testing to be carried out (see Table 9.2) and to reduce the risk of pasture contamination with resistant gut worms or liver fluke.

Quarantine strategies in this chapter have been rated according to the level of risk (see Table 9.2), with essential being the minimal expected level of quarantine or treatment, advisable as a useful addition to flock biosecurity and strategies for those aspiring to high health status flock. None of these quarantine strategies should be allowed to compromise the welfare of livestock, for example animals should not go without food or water and any that need treatment urgently must be attended to.

On arrival, new sheep should be put straight into a shed or yard, that is, off pasture and kept there with food and water. The timing of turn out depends on whether they have come from a farm with liver fluke and whether liver fluke is likely to survive on your pasture (see 'Liver fluke' in Chapter 7). See Table 9.2 for details.

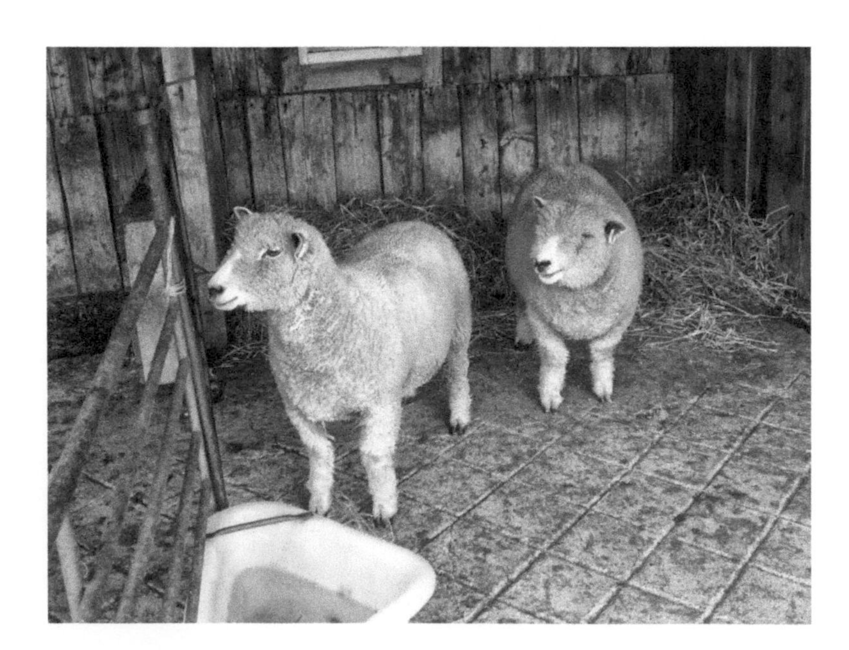

FIGURE 9.4 New sheep should be quarantined away from other livestock and monitored for disease, which may not be evident on arrival.

Table 9.2 The practicalities and diseases to consider during the quarantine period.

CONSIDERATION	ESSENTIAL	ADVISABLE	HIGH HEALTH STATUS
Duration of quarantine	A minimum of three weeks.	Four to six weeks.	Ewes until after their first lambing.
Isolation requirements	Minimum of 2 metres distance. Not in the same shed as other livestock. Do not allow stock to have contact with faeces or urine from quarantined animals.		
Hygiene	Feed and handle quarantined livestock after other stock. Wash and disinfect hands, overalls, equipment and handling facilities after handling quarantined stock.	Use separate boots and overalls when handling quarantined animals.	
Sheep scab	Check for itchy sheep and/or missing patches of wool. Give one of: • Moxidectin injection • Doramectin injection • Two ivermectin injections seven days apart. Farm stock should not go into an area that has been inhabited by quarantined stock in the preceding three weeks.		Treat with diazinon sheep dip instead. Blood test.
Resistant gut worms	House on arrival. Give two wormers on the same day but not mixed together: • Moxidectin[1] or doramectin; and • Monepantel or derquantel Turn out at least 48 hours after treatment onto pasture grazed by sheep within the last six months.	Give three wormers: • Moxidectin[1] or doramectin; and • Monepantel *and* derquantel Test faeces before and 14 days after treatment.	
Liver fluke and resistant liver fluke	Find out whether the farm of origin has liver fluke. If positive, give triclabendazole, followed by closantel, on the same day but not mixed together. Turn sheep out at least 14 days after treatment, preferably onto dry pasture.	Blood test. Test faeces before and 21 days after treatment. Eight weeks after the first treatment give nitroxynil or closantel. Keep quarantined animals away from wet areas until after the second liver fluke treatment.	

Table 9.2 continued.

CONSIDERATION	ESSENTIAL	ADVISABLE	HIGH HEALTH STATUS
Footrot and CODD (contagious ovine digital dermatitis)	Do not buy lame sheep. Look at all feet of new sheep upon arrival. Treat affected sheep and reassess three weeks later. Do not keep sheep that do not recover or with CODD if it is not already in the flock.	Footbath at the start and end of quarantine (see Chapter 8).	Test swabs from sheep's feet. Note these are very likely to be positive for sheep sourced in the UK.
Maedi visna	Do not buy thin sheep or sheep with breathing difficulties.	Buy sheep from accredited MV-free flocks. Blood test.	Blood test sheep from accredited flocks.
Johne's disease	Do not buy thin sheep.	Blood test.	Buy sheep from flocks that are known to be free of Johnes' disease. Test faeces samples from all new sheep.[2]
OPA (ovine pulmonary adenomatosis)	Do not buy thin sheep or those with breathing difficulties.		Ultrasound scan lungs – few vets are confident with this technique, so test availability is limited.
Border disease virus	Do not buy thin sheep, or particularly small lambs.	Blood test all new sheep.	
CLA (contagious lymphadenitis)	Monitor for lumps especially behind the angle of the jaw, along the neck and inside the back legs. Test lesions that appear during quarantine.		Blood test.
Enzootic abortion of ewes (Chlamydophia abortus; EAE)	Vaccinate all ewes before breeding, unless aiming for EAE-free status.	Keep new ewes separate until after their first lambing.	Blood test – only unvaccinated ewes.
Scrapie			Blood test for genetic susceptibility.
Orf	Monitor heads, ears and legs for orf throughout quarantine. Keep affected groups quarantined until all of the lesions have resolved. Wear gloves. Disinfect indoor surfaces once it has been vacated.		

CONSIDERATION	ESSENTIAL	ADVISABLE	HIGH HEALTH STATUS
Ringworm	Monitor heads, ears, legs and bodies for ringworm throughout quarantine. Keep affected groups quarantined until all the lesions have resolved. Wear gloves. Disinfect indoor surfaces once it has been vacated.		
Infectious kerato-conjunctivitis	Monitor eyes for weeping, inflammation, swelling or being closed due to pain throughout quarantine. Treat affected sheep according to veterinary advice and/or remove them from the flock.		Swab eyes for culture.
Louping ill	If the farm of origin has ticks, apply tick treatment to all new sheep. Check all sheep for ticks before and after treatment.		Treat with diazinon sheep dip to remove ticks.
Chorioptic mange	Monitor for itchy sheep with roughened, moth-eaten hair above the feet and on the scrotum.	Treat with diazinon sheep dip.	
Keds	Look for keds before purchase.	Treat with diazinon sheep dip.	

1 Do not use an injection that contains 1% moxidectin in sheep that have been vaccinated with 'Footvax' (MSD Animal Health™); check this with the vendor.
2 It is difficult to remove all risk of buying in Johne's disease. Other species can carry the infection, e.g. cattle, goats, deer, rabbits.

Diseases to consider

The importance of excluding these diseases from your flock will depend on whether they are already present or not, except for:

- Gut worms, for which levels of resistance to worm treatments vary from farm to farm
- Liver fluke, because only certain farms have liver fluke that are resistant to certain treatments
- Footrot, of which there are many strains; most flocks have two or three of these strains, so bringing in new strains can cause additional lameness

Treatment can remove some of these diseases. However, it is important to check that the treatment has been effective using follow-up tests; a vet will be able to advise on follow-up tests.

Hereditary diseases

When buying new livestock, infectious diseases are the main concern; however, for breeding animals, genetic diseases should also be considered. If these diseases are passed on, they can compromise the welfare of the next generation, for example:

- Dental problems
- Leg conformation:

  - None of the legs should be twisted, bent inwards or bent outwards
  - The front legs should be almost straight from the elbow to the floor, with a slight bend at the fetlock
  - The back legs should not be too straight (post-hocked) or too bent at the hock

- Entropion may be indicated by excessive skin around the eyes or signs of surgical correction
- Temperament is strongly heritable, so calm animals are likely to produce calm offspring, however, flighty or aggressive animals will have similarly problematic offspring

Showing sheep

Infectious diseases can be spread at livestock shows, therefore farmers with flocks of high health status (those with few significant infectious diseases) should consider extremely carefully whether or not to show their stock (Fig. 9.5).

If showing livestock is a high priority, minimise the risk of importing disease by:

- Keeping show animals separate from the rest of the flock
- Continuing to quarantine show sheep for a month after the showing season or sell them
- Foot bathing show sheep between shows
- Testing show sheep for maedi visna at the beginning and end of the showing season
- Treating for gut worms and liver fluke as described for quarantined sheep, if show sheep have eaten grass or forage from another farm

Exotic diseases

There are many diseases that are not normally present in the UK, some of which must be reported to the government's department for agriculture if they are found in the UK; these are known as 'notifiable diseases'. This allows the spread of these diseases to be limited by preventative measures.

Many notifiable diseases spread quickly between animals and cause severe symptoms. Descriptions and pictures of them are available on the Internet. Notifiable diseases that have made a significant impact in the UK in recent years include foot-and-mouth disease and bluetongue, both of which cause mouth lesions, excessive drooling and severe lameness; bluetongue virus can also cause swelling of the head and face.

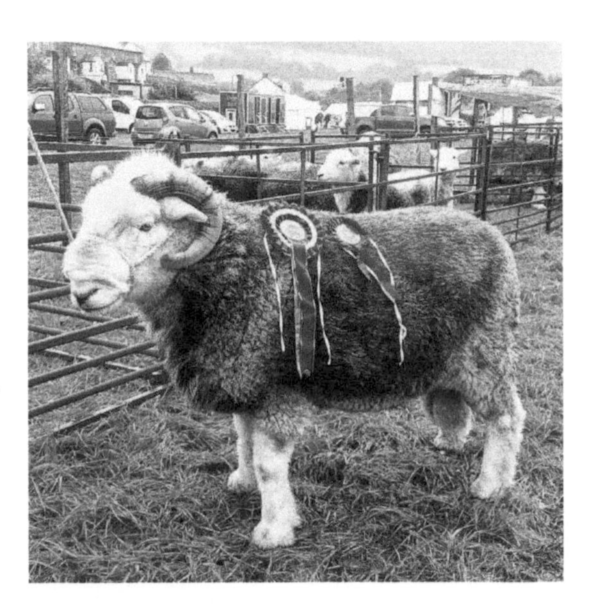

FIGURE 9.5 Showing sheep can be an enjoyable pastime, but the health implications for the rest of the flock must be considered carefully.

Photograph courtesy of Lizzy Wilcock.

In Scotland, sheep scab is a notifiable disease and requires immediate action when suspected.

If any animals in the flock are suspected of having any of these diseases, your local veterinary surgeon should be contacted immediately.

THE SHEEP FARMING YEAR

10

CALENDAR INTRODUCTION

In this section, there are two calendars that have been produced as a quick guide to the key management and disease prevention strategies discussed in this book. There are several factors that need to be considered when planning these activities in the sheep farming year:

- Seasonal dependency
- Timing of the breeding cycle
- Type of flock
- Location of the flock

Instructions to assemble it

The second calendar, with lambing-related events, is intended to be photocopied on clear paper, cut along the scissor-dotted lines and fit on top of the monthly calendar, which can also be photocopied and cut along the dotted lines. This clear paper calendar should then pivot at the centre so that it can be turned to the correct position, to move the lambing date to the correct month for each flock.

The two calendars are now superimposed on top of each other; according to your breeding plan the calendar for the breeding cycle can be rotated to fit your flock. For example, if you lamb your ewes in March, rotate the top calendar until 'Lambing' sits in the 'March' position; this will help you to work out when to breed and vaccinate your ewes to achieve the best results for a March lambing.

Once your preferred cycle has been identified, management practices should be added to a wall calendar or diary to act as reminders. For example, a note should be made to collect faecal samples from lambs once a month during the summer, such as: 'Take lamb stool samples to vet'; it is useful to have a tick box next to activities to indicate when each task has been completed.

In addition to management tasks, it is good practice to make a reminder of when preventative treatments are due to run out, so that additional tasks can be planned well in advance. For example, when applying blowfly preventative treatments, check the longevity of the product used and place a reminder in your diary or calendar at the start of the expiry week; this gives you time to assess whether further treatment is necessary, which will vary depending on the product used, the time of year, weather, number of flies and veterinary advice.

This calendar is intended as a guide only; some management protocols will need to be adjusted according to geographical location and annual weather patterns and it is important to work with your local vet to adjust the sheep farming calendar to suit your flock's needs.

BOTTOM WHEEL

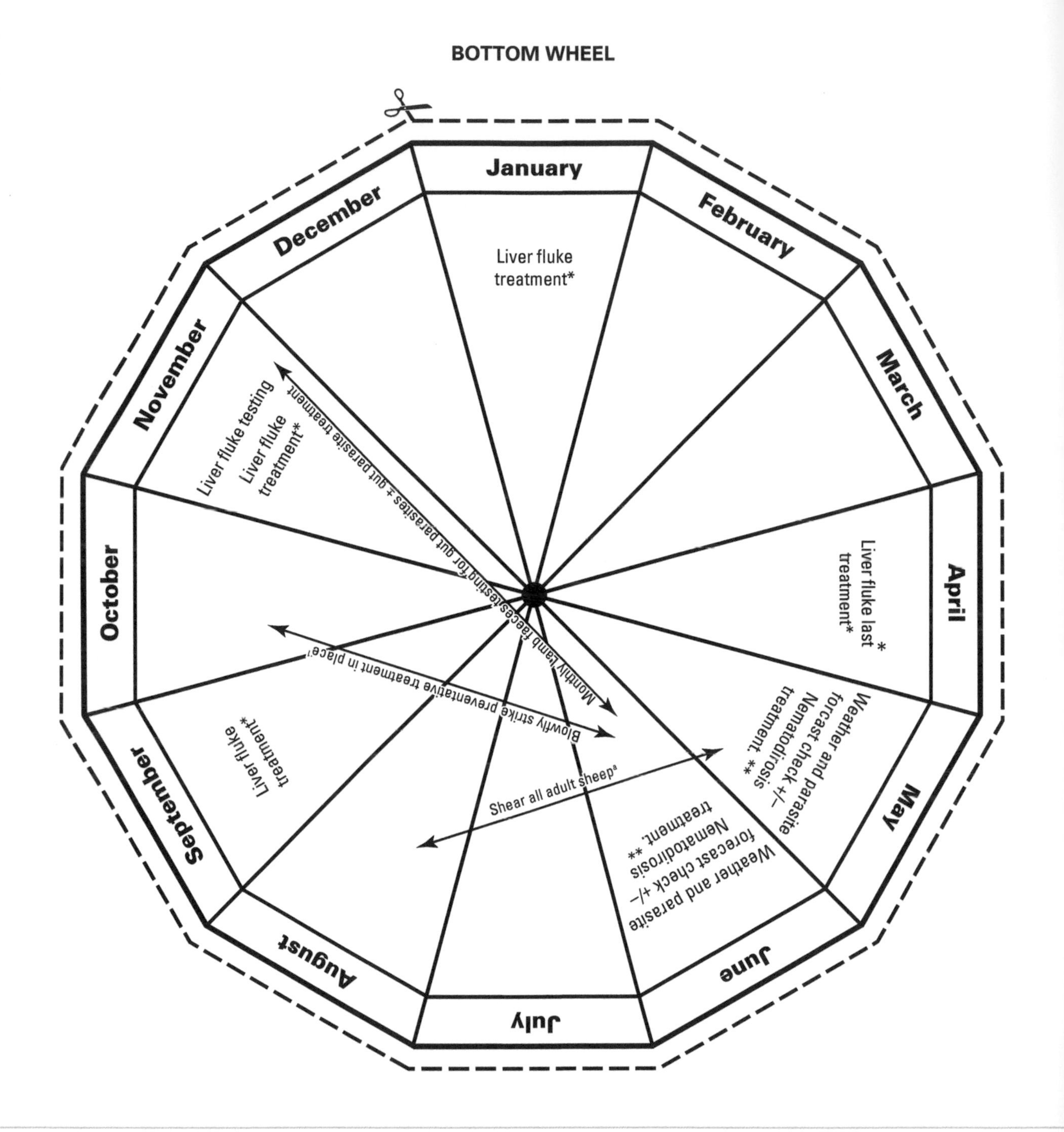

* Only if liver fluke is present; the frequency of treatments will depend on the level of infection on your farm; see 'Liver fluke' in Chapter 8. Liver fluke normally affects flocks in autumn, winter and spring.

** Monitor the weather and parasite forcasts for nematodirosis from March until June, in case of an unusually early warm spring or particularly late cold spring.

[a] Timing depends on local climate and fly populations.

TOP WHEEL

please use clear paper

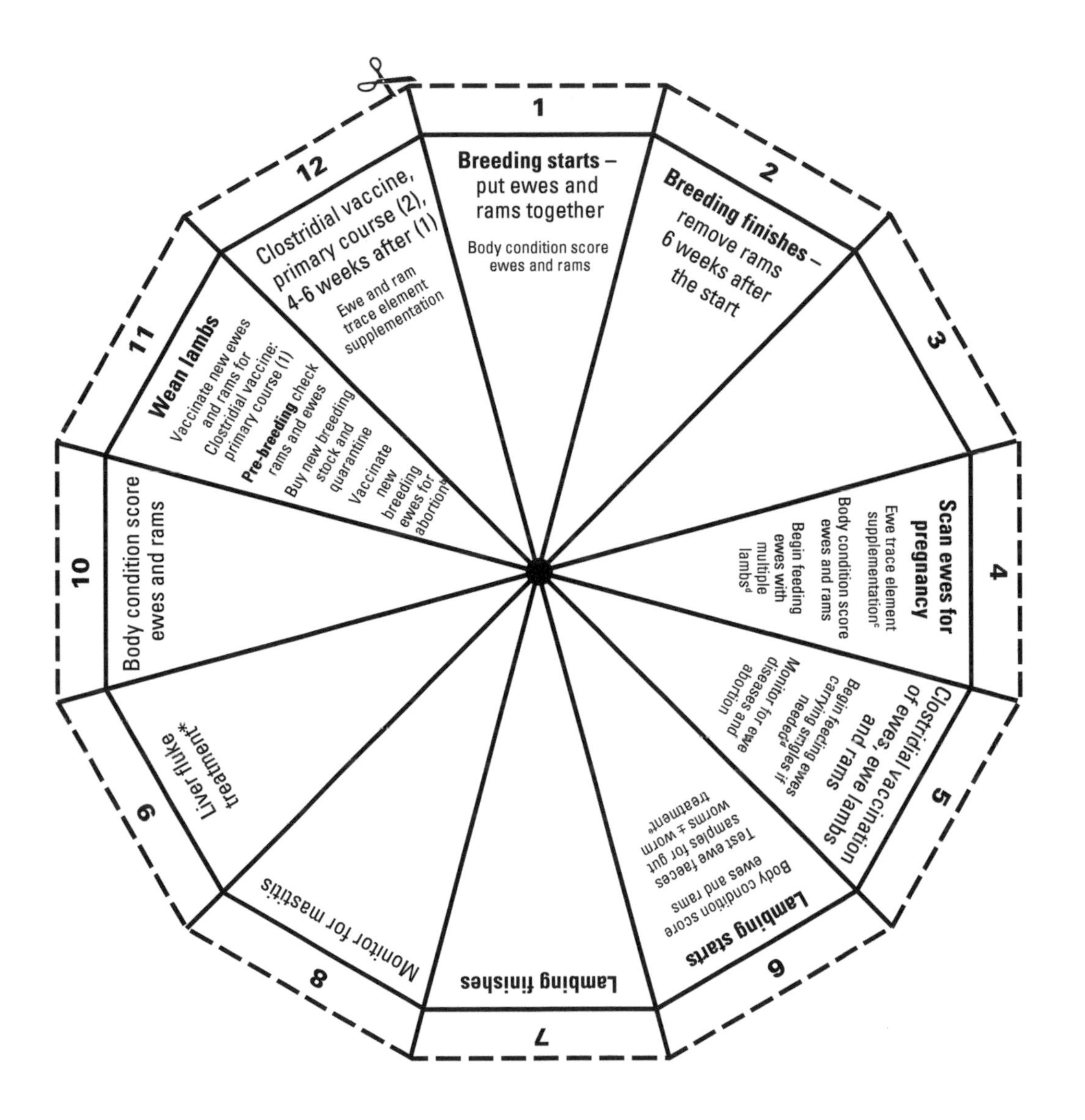

[b] Leave a two-week gap between clostridial vaccination and abortion vaccination.

[c] If testing shows that it is needed.

[d] Pregnant ewes need additional concentrate feed before and after lambing unless they have grass 4–6 cm in height to eat.

[e] Ewes are more likely to need worming at lambing time if they:

- Are thin
- Have low protein in their diet
- Are carrying multiple lambs – ewes with single lambs probably do not need to be wormed

INDEX